Aerobics
THEORY & PRACTICE

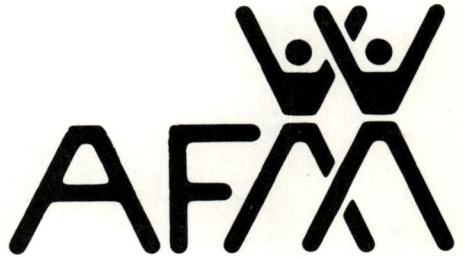

**AEROBICS AND FITNESS
ASSOCIATION OF AMERICA**

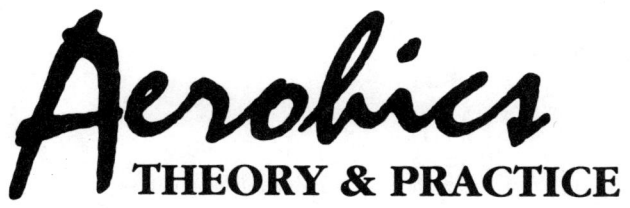
THEORY & PRACTICE

Edited by Phyllis Gorney Cooper, RN, MN

Foreword by Jack Kelly, President
United States Olympic Committee

Published by the AEROBICS AND FITNESS ASSOCIATION OF AMERICA
in association with CAMPBELL'S INSTITUTE FOR HEALTH AND FITNESS

AEROBICS AND FITNESS ASSOCIATION OF AMERICA, Sherman Oaks, CA

Acknowledgements

Production Editor:	Catherine Chambers
Assistant Production Editor:	Nora Galvin
Copy Editor:	Mary Beth Ferrari
Editorial and Content Input:	Peg Angsten
Creative Services:	Pati Kern
Cover Design:	Dave Whitaker
Body Shaping Photos:	Campbell's Institute for Health and Fitness
Triangle Health and Fitness Products:	Frank Dudowicz Triangle Health and Fitness Systems
Illustrations:	Tony Penido
Word Processing:	Peggy Paige
Typesetting:	Freedmen's Organization
Special Contributions:	Dan Cooper, Lauren Cooper, Marti Steele West, Linda West Abrams, Linda Shelton, Peter Grove
	AFAA office staff

Copyright © 1985 AEROBICS AND FITNESS ASSOCIATION OF AMERICA
All rights reserved

No part of this publication may be reproduced or reprinted in any form without the express written permission of the AEROBICS AND FITNESS ASSOCIATION OF AMERICA (AFAA).

1st Printing 1985

AEROBICS AND FITNESS ASSOCIATION OF AMERICA
15250 Ventura Blvd., Suite 802
Sherman Oaks, CA 91403

Printed in the United States of America

ISBN 0-9614719-0-5 Perfect Bind

Contents

Foreword ... ix
Preface ... xi
Basic Exercise Standards and Guidelines of
the Aerobics and Fitness Association of America ... xiii

Part A Essentials of Aerobic Exercise

Chapter 1: What is Aerobic Exercise? ... 3
Chapter 2: Anatomy and Physiology of Aerobic Exercise ... 11
Chapter 3: Medical Considerations of Aerobic Exercise ... 41
Chapter 4: Applied Physiologic Principles of Aerobic Exercise ... 51
Chapter 5: Body Composition ... 67
Chapter 6: General Nutritional Needs ... 81
Chapter 7: Developing Endurance ... 97
Chapter 8: Nutrition for Endurance and Training ... 113
Chapter 9: Strength Training ... 123
Chapter 10: Developing Flexibility ... 129
Chapter 11: Neuromuscular Power and Plyometrics ... 133
Chapter 12: Applied Sports Psychology ... 137
Chapter 13: Sports Injury Prevention ... 143
Chapter 14: Common Injuries in Aerobics and Their Treatment ... 147

Part B Developing an Aerobic Program

Chapter 1: Fitness Testing and Exercise Prescription ... 159
Chapter 2: Class Design and Conduct ... 169
Chapter 3: Body Shaping ... 187
Chapter 4: Motivation and Habit Training ... 211

Part C Professionalism and Aerobics

Chapter 1: Professional Conduct ... 221
Chapter 2: Certification ... 225
Chapter 3: Continuing Education ... 229
Chapter 4: Instructor Training ... 233

Part D The Aerobics Business

Chapter 1: Starting Your Own Business ... 239
Chapter 2: Legal Considerations ... 249
Chapter 3: Equipment for the Aerobics Business ... 257
Chapter 4: Common Sense Guide to Success ... 265
Chapter 5: Aerobics: Past, Present, and Future ... 273

Appendices

A Basic Exercise Program Outline ... 279
B Correct and Incorrect Exercise Positions ... 281
C Medical Emergencies ... 293
D Glossary of Terms ... 307

Editor
Phyllis Gorney Cooper, RN, MN,—*Independent Educator and Consultant; Acting Continuing Education Specialist, UCLA Extension, Department of Health Sciences; Trustee, Aerobics and Fitness Foundation of America, Los Angeles, CA*

Reviewers
Neil Sol, Ph.D.—*Director, Department of Health Promotions, Methodist Hospital, Memphis, TN; President-Elect, Association for Fitness in Business; Co-author and Co-editor, Presidential Sports Award Fitness Manual; Certified Preventive and Rehabilitative Exercise Program Director, American College of Sports Medicine; Editor,* Optimal Health: Publication for Health Promotion Professionals.

David E. Abrams, MD—*Publisher,* Aerobics and Fitness; *Physician, Internal Medicine and Nephrology; President and Chief Executive Officer, Valley Dialysis Associates, Van Nuys, CA*

John Black, RPT, MA—*Physical Therapist, Valley Presbyterian Hospital; Director, Human Performance Testing Center for Sports Medicine, Valley Presbyterian Hospital, Van Nuys, CA; Member, American College of Sports Medicine; Member, AFAA Advisory Board*

Stephanie Ben, MA—*Coordinator of Research, Campbell's Institute for Health and Fitness,* Campbell Soup Company, Camden, NJ; *Independent Consultant for Corporate Fitness, Chapel Hill, NC.*

Contributing Authors
Donald Chu, Ph.D.—*Director and Owner, ATHER Sports Injury Clinic, Hayward, CA; NATA Certified Athletic Trainer*
Sheila Cluff—*Owner and Director, Oaks at Ojai and Palms in Palm Springs, CA*
William C. Day, Ph.D.—*Executive Director, Health and Fitness Services, Canyon Ranch Health and Vacation Resort, Tucson, AZ*
Barry M. Devine, Ph.D.—*Professor, Exercise Science, California State University, Northridge, Northridge, CA*
Patricia Eisenman, Ph.D.—*Director, Department of Health, Physical Education, and Recreation, University of Utah, Salt Lake City, UT*
Randi Lewis, J.D.—*Associate Attorney, Breidenbach, Swainston, Yokaitis and Crispo; AFAA Member and Certified Aerobics Instructor, Los Angeles, CA*
Lauve Metcalfe, M.S.—*Director, Program Development, Campbell's Institute for Health and Fitness, Campbell Soup Company, Camden, NJ; Consultant, Employee Fitness, President's Council on Physical Fitness and Sports*

Terence Moffatt—*Freelance Writer, Author of Consumer and Business Articles on Exercise Equipment, New York, NY*
Michael Nicola—*Owner, Body Express, Los Angeles, CA; Business Member, AFAA*
Laura L. Pawlak, RD, Ph.D.—*Consultant Dietitian, Cathedral City, CA; Educator and author; Member AFAA*
Linda Erickson Shelton, BA—*AFAA Coordinator of Training Services; AFAA Certified Instructor and Consultant; Independent Aerobics Training Consultant, Thousand Oaks, CA*
Arthur J. Siegel, M.D.—*Medical Director, Hahnemann Hospital, Brighton, MA*
Joanne L. Smith, MS—*Assistant Professor, East Stroudsburg University, East Stroudsburg, PA; Certified Exercise Specialist, American College of Sports Medicine; Aerobic Consultant, AFAA*
Rose Snyder, MS—*Head Athletic Trainer, Center for Athletic Medicine, Henry Ford Hospital, Detroit, MI*
John E. Thiel, M.Ed.—*Coordinator, Exercise Programs, Emory Health Enhancement Center, Atlanta, GA*
Marti Steele West, BA—*Vice-President and Director of Certification, AFAA; AFAA Certified Instructor and Consultant; Independent Aerobics Training Consultant, San Diego, CA*
Gerald P. Whelan, MD, FACEP—*Associate Director and Director of Resident Training, Department of Emergency Medicine, Los Angeles County/USC Medical Center; Assistant Professor of Emergency Medicine, School of Medicine, University of Southern California, Los Angeles, CA*

Foreword

For years, physical fitness was the concern only of athletes who were seeking every possible tool to sharpen their competitive skills. Conditioning, strength training, and flexibility exercises were relegated to the gymnasiums and training fields.

Even there, the importance of total fitness was slow to be recognized. In recent years, coaches and trainers have begun to understand the importance of developing the total physical being.

The fitness movement has now moved far beyond organized athletics, and, to some degree, millions of Americans have become athletes in the sense that they wish to sharpen their physical abilities to compete in a fast-paced society. They are competitors whose playing fields include the office, the weekend road race or softball game, and social events.

What is physical fitness? Some authorities suggest that it is the capacity to carry out everyday activities—both work and play—without excessive fatigue and with enough energy in reserve for emergencies. But is that sufficient? Is not almost everyone physically fit under that definition?

If we believe that good health is more than an absence of illness, then we must also recognize the role of the individual in caring for his or her own body. Exercise is one of the key components to a personal commitment to well-being. Along with good nutrition, abstinence from smoking, proper rest, and moderation in other areas of life-style, exercise can help us maximize our physical capacities.

The level of fitness determines the operating capacity of each and every component of the body's system. When you're in good shape, your heart, lungs, and blood vessels work the way they are designed to work. Your muscle strength and endurance is increased, flexibility is enhanced, lean body mass is maintained, and overall body fat is decreased.

What happens when we do not take responsibility for our health? In 1968, Americans spent $58 billion on health, and by 1983, the figure had rocketed to $355 billion annually. Medical and health costs are 11 percent of the gross national product.

The good news is that people are recognizing their opportunities to improve their quality of life, their health, and even their happiness. The fitness movement that began to snowball in the 1970s shows no signs of slowing down. The way people pursue fitness—marathons, triathlons, racquet sports, etc.—will change. However, too many people are experiencing positive changes in their bodies and minds to allow the movement itself to die. Physical fitness has become a way of life.

The movement knows no age limits, having begun with the growing-up "baby boomers," and now spreading into the young and the aging populations. Advertisers are incorporating fitness activities into their promotions, with the emphasis that an active life-style is not only healthy, it's vogue.

I congratulate the Aerobic and Fitness Association of America, Triangle Health and Fitness Systems, and Campbell's Institute for Health and Fitness for joining efforts to provide this comprehensive guide. In the hands of those who provide leadership in the fitness movement, it will be an invaluable resource.

I congratulate you, also, for your desire to increase your knowledge in the ever-changing study of how our bodies can function at maximum capacity. I challenge you to share your active life-style with those around you, and to share your experiences with those who have a whole new world yet ahead of them.

Jack Kelly
President
United States Olympic Committee

A postscript of sorrow must be added. Before this book could be published, Jack Kelly died. His untimely death stunned those close to him who appreciated his strength, leadership, and humanity. He led a life immersed in action; his unwritten will: the spirit to continue. It is to that spirit, and his memory, that we dedicate this book.

Preface

Fitness is an elusive state. What is here today may very well be gone tomorrow without continual hard work, determination and discipline. For many (particularly those who are instructors) this way of life is the only way of life. Because instructors are fit, they are role models in an age of health awareness. In sharing with others their enthusiasm, sense of well-being, and love for fitness, they are often regarded as fitness "experts." But is an exercise instructor prepared for the more encompassing task of fitness education? Has he or she the knowledge and tools to do a good and safe job? Or, have the guidelines for instruction been as elusive to instructors as fitness itself is to most of the population? Up until now, the aerobic exercising professional has not had a hands-on workbook to advise and guide her/his daily quest for the best injury-free exercise program. Using the combined talents and expertise of the advisors, AFAA has written the first complete set of these long overdue guidelines.

In **Aerobics: Theory and Practice**, thirty accomplished fitness researchers and practitioners elucidate upon AFAA's "Basic Exercise Standards and Guidelines." Bringing their unique expertise to this anthology, the authors created a practical and valuable composite. A project of this ambition required the cooperative effort of both authors and reviewers. Among the reviewers, special recognition is extended to Neil Sol, Ph.D., for his diligence in coordinating these efforts. He and the editor, Phyllis G. Cooper, R.N., spent countless hours that only come from a professional's deep commitment to excellence.

The emphasis of this book is on the exercise considerations for adult, able-bodied participants. Special needs of persons with disabilities, pre-and post-partum women, children and seniors, could not be adequately covered in this text. Subsequent publications from AFAA will cover specific concerns and precautions for these groups.

A project of this kind arises from public necessity for the dissemination of sound and accurate information on exercise. Lee Dukes and Campbell's Institute of Health and Fitness have recognized this pervasive need and we at AFAA appreciate their support. In the hope that each exercise instructor who owns this book will incorporate the principles contained within it, **Aerobics: Theory and Practice** is presented to encourage a professional stance in fitness instruction.

Linda Pfeffer, RN
President,
Aerobics and Fitness
Association of America

Basic Exercise Standards and Guidelines of the Aerobics and Fitness Association of America

Introduction by Marti Steele West, BA

Professionals and researchers in the field of exercise science have literally written volumes on the physiological implications of most popular sports, such as tennis and football. Aerobic exercise, however, is a relative newcomer to the fitness scene and has yet to be the focus of prolonged scientific study. Much has been written about the different forms of exercise such as running, cycling, cross-country skiing, and swimming. How do the demands of aerobic exercise as it is performed in a class setting differ from these sports?

Aerobic exercise classes are increasing in popularity with every passing day. So, too, unfortunately, are the misconceptions and the numbers of related injuries. What we have in fact been witnessing is a sport being played with no rules. Attend one class and the instructor will perform an exercise in one manner. Attend another class and that instructor will do just the opposite. The consumer and the instructors alike have been generally performing in an educational void, relying largely on exercises borrowed from other disciplines such as dance or running. What we have discovered, of course, is that the safe and effective execution of an aerobic exercise class is a discipline unto itself, requiring its own set of rules. Thus, the Aerobics and Fitness Association of America was created in 1983 to provide the supportive framework from which the standards for this exercise form could grow.

The printing of our first *Basic Exercise Standards and Guidelines* was a landmark for the profession, as it was the first time that data relevant to an aerobic exercise class had been gathered into one document. The AFAA *Standards and Guidelines* are the result of countless hours of research, discussion, and revision by members of our board of advisors and other exercise professionals. In their present form, the *Standards and Guidelines* present a conservative approach to instructing a freestyle aerobic exercise class. In freestyle aerobic exercise, the individual exercises are not rigidly choreographed to fit a particular piece of music as they are in aerobic dance. However, the principles discussed in the *Basic Exercise Standards and Guidelines* are applicable to aerobic dance and many other types of exercise class as well.

It is the purpose of the *Standards and Guidelines* to provide the professional instructor with up-to-date information presented in an easy-to-follow format on how to teach a class that is both safe and effective while still allowing for the individual creativity inherent in this exciting exercise form. With the printing of the *Basic Exercise Standards and Guidelines* we witness the establishment of the rules of play, if you will, and a first step in creating a consistent standard of performance, acceptable to both the public and the professional, against which an instructor's competency can be tested through AFAA certification. In the months and years to follow we anticipate an ever increasing interest in aerobic exercise. This will in turn stimulate much needed scientific research in the field and allow AFAA the tools necessary to further expand and refine our *Standards and Guidelines*.

Throughout this book the *Standards and Guidelines* will be used to emphasize specific areas of content. Since it is useful to keep these standards in mind as content is reviewed, they will be cited in the text. When a standard or guideline is cited, it will be done by designating the roman numeral, then letter and title of the specific area.

For example, content on daily workouts might cite the standard related to Basic Principles and appear in the text as **[I.A: Frequency of Workouts]**.

The AFAA *Standards and Guidelines* are reprinted below in their entirety. They serve as the framework of this book and are here to enhance your use of the content.

Basic Exercise Standards and Guidelines of the Aerobics and Fitness Association of America™

I. Basic Principles, Definitions and Recommendations

All standards and guidelines outlined as follows apply to an average adult without known physiological or biological conditions that would in any way restrict their exercise activities.

A. Frequency of Workouts

Your body can't store fitness. We recommend at least three workouts, evenly spaced, throughout the week. As an instructor, be aware of overuse syndromes that may manifest themselves in several of the body's systems. Example: stress fractures, fatigue, certain tendonitis and bursitis problems, and often shin splints. The body needs time to recover and strengthen. Teaching 12 classes a week, and no more than three classes per day, should be considered the maximum for the experienced instructor.

B. Muscles to be Exercised

For every major muscle worked, the opposing muscle should also be worked. Example: biceps/triceps. By exercising opposing muscles one is lessening the possibility of muscular imbalance. Any time a muscular imbalance is present, the potential for injury is greater. Repeating the same exercise month after month works the muscles and wears the joints in exactly the same areas and through the same planes. A variety of exercises that seek to provide toning potential to opposing muscles will provide more balanced wear to the joints and strengthening to the muscles.

C. Body Alignment

Throughout all exercises be conscious of body alignment and posture. Stand tall and yet keep posture relaxed, not tense. Imagine a "midline" running from the top of your head down through the middle of your body. Try to keep your body balanced in relation to this imaginary midline. Abdominal muscles should be held firmly in and up, shoulders back and down. Do not hyperextend (lock) your knee or elbow joints. Hyperextension places excess stress on the ligaments in the joint and decreases the effectiveness of stretching or strengthening activities. Hyperextension of the knee while standing also causes an unnatural arch and excessive stress in the lumbar spine (lower back). Arching or back bends should be avoided as this may cause pain or damage to the discs which separate the vertebrae.

D. Speed, Isolation, and Resistance

Exercises should be performed at a moderate speed that will allow full range of motion and concentrated work within the isolated muscle or group of muscles which are the focus of the exercise. Performing an exercise too quickly will often make this type of controlled movement impossible and can also lead to injury. Strengthening a muscle involves controlled, deliberate muscular strengthening exercises without the use of weights. Resistance is accomplished by the concentration of tension through muscular contraction working against gravity. Exercises performed too quickly often rely on momentum instead of actual muscle work. Slow, controlled, resistive movements demand more work of the muscle than those movements which are fast and ballistic in nature.

E. Training Effect

The training effect refers to the changes in the body achieved through exercise. Exercise must be of sufficient duration, intensity, and frequency in order to create a training effect.

F. Overload Principle

The overload principle states that the body, when regularly stimulated by an increasing intensity and duration of exercise, will respond with an increased capacity to perform physical work. The body is being trained to adapt to increasing physiological demands. This principle applies to all types of physical conditioning, muscular endurance, muscular strength and cardiovascular endurance. This does not mean that you must "go for the burn." A training effect will occur when a muscle is worked *just a little* beyond its point of fatigue on a regular basis with increased intensity and duration.

G. Full Range of Motion

The working muscle(s) should extend through the fullest range of motion as provided by the dictates of the particular exercise and the flexibility of the muscles and joints involved. Example: If instructed to reach high above head with both arms and then lower arms to sides of body, don't reach halfway with bent elbows and then just let the arms drop down. *Work* the muscles through the range of movement provided by the exercise.

H. Danger Signs

Know the following danger signs. Should you observe any one of these or should a class participant complain of any one of these, they should be advised to stop vigorous exercise immediately!

- Unusual fatigue
- Nausea
- Dizziness
- Tightness or pain in chest
- Lightheadedness
- Loss of muscle control
- Severe breathlessness
- Allergic reactions, i.e., rash/hives

Individual should contact his/her physician or obtain immediate medical advice. Always maintain your CPR certification at an up-to-date status.

II. Class Format
A. Sequence
In the case of certain exercise categories such as cool-down and stretching, the order in which exercises are performed is important. The following is the recommended sequence as adopted by AFAA for a one-hour class:
1. Pre-class instruction
2. Warm-up: A balanced combination of static stretching and rhythmic limbering exercises.
3. Exercises from the following groups, performed in a standing position, in order of preference:
   a. Standing leg work
   b. Arms, chest and shoulders
   c. Aerobics and cool-down
   d. Waist work
4. Dropping to the floor for the remainder of the class, exercises from the following groups may be performed in order of preference:
   a. Legs
   b. Buttocks
   c. Hips
   d. Abdominals
5. Static stretching

B. Purpose of Sequence
The above sequence is desirable because it will help to keep the flow of the class smooth. Getting up and down off the floor repeatedly creates "exercise gaps." Strive for smooth transitions. Stopping the class for explanations or changing a record is a sure way to lose a class. Keep the class moving and the energy and interest level high.

If the above sequence does not fit the policy of the exercise studio or your personal preference, there is no physiological reason for following this order as long as the following rules are observed:

1. Always begin class with "warm-ups."
2. Always end class with static stretching.
3. Always follow aerobics with a sufficient cool-down period.
4. Upon completion of strengthening exercises within a specific muscle group, always stretch those muscles before proceeding to the next group.

C. Class Level
Unless class level is specific, i.e., beginner/advanced, it is best to teach at an intermediate level and explain to class how to adjust the individual exercises to their particular level of fitness and experience. In other words, try to give both a beginning and advanced version of your exercises, while performing at an intermediate level. Motor skill, intensity, and duration capability of individuals must be considered.

III. Pre-Class Procedure

A. Medical Clearance
Before class determine if there are any new class members and the level of their experience. Ask the date of their last physical. We recommend a medical physical examination for all students who have not been exercising regularly, unless they are under 30 years of age and have had a satisfactory check-up within the last year. If between ages 30 and 34, the check-up should have been within the last three months and should include a resting EKG. For participants ages 35 and over, a medical examination and testing should include a stress EKG where the pulse reaches the level it would during aerobic workouts. Anyone with a preexisting medical condition should be screened by his or her physician prior to beginning an exercise program.

B. Introductions
Introduce yourself and announce the level of the class.

C. Attire
If some class members are without shoes, AFAA strongly recommends they obtain and use proper shoes as a means of reducing the risk of injury to feet, knees and shins. This should be explained to the class, and the criteria for appropriate shoes discussed.

D. Level of Participation
Explain that the class is non-competitive and that all participants should work at their own level. Make sure the class is aware of danger signs as outlined in I.H. above. In case of any other sharp

pain experienced while exercising, the activity should be discontinued immediately and be discussed with the instructor following class.

   E. **Breathing**
Explain that breathing should follow a consistent rhythmic pattern throughout the class. The activity will reflexly dictate rate and depth of ventilation. Do not restrict inhalation to the nose. Inspire and expire through the nose and mouth in a relaxed fashion.

   F. **Orientation to Aerobics**
Define aerobics for new members. Explain before class how they can find their own target zone for aerobic work.

IV. **"Warm-Up"**

   A. **Purpose**
Prepares the body for vigorous exercises and reduces the risk of injury.

   B. **Time**
Class should begin with 7-10 minutes of a balanced combination of static stretches and smoothly performed, rhythmic limbering exercises.

   C. **Stretching**
Correctly performed stretching is important because it increases flexibility and your capacity for full range of movement. This allows one to perform more smoothly with less risk of injury.
     1. Muscle length
        a. Resting length—length of a muscle at rest
        b. Maximum length—the limit of the length of the muscle that it can be stretched at any particular time.
        c. Increasing length—repeated stretching of a muscle over a period of time will gradually increase the resting length of the muscle fibers.
     2. Static stretch
Stretches should always be static, non-ballistic. Static stretches are sustained stretches with the muscle relaxed. Ballistic movement is forcefully executed and cannot be accomplished with the muscle relaxed. Ballistic movement such as bouncing during a stretch, invokes the stretch reflex.
     3. Stretch reflex
The stretch reflex is the body's automatic protective mechanism against severe injury and abuse. Whenever a muscle is stretched quickly and with force, a reflex is initiated

which causes the stretched muscle to contract to protect and prevent injury. Stretching is most effective if it is done slowly and gently with the muscle relaxed.
4. Position
Always assume a position with the body correctly aligned and the stretch occurring along the longitudinal line (the long way of the muscles to be stretched). Example: in a calf stretch do not turn the toes of the back foot out.

D. Sequence
In order to maintain a smooth flow of your warm-up, one should follow a specific order. Warm-up from either the head to the toes, or vice-versa, i.e., don't skip from the neck to the ankles, to arms and back to the calves.

E. Muscle Groups
We recommend that all of the following muscle groupings be warmed-up at the beginning of class:
1. Head and neck (suboccipital group)
2. Shoulders, upper back, arms and chest (trapezius, deltoid, biceps, triceps and pectoralis).
3. Rib cage, waist and lower back (external oblique, latissimus dorsi)
4. Front and back of thigh (quadriceps and hamstrings)
5. Inner thigh (adductor longus, gracilis)
6. Calf (gastrocnemius, soleus)
7. Feet and ankles

F. Rhythmic Limbering Exercises
These exercises help prepare your body for more vigorous exercise by providing an increase in the flexibility of tendons and ligaments, raising muscle temperature and maximizing the mechanical advantage of muscle function.

Example: arm circles, leg circles, small kicks, knee lifts, high reaches. Exercises that directly involve different types of movement of the bones in the joints. Should be smoothly performed at a moderate pace.

G. Special Warm-up Do's and Don'ts
1. Do warm-up and stretch the lower back before attempting any lateral movement of the upper torso, i.e., side bends.
2. Don't do traditional toe touches to stretch the hamstrings. Roll down with knees bent, partially straighten one leg keeping

hips square and hold relax. Alternate legs. Come up from this position by uncurling with knees bent.
3. Don't do full deep knee bends (grand plies), as this strains the cruciate ligaments in the knee.
4. Don't do "the plow," as this position could cause injury to the neck. The vertebrae and discs in the cervical area were not designed to withstand this type of pressure.

V. Arms, Chest and Shoulders

A. Purpose
To strengthen the muscles of the arms, chest and shoulders.

B. Time
5–7 minutes

C. Arms, Chest and Shoulder Exercises
May be performed with either limited movement in the lower body or they may be incorporated with the aerobics. If performed during aerobics, keep the footwork simple in order that the arms and/or chest and shoulders may be the area of concentrated work.

D. Arm Work Versus Arm Movement
Arm movement that does not involve a conscious contraction of the working muscle(s) will not provide the same training effect as arm work. Arm work involves the concentration of tension through muscle contraction within a specific muscle or group of muscles. Arm movement involves the movement of the arm from point A to point B without specific, repetitive work necessarily being accomplished.

E. Position
Maintain correct body alignment. Abdomen should be held firmly. Do not pull backwards or forwards with the shoulders, as this can cause unnecessary strain on the back.

F. Push-ups
Push-ups performed with either straight legs, or on the knees, can be an excellent exercise for strengthening the muscles of the arms and chest. In order to perform push-ups safely the following should be noted:
1. In order to protect the lower back it is advisable to slightly raise the buttocks.
2. Elbows should not lock or overbend.
3. Head should be held straight out at a natural extension of the spine.

xxii BASIC EXERCISE STANDARDS AND GUIDELINES

VI. Aerobics

A. Aerobics
A variety of exercise which creates an increased demand for oxygen over an extended period of time, as opposed to anaerobic exercise, which means exercise without oxygen. Aerobic exercises train the heart, lungs and cardiovascular system to process and deliver oxygen quickly and efficiently to every part of the body. As the heart muscle becomes stronger and more efficient, a larger volume of blood is able to be pumped with each stroke and with fewer strokes, thus facilitating the rapid transport of oxygen to all parts of the body, an aerobically fit cardiovascular system will allow the individual to work longer, more vigorously and to recover more quickly.

B. Time
14-20 minutes

C. Sequence
Start slowly and gradually increase the intensity and range of motion of your aerobic movements. Try to avoid lateral (side to side) moves during the first three minutes, allowing ankles and feet to become sufficiently warmed up. Peak movements, that is, large movements using both arms and legs and requiring that a greater amount of oxygen be delivered to the muscles, should be interspersed with smaller aerobic movement. These peak movements should not be attempted during the first three minutes.

D. Position
Correct posture with the abdominals held firmly should be maintained throughout aerobics. Heels should always come all the way down to the floor. Don't jog on your toes, as this shortens the calf muscles and Achilles tendon. Do not lean forward, as this can contribute to shin splints, but do keep body weight balanced forward over entire foot and not backwards on heels.

E. Type of Movements
Try to vary your movements in order to both maintain interest level and effectively work as many muscles as possible. Combination moves requiring coordination of both arms and legs should be entered into slowly, starting with either the arms or the

legs and then adding the other. Build upon your moves instead of trying to teach a complicated combination movement all at once.

F. Breathing
Steady, rhythmic breathing, using both nose and mouth which fits the exercise and does not impede mechanics should be used. Breath holding should be avoided in aerobic-rhythmic exercises.

G. Surface
Aerobics should ideally be performed on a good floor with a cushion of air beneath, not wood directly laid on concrete. This type of wood floor has a certain amount of "give" to it and is much less stressful on the bones and ligaments of the feet, ankles and legs. If jogging on concrete is unavoidable, mats should be used. In any case, well-fitting shoes designed for aerobics that provide sufficient lateral support and cushion should always be worn.

H. Heart Rate
Monitoring heart rate indicates to an individual a safe and effective intensity of aerobic exercise.
1. Where to take your pulse
   a. Carotid artery: Place index and middle finger by outside corner of eye and slide them straight down to the neck. *Do not* press hard or place thumb on opposite side of neck at the same time as the blood flow could be impeded.
   b. Radial artery: Place the index and middle fingers only on the inner wrist, just below the wrist bone, straight down from the base of the thumb. This method is preferred to the carotid pulse due to the possible depressant effect of the carotid reflex during palpation.
2. How to determine your heart rate
   a. Count—Count your heart rate for 10 seconds
   b. Multiply—Multiply this number by 6, and you will know what your heart rate is for one minute at that particular point in time.
3. Resting heart rate
   a. Average—Average for women is 78–84 beats per minute. Average for men is 72–78. A person in good aerobic condition generally has a lower resting heart rate.
   b. How to determine your resting heart rate—Take pulse for three mornings while still lying down, but after the heart

has settled down if awakened by an alarm. Add these three numbers together and then divide the answer by three. This number is your resting heart rate.
4. Maximum heart rate
Theoretical maximum rate at which your heart can beat at your age. 220 minus your age equals your maximum heart rate. *Do not* exercise at this rate!
5. Target heart rate
    a. Purpose: Provides an easily identifiable gauge of an individual's level of aerobic work and whether or not the intensity of their aerobic activities should be increased or decreased.
    b. To determine target heart rate: Subtract your age from 220 and multiply this number by .7 and .8. This is your target heart rate range or zone that you shall "target" for during aerobic exercise. Individuals with special needs (i.e., pregnant women or anyone with a history of any cardiopulmonary problem) should consult their physician regarding the rate they should target for. When beginning an aerobics program, it is recommended that all individuals train at the lower end of their range for the first eight to ten weeks.
6. Application
The pulse should be quickly located after vigorous exercise. Keep walking and take a 10-second count. Multiplied by six, this number should be in your individualized target zone. If it is higher or lower than the acceptable limits of your range, you will need to adjust the intensity of your exercise accordingly by being more or less vigorous.
7. Monitoring heart rate during aerobics
In the most ideal of situations, AFAA recommends the taking of heart rate five minutes after the beginning of active aerobic work to determine if participant is working within his/her target zone. However, as taking heart rate at this time is not always feasible, heart rate should be checked at the completion of aerobic work rather than not at all.
8. Recovery heart rate
    a. Purpose: Taking a recovery heart rate can show if the cool-down period has been sufficient and if you were exercising at a level that was too intense. After five minutes, your heart rate should equal less than 60 percent of your maximum (220 minus your age, multiplied by .6).

VII. Post-Aerobic Cool Down

A. Purpose
To provide a transition period between the vigorous aerobic work and less aerobically taxing muscular strengthening exercises or stretches. Without a gradual cool-down period, the blood which is pooled in the extremities immediately after an aerobic workout does not return to the heart as quickly or efficiently. By stopping abruptly, the large muscles which were pushing the blood back to the heart during exercise are no longer doing this job and the blood remains in the arms and legs. Stopping motionless after an aerobic workout could result in fainting or undue stress on the heart.

B. Time
2–3 minutes of decreasing aerobic work, such as walking.

C. Breathing
Should be relaxed with rate and depth dictated by physiological reflexes. Students should learn to be aware of their own oxygen requirements and learn to regulate their breathing accordingly.

D. Stretches
After 2–3 minutes, the calves and hamstrings should be stretched before proceeding with other exercises or rest.

E. Heart Rate
As an added precaution, we recommend that the heart rate be again checked before beginning floor work. Heart rate should not exceed 60 percent of maximum (220 minus age multiplied by .6), five minutes after aerobic work. If heart rate is too high, individual should continue walking slowly until heart rate has lowered sufficiently.

VIII. Standing Waist Exercise

A. Time
5 minutes

B. Muscular Strengthening versus Rhythmic Movement
Exercises for the waist generally involve working the abdominal (rectus abdominis, external oblique, internal oblique, and transverse abdominis) muscles. Standing waist exercises that involve lateral bending or trunk rotation (twisting) are not the best exercises for these muscles as isolation, and resistance are difficult in this position. Abdominal curls with a twist (opposite elbow towards knees) are more effective for working the external

oblique. However, if standing waist exercises are performed, work should be done at a moderate speed with an effort made to create resistance for the working muscles.

C. **Body Alignment**
In order to protect the back from possible injury, care should be taken to correctly align the body as described in I.C. Head should be in midline position with shoulders square. When working to side, shoulder should drop directly to side, not to front or back, as this can cause unnecessary strain on the lower back.

D. **Twisting**
If twisting the upper torso, knees should be slightly bent and be aligned over the feet, not rolled in. Weight should be over the balls of the feet. Twisting exercises should be performed smoothly, not forcefully.

IX. Legs, Hips and Buttocks

A. **Purpose**
To strengthen the muscles of the legs and buttocks

B. **Time**
10–15 minutes

C. **Outer Thigh, Lying on Side**
Body should be in a straight line with the top arm positioned squarely on floor in front of body. Lower leg should be relaxed. Hip bones should be square and not leaning to the front or to the back. When extending leg, extend completely without locking the knee.

D. **Inner Thigh, Lying on Side**
Again, body should be in a straight line with hips square. When bringing top leg over working leg, keep foot on floor and lower leg in a straight vertical line.

E. **Upper Body**
Upper body should not move or jerk back and forth while performing leg, hip, and buttock exercises.

F. **Hips and Outer Thigh, "Doggy Position"**
Head should be held in a natural extension of the spine, not dropped forward. Hands should face forward. Weight should be balanced. Do not lean to side to compensate for work of muscles, do not allow lower back to arch inwards.

G. Buttocks
  1. On knees
     When working one leg to the back, the hips should be square, and the back straight, not swayed. Leg lifts should be small and resistive. Avoid jerking or throwing the leg up, as this can injure the lower back. If leg extends higher than hips, drop to elbows.
  2. Pelvic lifts
     When lying on back with knees bent and feet flat on floor, back should not arch or sway in. Pelvis should be tilted and the abdominals tight. The gluteus maximus should be contracted and released without bouncing or jerking the pelvis up and down. The mid-back should not leave the ground.

X. Abdominals
A. Purpose
To strengthen the abdominal muscles and thus help provide support for the internal organs and the back.
B. Time
4–8 minutes
C. Sit-Ups
Generally, abdominal work should not be performed with straight legs. Keep knees bent and lower back pressed into floor. Do not lift with the neck and push the head out of alignment. Head should be fully supported without any neck movement. To come to a full sitting position is not necessary and can risk injury to the back.
D. Leg lifts
Never lie on back and lift both legs straight up. Even with the hands under the buttocks one risks injury to the lumbar spine. In addition, leg lifts are *not* an effective abdominal exercise as the hip flexors, not the rectus abdominus, lift the legs through more than half of the lifting movement.
E. Position
No abdominal exercise should be performed in a manner that the lower back arches up off the floor. Body should be straight with lower back pushed firmly into the floor.
F. Breathing
Breathing is especially important while performing abdominal exercises. Exhale while contracting the abdominals at the point of

finishing your greatest exertion. Example: Exhale at the top of the sit-up, inhale when you lie back down.

G. Variety
Vary your abdominal exercises. Six minutes of bent knee sit-ups is not only boring, but insufficient to work the entire abdominal area. Adding a twist (opposite elbow towards knee) to your abdominal curl will effectively work the external oblique muscle and provide another base exercise for variation.

XI. Cool-Down Stretches
A. Purpose
To stretch muscles involved in strengthening exercises.

B. Time
3–7 minutes at the very end of your class.

C. Mode
Follow the same basic guidelines as outlined for the stretches at the beginning of your class. Again, no bouncing—static stretching only.

D. Muscle Groups
Particular attention should be paid to the calves, hamstrings and quadriceps. Stretches for the back are also recommended. Stretches should be appropriate to the exercises performed during class.

E. Breathing
Inhale as you begin the stretch, and simultaneously relax the muscles as you are stretching as you exhale.

XII. Final Heart Rate
A. When
Should be taken as stretches are finished and class member prepare to leave.

B. Heart Rate
Again, the recovery heart rate equals 60 percent of maximum (220 minus age, multiplied by .6). If not below this level, the individual was probably exercising too intensely and should work at a less vigorous level during the next class. Cool-down stretches should be continued until heart rate was lowered.

C. Saunas and Hot Tubs
Saunas and hot tubs, even hot showers, should be avoided immediately following exercise. The heat causes the blood vessels to dilate and this, along with the fact that the blood tends to be pooled in the extremities following vigorous exercise, cause the heart and brain to receive less blood.

Part A

Essentials of Aerobic Exercise

Chapter 1

What is Aerobic Exercise?

John E. Thiel, M.Ed.

Very simply put, *aerobics* means to exercise. Everyone has heard the word aerobics. It's widely used today in connection with exercise, but it's often not well understood. We might be confused because back in the 1960s we learned, maybe in a life science or biology class, that aerobic meant *with oxygen* or *in the presence of oxygen*. It was also back in the 1960s that Americans woke up to headlines in the morning paper that read, "The United States Leads the World in Deaths Due to Cardiovascular Disease." On page two it read, "Americans Are Unfit and Overweight." With this news, Americans started turning off their sedentary life-style and turning on to aerobic exercise.

At first, most people didn't know what they were doing, but Dr. Kenneth Cooper, the father of modern physical fitness, helped to lead the way. He organized a system, kept it in simple language, and called it aerobics. He got Americans pumping oxygen again. This is only one example of the significant contributions responsible for generating in Americans a nationwide interest in physical activity and aerobics.

This current interest in aerobic conditioning is the result of many people wanting to improve their everyday life. In most instances this desire is directed toward sports participation and a variety of recreational and leisure activities that require a continuous, high level of energy expenditure. Participation in aerobic exercise classes, jogging, swimming, tennis, cycling, and many other forms of activity all require a conditioned cardiovascular system capable of supplying adequate amounts of oxygen to the working muscles.

The purpose of this chapter is to provide the aerobic fitness instructor and other exercise enthusiasts with a better understanding of aerobics. An overview of the body's oxygen transport system and aerobic and anaerobic energy pathways will be presented. Discussion will include the physiologic changes that occur in the oxygen transport system and in the muscle cells as a result of aerobic conditioning. Finally, we will examine the factors that affect aerobic training and their recommended guidelines.

The Oxygen Delivery System

Aerobic energy production requires a constant and adequate supply of oxygen. To meet this demand, we must first have the ability to transport oxygen from the environment to the cells of the body. This ability comes from the oxygen transport system, which consists of the respiratory and cardiovascular systems.

The respiratory system begins with the lungs, which bring oxygen from the outside environment, across the alveolar membrane, and into the circulatory system. This process is called pulmonary ventilation. The movement of oxygen into, and the removal of carbon dioxide from the blood takes place through a process called diffusion. Oxygen is carried predominantly in the blood stream by its attachment to hemoglobin, an iron-containing protein molecule. The red blood cells then transport the oxygen by the cardiovascular system to the working muscles and all the rest of the body's cells.

The Cardiovascular System

Oxygenated blood is pumped by a strong left ventricle chamber into the aorta, which then branches out, delivering oxygen-rich blood and nutrients to the body's organs and tissues. At rest, the heart beats about 70 times a minute in adults, or more than 100,000 times a day. The two hollow chambers, atrium and ventricle, of the right side of the heart receive deoxygenated blood returning from all parts of the body and pump this blood to the lungs for removal of the end products of metabolism. A complex network of small blood vessels, called capillaries, delivers the oxygenated blood to the tissues.

With each contraction of the heart, blood surges out of the left ventricle into the aorta, distending it and creating pressure on the vascular wall which travels through the entire system. This pressure is called systolic blood pressure and represents the contraction or systole of the left ventricle. During the relaxation phase of the cardiac cycle there remains a blood pressure in the arterial system. This remaining pressure is known as diastolic blood pressure.

The amount of blood the heart pumps per minute is referred to as cardiac output, which is determined by multiplying the heart rate by the amount of blood pumped out of the heart per beat—*stroke volume.* Cardiac output relates to the functional capacity of the circulatory system to meet the demands of aerobic endurance activity. As the exercise intensity increases, the demand for oxygenated bloodflow to the exercising muscle increases. The increases in cardiac output are met by both an increase in heart rate and in stroke volume.

At rest, the cardiac output of trained individuals and sedentary people is about the same. There is, however, a difference in the stroke volume between the trained and untrained while at rest. The *trained individual* will have a *higher resting stroke volume* and a *lower heart rate,* thus having a cardiac output similar to the untrained person. This is desirable. The lower the resting heart rate, the healthier the individual, because the heart simply does not have to beat as fast to deliver the necessary blood to the body.

Physiologic changes that take place in the cardiorespiratory system as a result of aerobic training will be discussed in more detail in the chapters on Anatomy and Physiology of Exercise, and Endurance Training.

Overview of Energy Pathways

Energy comes into the body in the form of carbohydrates, fats, and proteins. These nutrients that are consumed in the diet, however, cannot be used for immediate energy production. Instead, the human body produces and stores its own form of energy to perform the many thousands of complex chemical functions required for biologic work. This biologic work takes place in all the body's cells and organ systems. The main storage sites for energy in the body are in muscle, liver, blood and fat tissue. We will focus our attention only on an understanding of the aerobic and anaerobic energy systems used during muscle contraction.

Food in a carbohydrate form is stored in the muscle, liver, and blood in the form of a muscle glucose called glycogen. During muscle contraction, stored glucose is broken down into carbon dioxide, lactic acid, and water. During this breakdown, chemical energy is released. This liberation of chemical energy from glucose is called cellular respiration or metabolism. The primary purpose of metabolism is to supply the energy needed to carry out the mechanical work of muscular contraction.

ATP—The body's fuel

The energy liberated during the breakdown of glucose is not directly used in muscle contraction. Rather, it is employed to manufacture another chemical compound known as adenosine triphosphate, ATP. ATP is stored in all cells, and is used for all the energy-requiring processes within the cell. There is a considerable amount of energy stored in the bonds that link the phosphate molecules. When ATP in a muscle cell is broken down, the energy released activates the contractile elements in the muscle fibers. The contractile elements, once activated, slide past each other and cause the muscle to shorten—that is, to contract.

Sources of muscle ATP

There are three ways in which ATP is an immediate source of energy for muscle contraction. They are the ATP-creatine phosphate (CP), and the two chemical or metabolic pathways of lactic acid and the aerobic energy system. The amount of available ATP for immediate use that is stored in our body at any one time is about three ounces. This amount of ATP provides enough energy to run all-out for only a few seconds. ATP is constantly being resynthesized in the cells, providing a continuous supply of energy. Cells store more creatine phosphate than ATP. Energy released from the breakdown of ATP and creatine phosphate (without the presence of oxygen) will allow all-out exercise, such as sprinting, for about five to eight seconds. If we are going to maintain activity, we need additional energy.

The anaerobic energy system (lactic acid system)

When a molecule of glucose enters a cell to be used for energy, it undergoes a series of reactions known as *glycolysis*. Glycolysis simply means the "dissolving of sugar." Oxygen is not required in this anaerobic series of reactions. As the glucose molecule is broken down, ATP is produced. The end product in this breakdown is lactic acid. The ATP produced through this anaerobic energy pathway provides a rapid, but limited amount of energy for muscular activity. Activities that are high intensity, but short in duration are fueled from the anaerobic reactions of glycolysis.

The aerobic energy system

Energy-releasing reactions that are dependent on a constant supply of oxygen are aerobic. Above we said that only about 5% of the energy contained within a molecule of glucose is released during the anaerobic pathway. It would be a big waste of glucose if there were not an additional means for harnessing the remaining energy available. The aerobic energy pathway provides for a complete breakdown of a glucose molecule to carbon dioxide and water. The end product of this breakdown is the release of 38 molecules of ATP. During the breakdown of glucose and in the presence of oxygen, large amounts of energy are released.

These aerobic reactions occur within the mitochondria of the muscle cell. Through a complex series of chemical reactions, glycogen and fats are broken down in the presence of oxygen to provide energy. As exercise intensity diminishes from a maximal effort and as duration extends to four minutes or longer, the energy required for muscle contraction comes almost totally from the aerobic production of ATP. During prolonged exercise, more than 99% of the energy requirement is generated by aerobic reactions. These aerobic energy pathways provide the major supply of energy to all the cells of the body. One of the more important characteristics of the aerobic energy pathway is the ability to utilize stored body fat as a primary source of energy.

Table A.1 Summary of Aerobic and Anaerobic Pathways of Energy Production

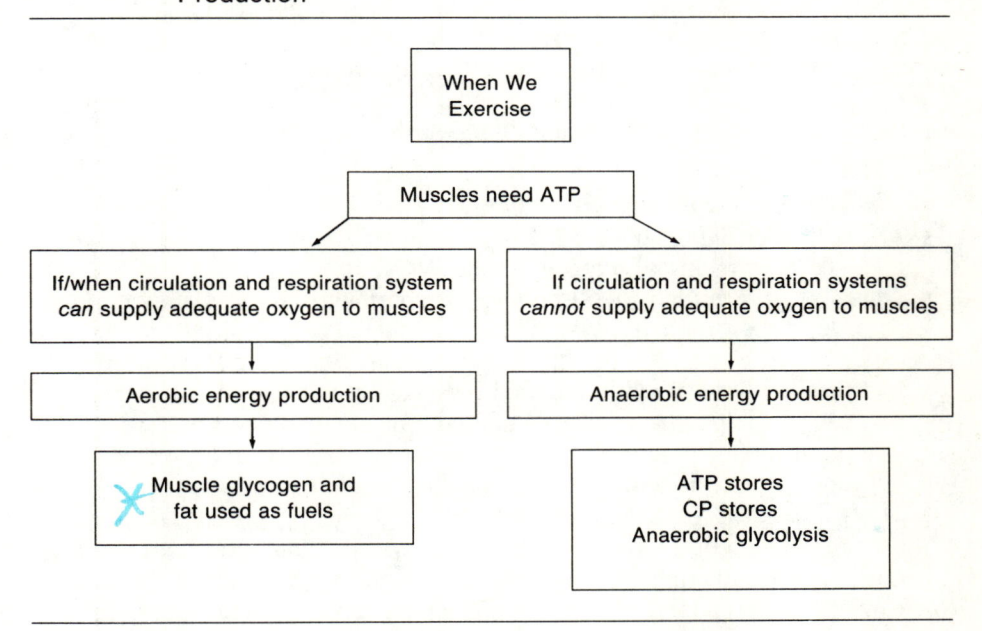

```
              When We
              Exercise
                 |
          Muscles need ATP
          /              \
If/when circulation and      If circulation and respiration systems
respiration system           cannot supply adequate oxygen to muscles
can supply adequate
oxygen to muscles
         |                              |
Aerobic energy production        Anaerobic energy production
         |                              |
Muscle glycogen and              ATP stores
fat used as fuels                CP stores
                                 Anaerobic glycolysis
```

Cardiorespiratory Changes Resulting From Aerobic Conditioning

Improvements in cardiorespiratory function as the result of continuous aerobic conditioning account for approximately 50% of the increase seen in maximal oxygen uptake, i.e., the maximum capacity to generate energy aerobically. *The most significant improvement in cardiovascular function due to aerobic training is the increase in maximum cardiac output.* This is due to the significant increase in stroke volume. *Total blood volume and the amount of hemoglobin present in the blood tend to increase with aerobic conditioning.*

The other 50% improvement in maximal oxygen uptake comes from the site of energy utilization inside the muscle cell itself. With aerobic training there is an increase in both the size and number of mitochondria present within the muscle cell. Most important is the trained muscle's capacity to mobilize and metabolize fat. During submaximal aerobic activity, the trained person will use more free fatty acids for fuel than the untrained person.

Factors That Affect Aerobic Training

In order to get the most out of exercising and directing others to exercise, an aerobics instructor must consider the major factors that are related to aerobics training improvements. Based on the existing evidence concerning exercise prescriptions for healthy adults, the *American College of Sports Medicine* makes the following recommendations for the quantity and quality of training for developing and maintaining cardiorespiratory fitness and body composition:

- *Frequency of training:* three to five days per week.
- *Intensity of training:* 60%–90% of maximum HR reserve, or 50%–85% of maximal oxygen uptake (VO$_2$max).
- *Duration of training:* 15–60 minutes of continuous aerobic activity; thus, low intensity activity should be conducted over a longer period of time. Because of the importance of the "total fitness" effect and the fact that it is more readily attained in long-duration programs, and because of the potential hazards and compliance problems associated with high-intensity activity, low-to-moderate intensity activity of longer duration is recommended for the nonathletic adult.
- *Mode of activity:* Any activity that uses large muscle groups, that can be maintained continuously, and that is rhythmic and aerobic in nature, e.g., running-jogging, walking-hiking, swimming, skating, bicycling, rowing, cross-country skiing, rope skipping, and various endurance game activities.

Summary

An overview of the oxygen delivery system was presented. Aerobics is widely used today in connection with exercise, but it is often not well understood. The physiologic changes associated with aerobic conditioning that occur within the cardiorespiratory system and at the site of energy metabolism were reviewed. Improvements in cardiorespiratory endurance are dependent on the intensity, duration, and frequency of the aerobic programs.

Commonly Asked Questions

Q. Does aerobic fitness automatically decrease with age?
A. As one gets older there usually appears to be a decrease in aerobic

fitness. However, if a person were to stay physically active, the rate of decline in aerobic fitness may be smaller.

Q. Is jogging or running the best form of aerobic conditioning?
A. Studies were conducted where running, walking, and bicycling were used as different modes of exercise. Frequency, intensity, and duration were kept constant for 20 weeks. Changes in aerobic capacity and body composition showed similar improvements. If an exercise activity is the same intensity as jogging and is maintained for the same duration and frequency, there should be very little difference in the aerobic improvements between the two.

Q. Is the energy required for a tennis serve stored, or is it provided by the aerobic energy pathway?
A. Sudden maximum bursts of energy—such as the tennis serve, volleyball spike and the 40- or 50-yard dash—are provided anaerobically, that is, almost exclusively by stored ATP and creatine-phosphate high-energy phosphates.

Q. What is oxygen deficit?
A. This is the time period during exercise in which the level of oxygen consumption is below that necessary to supply all the ATP required for the exercise. It is also the time period during which an oxygen debt is contracted.

References

American College of Sports Medicine. "Position Statement on the Recommended Quantity and Quality of Exercise for Developing and Maintaining Fitness in Healthy Adults." *Medicine, Science and Sports.* 1978:10:vii–x.

Government of Canada. "The Measure of Energy—A Participation Kit for Fitness Leaders." Participation: Fitness Canada, 1984.

Katch, F. and McArdle, W. *Nutrition, Weight Control, and Exercise*, 2nd Ed. Philadelphia: Lea and Febiger Co., 1983.

McArdle, W. et al. *Exercise Physiology-Energy, Nutrition, and Human Performance.* Philadelphia: Lea and Febiger Co., 1981.

Mathews, D. and Fox, E. *The Physiological Basis of Physical Education and Athletics*, 2nd Ed. Philadelphia: Saunders College, 1971.

Pollock, M. "How Much Exercise Is Enough?" *The Physician and Sportsmedicine.* 1978:June:50–64.

Pollock, M., et al. *Exercise in Health and Disease.* Philadelphia: Saunders, 1984.

Chapter 2

Anatomy and Physiology of Aerobic Exercise

Patricia Eisenman, Ph.D.

The human body is a fantastic mechanism. It can take us hiking to the tops of mountains, skiing in the wilderness, diving in the ocean, running, jumping and cavorting in our local fitness centers, as well as allow us to fulfill the routine requirements of our daily lives. This diversity of accomplishment is possible because of the marvelous ability of our body—bones, muscles and other tissues—to adapt to the demands placed upon it.

Aerobics and fitness instructors need to be aware of how to best facilitate these processes, both in their own bodies and the bodies of their clients. Consequently, the material in this chapter will help you to better understand the anatomy and physiology of the body and how certain anatomical structures and physiological processes interact in order to execute physical activities in a safe and effective manner. Since anatomy refers to the structure of the body and physiology refers to how these various body structures function, the first sections of this chapter will discuss anatomy. Next will come the exploration of how the various organs and structures function as humans engage in physical activity. Finally, the chapter focuses on anatomy and physiology as it relates to aerobic exercise.

Anatomy

There are many structures that comprise the human body and as we learn more about exercise and physical activity, we are discovering that most anatomical structures are involved in the exercise process in some fashion. This chapter, however, will be limited to introducing you to key anatomical structures and sensitizing you to the need for aerobics and fitness instructors to have an appreciation for and awareness of the importance of anatomy.

The Living Skeleton

The skeleton of the body is frequently referred to as the framework of the body. Granted the 206 bones that make up the skeleton do support body weight, but they do much more than the steel beams that comprise the framework of a building. Those steel beams may lose some strength as the building ages, but for the most part they will remain unchanged. This is not true of bones. They are living, and therefore in a constant state of change. Bones are made up of cells, a hard material between the cells known as the matrix, and fibers that are found in the matrix. Although the cells are surrounded by the matrix, and calcium, phosphorus and other minerals are stored here, this does not mean that bone is a solid material. Quite the contrary is true. If you cut a bone in half (see figure A.1), you can see that while there is a layer of compact bone, a substantial portion of the bone has a sponge-like appearance. There is also a cavity-like area called the marrow in which blood cells are made. As long ago as the 1890s, an anatomist named Wolfe observed this sponge-like layer and speculated that it was caused by tiny pieces or spicules of bone forming along the stress lines in that bone. In other words, Wolfe was suggesting that bone has an internal structure that differs from individual to individual, depending upon the forces that the individual's bone must withstand. Researchers have compared the bones in the arms of tennis players and reported that the dominant arm—the arm that holds the racquet—has a larger diameter, and the bone is more dense than in the nondominant arm. Other investigators have noted that the bones in the legs of runners have more of these bone spicules than the bones in the legs of nonrunners. Older women who have been sedentary have been observed to experience an increase in the density of their bones if they initiate moderate physical activity programs.

These kinds of observations substantiate the fact that bone is not static, that it is living, and that new cells are constantly developing and laying down new spicules while older cells and their spicules are being removed (resorbed). These processes take place constantly, but when the body is subjected to new stresses, such as those that occur at the onset of an exercise program, these processes are stimulated. If nutrition is adequate, if the individual gets plenty of rest, and if the exercise is not too intense, the internal structure of the bone will be able to adapt to the new stresses placed upon it. The potential is there for a skeletal system that is stronger than it was prior to the physical activity program. In other words, the skeleton should be better able to do its job of supporting the body's weight. On the other hand, if nutrition is inadequate, if the person does not get adequate rest, or if the exercises or physical activities are too intense, the resorption of bone will exceed the production of new bone and the possibility of a stress fracture exists.

ANATOMY AND PHYSIOLOGY OF AEROBIC EXERCISE   13

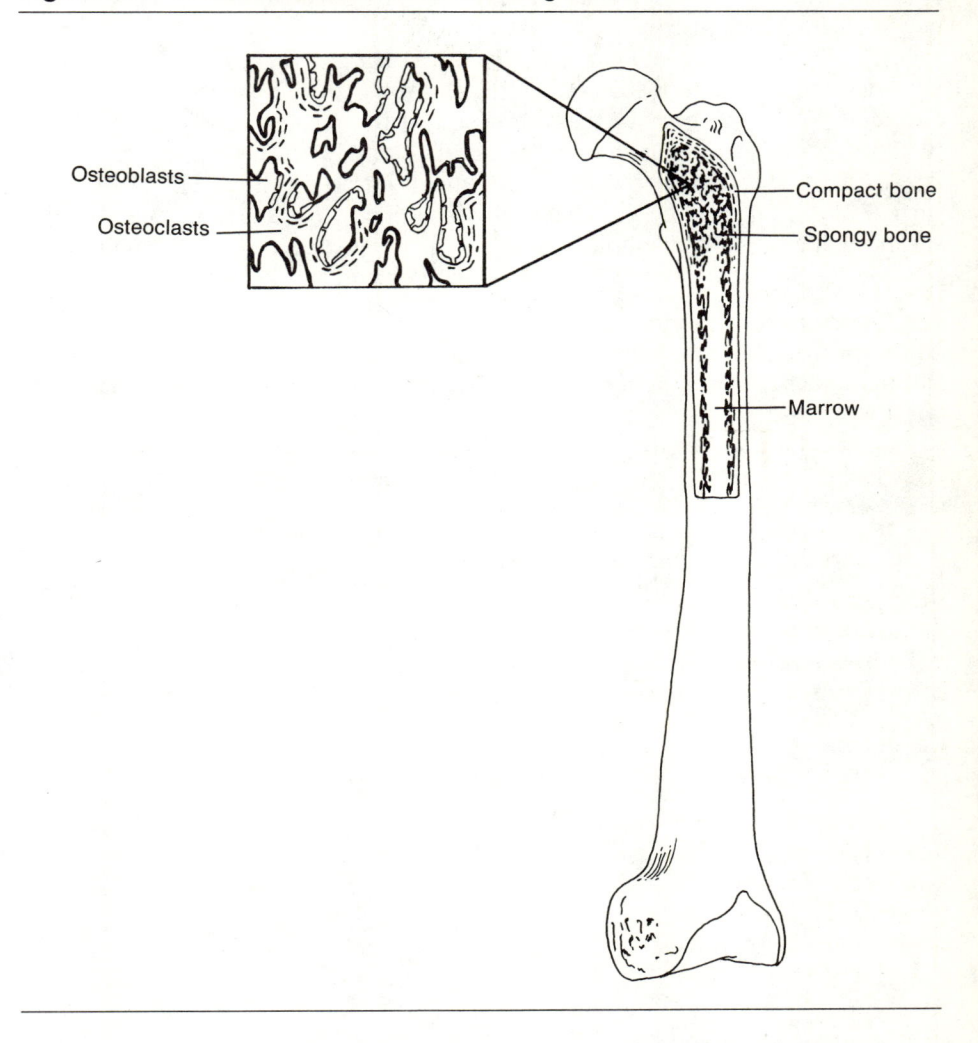

Figure A.1   A cross-sectional view of a long bone.

   There are a number of circumstances and/or situations which might result in this type of overstressing. That is why the AFAA *Basic Exercise Standards and Guidelines* have addressed the concept of how frequently one should workout.   [**I.A: Frequency of Workouts**]   Active participation in 12 classes a week and no more than three classes per day should be considered the maximum for the experienced instructor. Instructors who are just starting should not exercise this frequently. Similarly, application of the

14   ESSENTIALS OF AEROBIC EXERCISE

overload training principle requires that there be only modest, gradual increases in the intensity, frequency, or duration of any given exercise or activity. The type of footwear as well as the exercise surface are also important considerations for controlling the stress of the exercise. [**VI.G: Surface**]   Well-fitting shoes that are designed for aerobics and provide sufficient support and cushion are the goal.   [**III.C: Attire**]   Additional insoles may be required to help absorb shock in the forefoot. The floor surface should ideally be wooden with a cushion of air under it. Our living skeletons have a fantastic ability to adapt, if we just give some thought to controlling the total impact stress to which we subject our bones.

The Supportive Skeleton

The human skeleton may be divided into two major divisions: the axial and the appendicular (see table A.2). The axial skeleton consists of those

Table A.2   Bones of the axial and appendicular skeleton

Name	Number
Axial Skeleton	
Skull	
Cranium	8
Face	14
Hyoid	1
Auditory Ossicles	6
Vertebral Column	
Clavicle	24
Sternum	1
Appendicular Skeleton	
Shoulder Girdles	
Clavicle	2
Scapula	2
Upper Extremities	
Humerus	2
Ulna	2
Radius	2
Carpals	16
Metacarpals	10
Phalanges	28
Pelvic Girdle	
Coaxial, hip, or pelvic bone	2
Lower Extremities	
Femur	2
Fibula	2
Tibia	2
Patella	2
Tarsals	14
Metatarsals	10
Phalanges	28
	206

ANATOMY AND PHYSIOLOGY OF AEROBIC EXERCISE   15

bones surrounding the axis of the body, which is the imaginary line running vertically along the body's center of gravity. As may be seen in figure A.2, this line runs through the head and down to the space between the feet. The appendicular skeleton contains the bones of the arms, legs, fingers, and toes (appendages) plus the combination of bones called girdles (e.g., shoulder girdle), which connect the free appendages to the axial skeleton.

Figure A.2   The axis of the body.

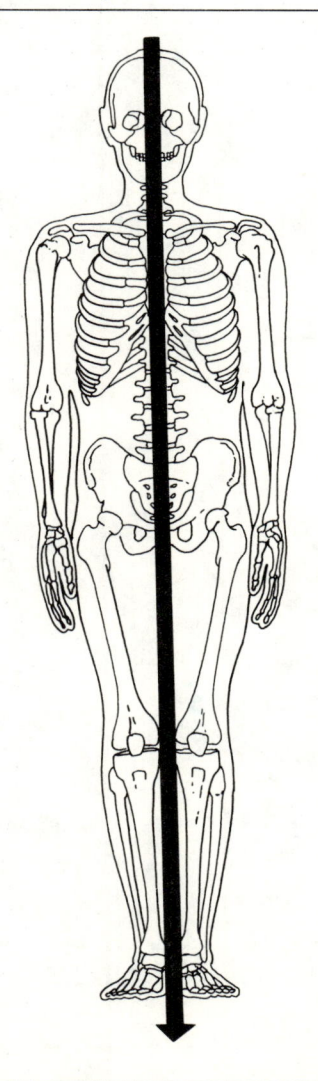

16 ESSENTIALS OF AEROBIC EXERCISE

The vertebral column or spine is typically made up of 26 vertebrae. Each vertebra has a body, several processes, and at least one opening or foramen (see figure A.3). Also, between the vertebrae there are intravertebral foramina (small passageways). The nerves that connect the spinal cord to various parts of the body pass through these openings. Because the vertebrae are arranged in a column, the vertebral foramina are aligned,

Figure A.3 The vertebrae.

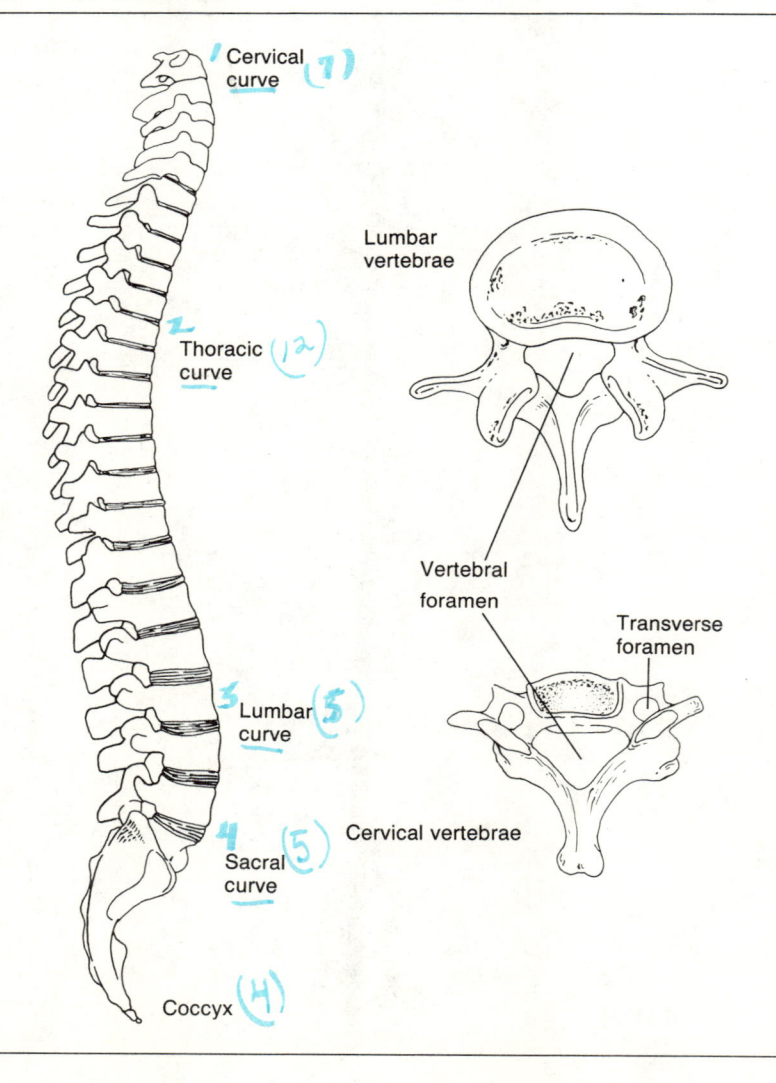

forming a protective passageway for the spinal cord itself. The transverse foramina of the cervical or neck vertebrae are also aligned, forming passageways for arteries and nerves. Now, while the term *aligned* has been utilized, this does not mean that the proper position for the vertebral column is a perfectly straight line. Quite the contrary; as can be observed in figure A.3 there are four distinct curves in the normal vertebral column. The cervical vertebrae form the cervical curve, the 12 vertebrae in the chest region form the thoracic curve, and the five vertebrae in the low back area form the lumbar curve. The fourth, or sacral, curve is formed by the sacrum (five sacral vertebrae that have fused) and four coccygeal vertebrae, which are fused into one or two bones called the coccyx. These curves provide resilience and help the body absorb the forces of walking, jogging, jumping, and other activities.

The appropriate body alignment is one in which the head, vertebrae, pelvic girdle, and legs are in a balanced position. The word *balance* is stressed to emphasize that with proper body alignment, the bones of the axial skeleton can efficiently support the body's weight. For example, if you were to take a series of boxes and stack them, you would quickly find that you must position the center of gravity of the boxes over one another, or the stack will succumb to gravity and topple over. The same would be true of the human body if it were not for the muscles. If you do not properly align your skeleton, the muscles will have to compensate to allow you to remain upright (see figure A.4). They can do this but not without paying a price—at the very least, muscle fatigue. At worst, the price of improper alignment may be muscle strain, low-back pain due to irritations to nerves passing through transverse foramina that are out of alignment, and uneven wear and tear to joint surfaces that are out of alignment.

The aerobics and fitness instructor should be aware of the proper alignment of the axial skeleton, provide feedback to students as to how well they are maintaining proper alignment, and encourage students to continually monitor their own bodies. **[I.C: Body Alignment]** Such monitoring should take place throughout the day as well as in exercise situations. Just because you are in the cardiovascular phase of your class does not mean that your students should allow their heads to fall forward, their shoulders to become rounded, or their stomachs to sag forward. The same is true for the execution of exercises designed to strengthen specific body parts; do not forget to maintain total body alignment.

Certain movements or actions will require temporary alterations in the alignment of the axial skeleton. If you understand the anatomy of the tissues involved in the movement, you will be better able to evaluate the safety of the move. Take the motions involved in head circling. The seven cervical vertebrae are the smallest and most delicate of the vertebrae. They also

Figure A.4 Skeletal alignment

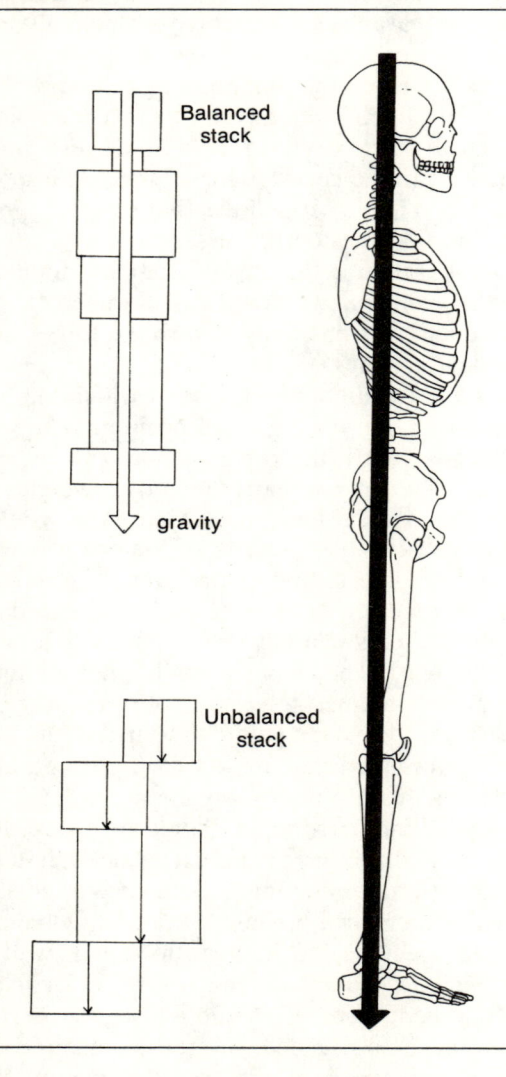

demonstrate the most degeneration with aging. Consequently, care should be taken to minimize the potential for damage to these relatively fragile vertebrae. Controlled movements of the head to the sides and forward are appropriate, but actions that require extreme neck flexion or extension are contraindicated. (Safety considerations indicate that these activities should not be done.) For example, many people when doing the plough or plow (see figure A.5) have all of their weight on the 7th cervical vertebra (the

Figure A.5 The plough

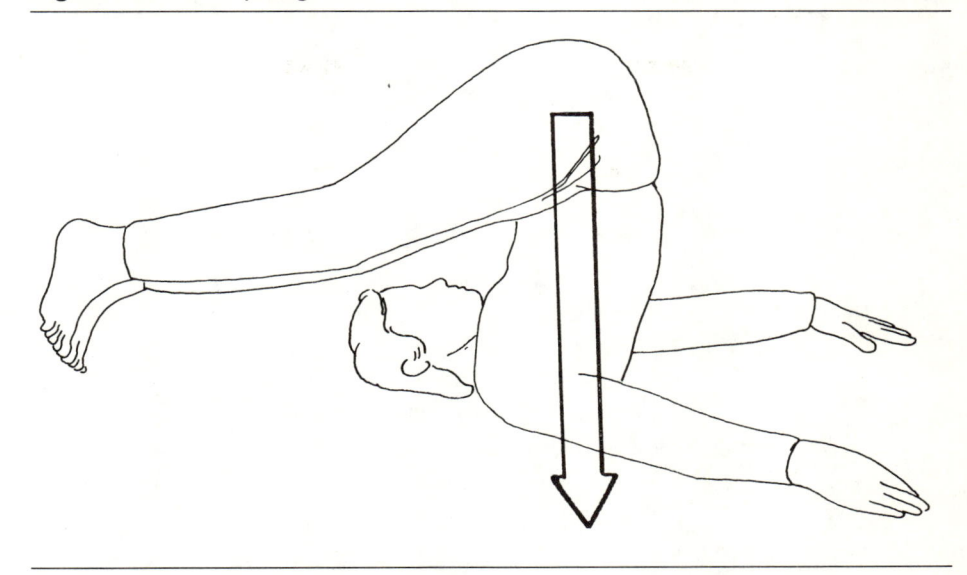

prominent vertebra at the base of the neck). This can result in excessive stress for this small vertebra, particularly if the exercise is performed repeatedly. Furthermore, in the neck flexion required for the plow or the neck hyperextension necessitated in the motion portrayed in figure A.6, there is the potential for pinching or kinking the vertebral artery that passes through the tranverse foramina of the cervical vertebrae. Although well designed to support movement, the integrity of the vertebral column should not be jeopardized by ballistic or uncontrolled motions of the trunk and/or head.

It is also important to remember that when we are in an upright posture, the bones of the axial skeleton are balanced one over the other and are therefore quite capable of supporting the body's weight because the pull of gravity comes down through the bones. However, this is not the case when we deviate from an upright position. For example, if we are standing and flex or bend forward at the waist. The downward pull of gravity is now working to pull the vertebrae apart. The ligaments (cordlike tissue which connect bones), tendons (cordlike tissue connecting muscle to bone), and muscles help to prevent this. However, the posterior longitudinal ligament that provides support for the vertebrae tapers down to its smallest size in the area of the lumbar vertebrae (see figure A.7). Consequently, this ligament is providing less support in the lumbar area. Standing toe-touching activities also place considerable compressive force on the intervertebral discs of the

Figure A.6 Hyperextension of the neck.

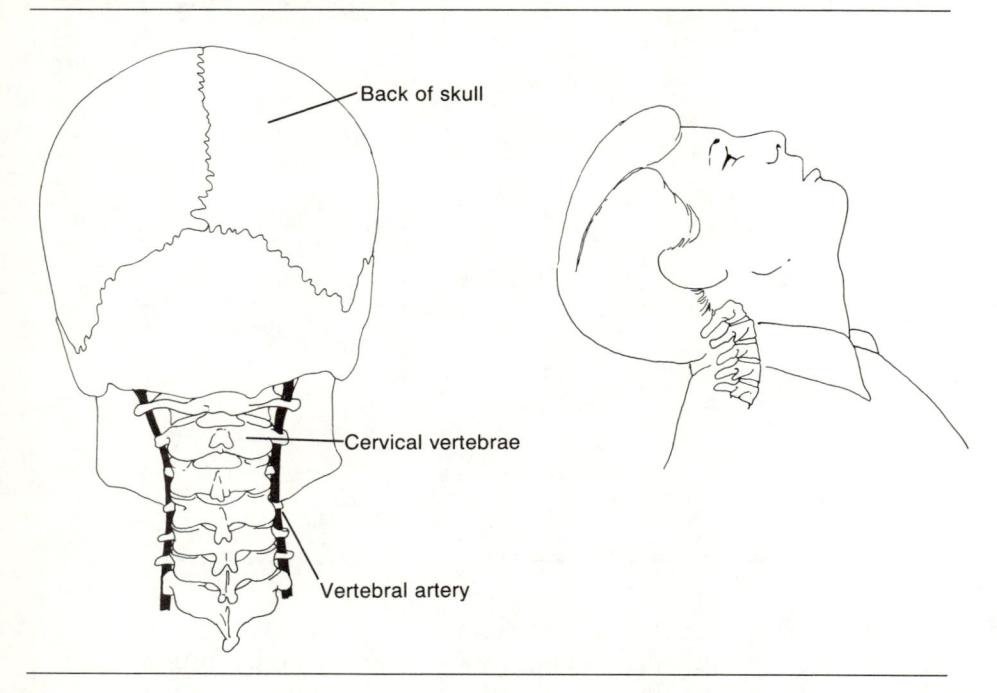

low back. Such toe-touching activities, particularly if they are ballistic, can aggravate existing low-back problems or even play a role in the development of disc problems. Most of these same toe-touching activities may be performed from a seated position with considerably less risk, so you may want to consider making some routine modifications for some of your students. In fact, such sensitivity to individual needs can go a long way toward preventing injury. Although we all have the same basic anatomy, there is considerable individual variability. Remember this potential for individual variability, particularly as we discuss interactions between the axial and appendicular skeleton in the next section.

The Moving Skeleton

In addition to supporting the body's weight, the bones act as a lever system. So, by having the muscles pull on the bones, we can move our body parts as well as our bodies, as in walking and running. Before further analyzing these processes, we need to define a few anatomical terms. A joint is the junction between two or more bones. Although we have a number of joints, they are not all alike. Since the different types of joints

ANATOMY AND PHYSIOLOGY OF AEROBIC EXERCISE   21

Figure A.7   Longitudinal ligament.

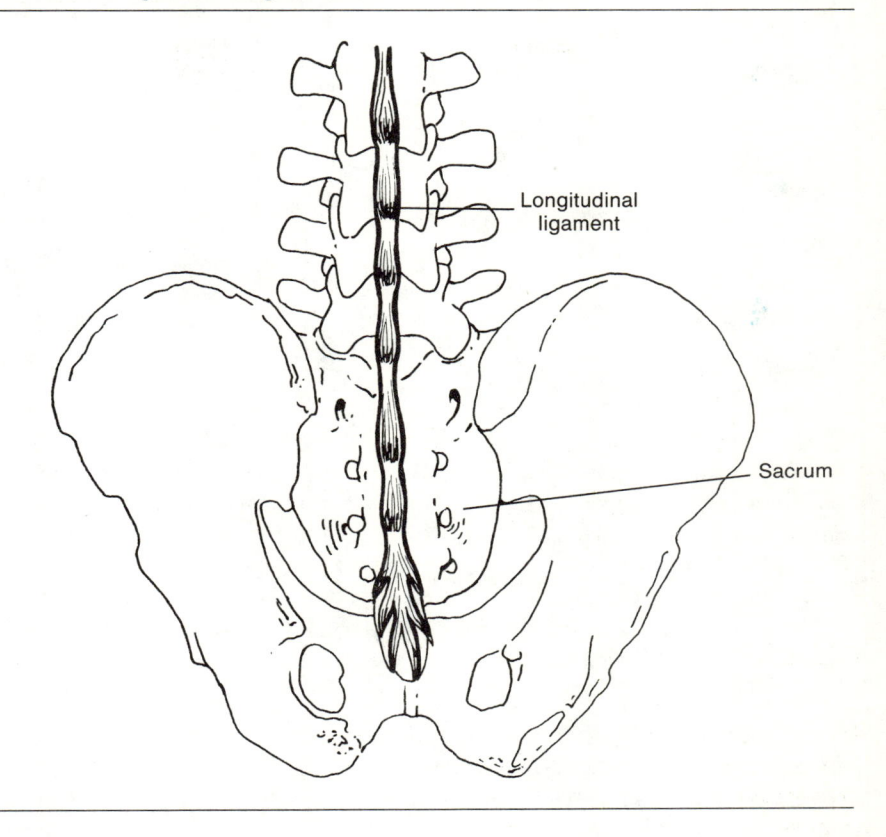

Longitudinal ligament

Sacrum

allow for different kinds of movements, examine the material contained in table A.3 and become familiar with the different types of joints and the scientific descriptions for the various joint motions.

Since muscles bring about these movements, a muscle that causes flexion of a joint is a flexor muscle; a muscle that extends a joint is an extensor; and so on. Because each of the joints has a number of muscles that facilitate its movement potential, the brain has the complex task of coordinating the contraction and relaxation of these muscles. Consequently, there is an elaborate communication system known as the nervous system (Figure A.8). The brain and spinal cord are connected to the muscles by way of efferent (carry signals from spinal cord to muscles) nerves and afferent (carry signals from muscle to spinal cord) nerves. The afferent nerves carry information about your body's position in space.

Table A.3 Types of joints and their movement potentials

Type	Movement(s)	Example
Gliding	Flexion and Extension Abduction (away from the mid-line of the body) Adduction (toward the mid-line of the body)	Intercarpal and intertarsal joints (as in the palm of the hand)
Hinge	Flexion and Extension	Elbow, knee, ankle and interphalangial (finger and toe) joints
Pivot	Rotation	Head-neck and the radioulnar joint (which allows for rotation of the forearm)
Saddle	Flexion and Extension Abduction and Adduction	Carpmetacarpal joint of the thumb
Ball-and-socket	Flexion and Extension Abduction and Adduction and Rotation	Shoulder and hip joints

While this elegant communication system coordinates the action at joints without our consciously thinking about it, there are some ways to enhance joint function and prevent injury to joints and the surrounding structures. We can select exercises and activities that result in the equal development of the muscles surrounding a given joint. Examination of the relationship between the lumbar vertebrae and pelvic girdle is an excellent way of illustrating this concept.

The Pelvic Area

Figure A.9 depicts the bones and muscles involved. The rectus abdominis flexes the trunk and can pull up on the pelvis, thus flattening the lower back. The erector spinae (ES) are a group of muscles that help to extend the spine and keep it erect. If they contract still more, they play a role in arching the back. Consequently, if these muscles are too short, they increase the normal lumbar curve, contributing to a "sway back" appearance. The iliopsoas muscle also attaches to the vertebrae, but it passes anterior to the spine and inserts on the femur (large bone in the thigh). Therefore, this muscle group flexes the trunk, and if it is shortened from use and continuously kept in a seated position, as is so true of people with desk jobs, the iliopsoas pulls the pelvis and lower back forward, increasing the lumbar curve. The rectus femoris and the quadriceps muscle attached to the pelvis can, therefore, also influence the tilt of the pelvis. Since the muscles of the hamstring group, at the back of the thigh, also attach to the lower part of the pelvis, they too influence the tilt of the pelvis. What we have is a situation that is somewhat analagous to placing guidewires on a sapling tree that we have just planted. If we place too much tension on one of the wires, the tree will be pulled too far in one direction and therefore be out of alignment. Similarly, if any of the muscles just discussed are too short, the

Figure A.8 Spinal column and nerves.

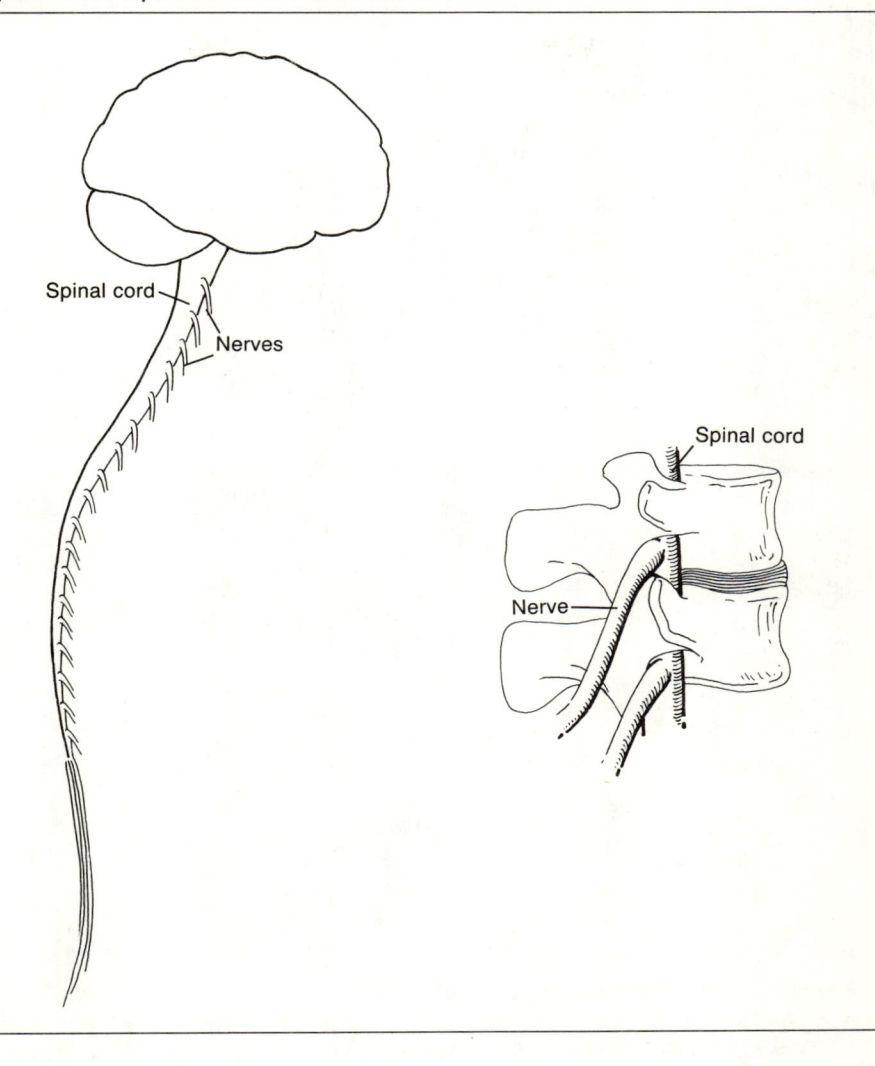

pelvis will be tilted. This forces the shortened muscle or muscles to work even harder because the skeleton is now out of alignment and less capable of supporting itself. The "overworked" muscles will be subject to frequent fatigue and perhaps injury. The poorly aligned skeleton can result in pressure on nerves entering and leaving the spinal area. In fact, there is quite a high incidence of low-back pain associated with individuals who have an excessive curvature in their lower backs.

24 ESSENTIALS OF AEROBIC EXERCISE

Figure A.9 Pelvic area and muscles.

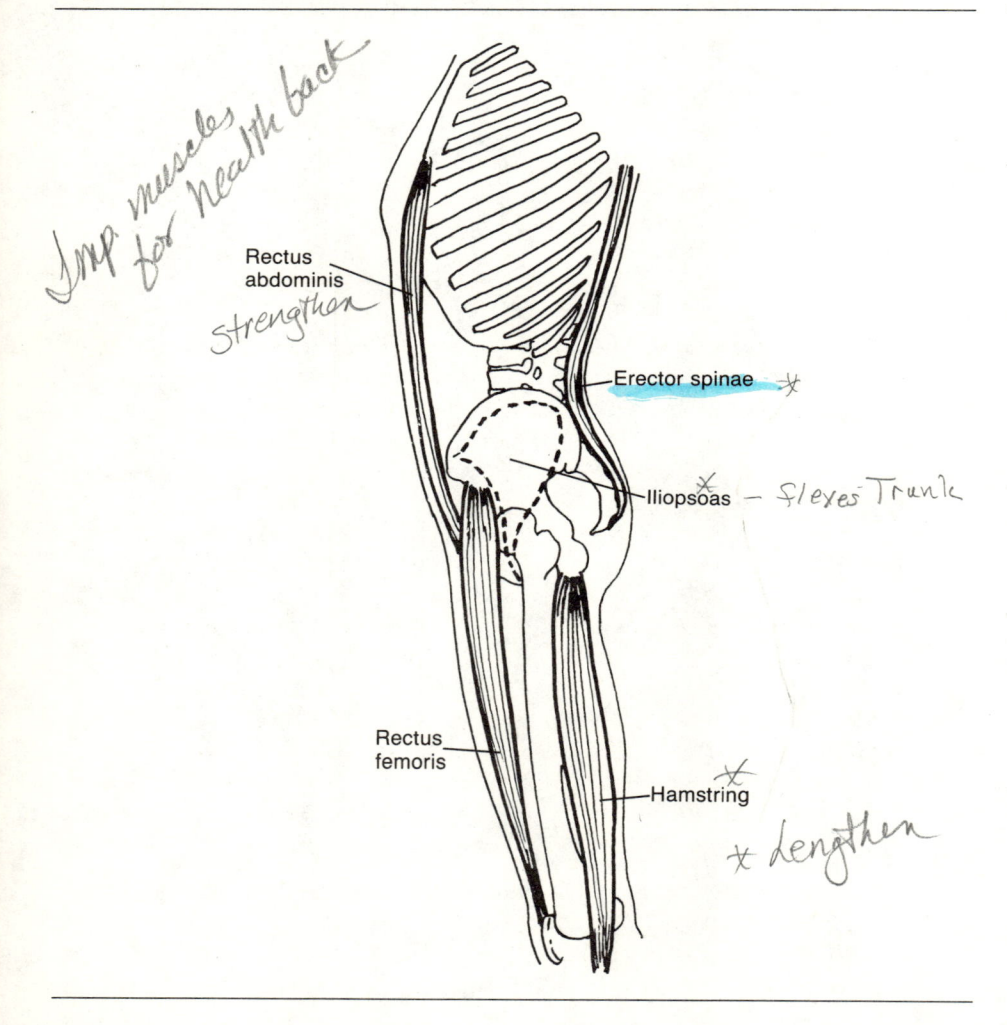

Imp muscles for healthy back

- Rectus abdominis — *strengthen*
- Erector spinae *
- Iliopsoas — *flexes Trunk*
- Rectus femoris
- Hamstring *

* lengthen

If you see that you have placed too much tension on one of the guide wires on your sapling, you can remedy the situation by readjusting the tension. Similarly, the position of the pelvis may be adjusted by strengthening muscles, which shortens them, or by stretching muscles to relax the pull being placed on the pelvis. The strengthening-lengthening process is frequently referred to as achieving muscle balance. Achieving this muscle balance should be the goal of all exercise programs for all of the joints of the body. Never overdevelop the muscles on one side of a joint. It may take several years for a problem to arise, but eventually muscle imbalances will cause difficulties. For example, baseball pitchers use primarily the muscles in their throwing arms and even then they utilize only some of these. If they do not strengthen the other muscles in the throwing arm and the nonthrowing arm as well, muscle imbalances are likely to result in injuries that shorten their careers. Similarly, fitness instructors need to select exercises that develop and maintain muscle balance. Obviously, not all your students will have the same needs, but there are some very common needs that you should be aware of. That is why so much time was spent explaining the anatomy of the pelvic area. Most of us sit at desks, drive cars with our arms and legs extended in front of us, and do tasks around the office, plant or house that require us to extend our arms and heads forward. All these situations increase the likelihood that our hamstrings, iliopsoas muscles, and erector spinae muscles will be overly tight, while our rectus abdominis is not as strong as it might be. Consequently, abdominal strengthening activities and activities to lengthen the hamstrings, iliopsoas, and erector spinae muscles are quite appropriate for aerobics classes.

The progressive exercises at the end of this chapter provide an example of a simple progression of exercises. They combine both strengthening and lengthening exercises.

Abdominal muscles portrayed in figure A.10 include the rectus abdominis, but there are other abdominal muscles as well. These other muscles are frequently neglected. They are best exercised by doing rotational or twisting movements with the trunk. So incorporate some sit-up variations requiring twisting actions; just be careful to avoid ballistic twisting actions when in a standing position. Those forces are much greater than forces experienced while doing more controlled actions on the floor.

The Knee

The knee is another example of a joint that is very much influenced by the balance of the strength of the muscles which surround it (see figure A.11). The actual knee joint lies between the femur and the tibia. These bones are held together by a very complex network of ligaments. The other small bone of the lower leg, the fibula, is not part of the joint. The muscles that cross the knee also help to maintain the integrity of the knee, the two major muscle groups being the quadriceps and the hamstrings.
Unfortunately, not all activities develop these muscles equally. For example, jogging tends to over develop the hamstrings, while sprinting emphasizes quadriceps development. Since most of us cannot do much sprinting, our quadriceps need strengthening. This is particularly true of women whose hips are relatively wide. The wider pelvis means that the quadriceps angle

Figure A.10 Abdominal muscles

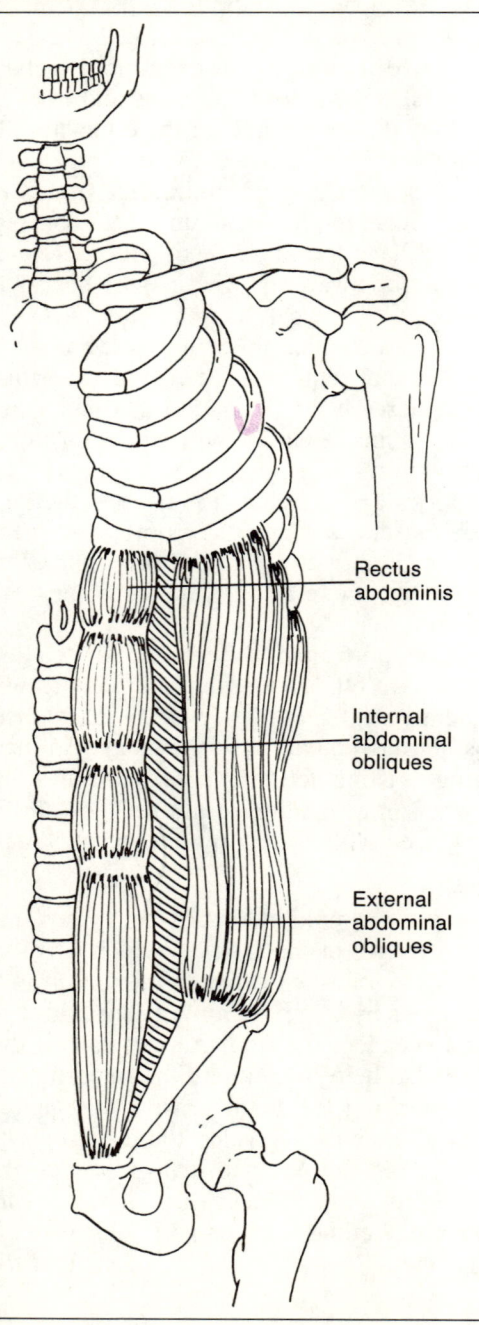

ANATOMY AND PHYSIOLOGY OF AEROBIC EXERCISE 27

Figure A.11 The knee.

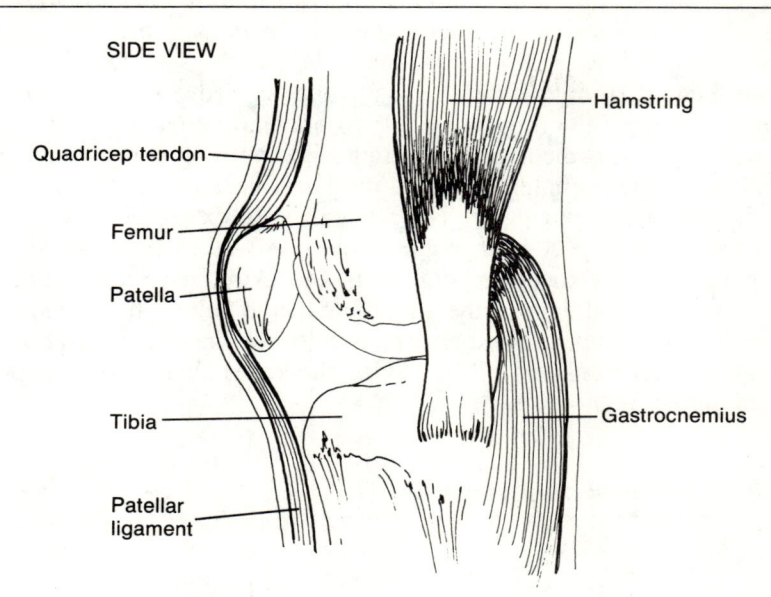

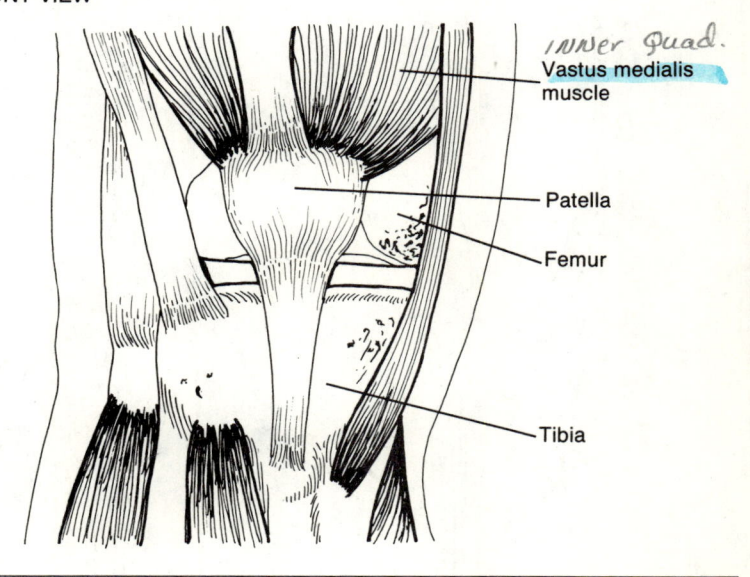

of pull at the knee is different than in an individual with a narrow hip (see figure A.12). Therefore, as the knee is flexed, the patella, the "knee cap," is pulled off to the side or dislocated. Since the patella is surrounded by the quadriceps tendon, strengthening the vastus medialis (the quadriceps muscle on the inner aspect of the thigh) can help to prevent the patella from dislocating. The vastus medialis is strengthened by doing knee extension activities. Be sure to completely extend the knee, because the vastus medialis is most active during the last 30 degrees of extension. Have students monitor their posture throughout class as well as throughout the day to make sure that their knees are slightly flexed. Also, have them notice what this knee position does to the alignment of the pelvis. It is almost impossible to have proper pelvic alignment with the knees locked in extension or hyperextension, but by having the knees slightly flexed, proper skeletal alignment is possible.

Figure A.12 Patellar dislocation.

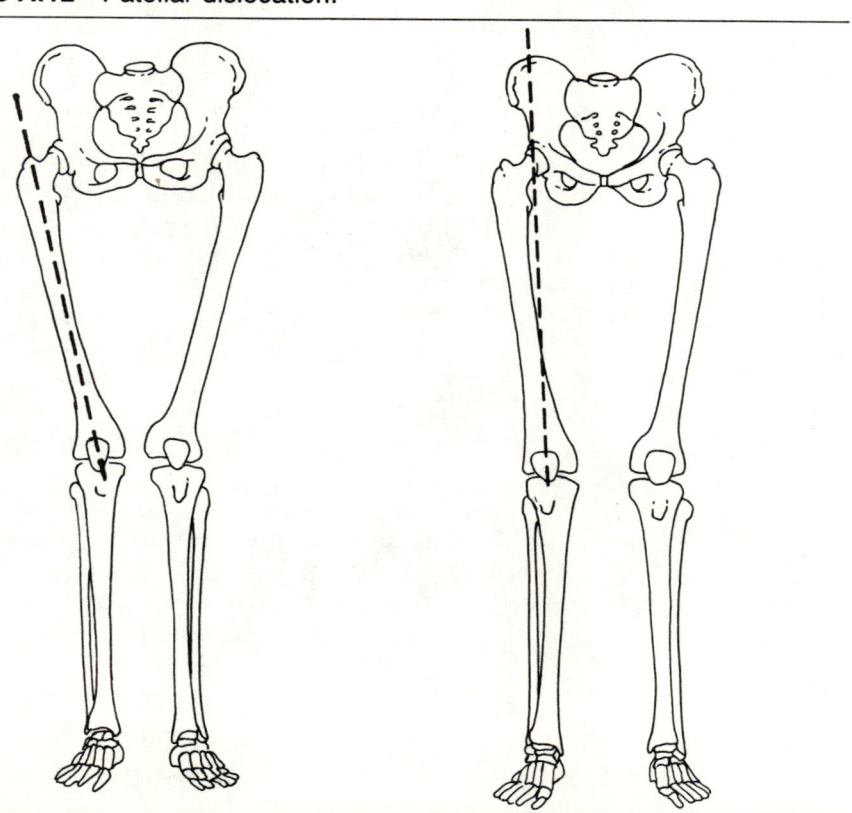

Anatomy Summary

Obviously, we have a very complex anatomy, but remember that structural foundation is what allows us to have the ability to accomplish so many functions. This section has discussed how anatomical information can be utilized by fitness instructors.

Physiology

This section refers to the study of body function. Although there are obviously many functions that must take place in order for us to engage in physical activity, none is more fundamental than the processes whereby the cells of the body obtain the energy to carry out their respective tasks. If you, as a fitness instructor, claim that you conduct a high energy class, what does that mean? Or, if one of your students comments that he or she just doesn't have the energy to workout today, what does that mean? These and a myriad of other topics related to energy metabolism will be addressed in this section on physiology.

Energy Metabolism

The word *energy* may be defined as the ability or capacity to do work. Typically, we think of work as force applied through a distance. When we contract our muscles to move our bodies or body parts, we are doing positive or concentric work. When we lower our bodies, as in the lowering phase of a push-up, we are doing negative work or eccentric work, and if we contract muscles to hold or maintain a static or isometric contraction, we are still using energy even though no visible movement has taken place. When we send signals along nerves, pump blood through the circulatory system, and conduct any of the other life-supporting functions that go on from moment to moment, biological work is being done and energy is being utilized. The word metabolism refers to all the chemical reactions that take place in the body, therefore the phrase *energy metabolism* refers to all the chemical reactions associated with the release of energy. Sometimes the phrase *energy production* is utilized instead of *energy release*, but actually the phrase energy release is more accurate because energy cannot be made or destroyed. Energy can only be transformed from one form to another. The basic forms of energy are electric, light, nuclear, heat, mechanical, and chemical. The basis of energy metabolism as it will be presented in this chapter will be the transformation of chemical energy from the food we eat to the mechanical energy required for muscle contraction.

The Source of Energy

The chemical energy in food is contained in the bonds between the molecules. Actually, plants utilize the process of photosynthesis to store light energy from the sun in the bonds of carbohydrate, fat, and protein.

This energy is not directly usable in our bodies. Similarly, if you have a diesel engine, it will not run on regular unleaded gas. The diesel engine simply cannot utilize the chemical bonds in the unleaded gas. The same is true of the cells of the body. They may be thought of as tiny engines, and the only fuel that they are capable of using directly is the energy held in a special high energy bond in a chemical called adenosine triphosphate, ATP. If a nerve signal is to be sent, a muscle is to contract, or some damaged tissues are to be repaired, ATP must be available for conversion to ADP (adenosine diphosphate). ADP is the "usable" energy made available to the cell. So, as long as sufficient ATP is available for conversion, cells will function. Unfortunately, just as automobiles have a limited ability to store fuel, so, too, do the cells have a limited ability to store ATP. While you can periodically fill your car up with fuel, the replenishment of ATP is a bit more complicated because the food that we eat cannot be used directly. When bonds in that food are broken, energy is released to resynthesize ATP from ADP. Our cells have three major systems or pathways that may be utilized to replenish ATP, creating a fairly complicated network. However, it is essential that the fitness instructor be familiar with energy metabolism because it is the basis for such terms as *aerobic exercise* and *anaerobic exercise*.

Replenishing ATP

As was previously mentioned, cells have three ways of getting the energy to resynthesize ATP from ADP + P. These three processes differ regarding how rapidly they can replenish the ATP stores and regarding how long they can continue to function. For example, sprinters can achieve running speeds of 25–27 mph for a few yards in the course of a 100-yard sprint. To do this requires many thousands of ATP molecules per second, representing a very high rate of energy release. Such sprint speeds can only be sustained for a few seconds, representing a very short duration. On the other hand, if the sprinter runs at a slower speed, say 20 mph, he or she will not require as many ATP molecules per second, and that 20 mph pace can be maintained for longer than the 25–27 mph pace. Finally, if the runner slows still more, to 10 mph let's say, even fewer ATP molecules per second are required, and the pace may be maintained for several miles. These three different intensities of activity are possible because of the three different energy metabolic pathways depicted in figure A.13. Some of the specifics of these pathways will be explained in the following sections.

ATP-PC System

The fastest way that cells have to provide the energy to resynthesize ATP is by using the stored energy in another chemical called creatine phosphate or CP. The chemical reaction in which CP breaks down to C + P can take place very quickly, almost as soon as any ADP appears. The only problem

ANATOMY AND PHYSIOLOGY OF AEROBIC EXERCISE   31

Figure A.13 The three metabolic systems for the resynthesis of ATP from ADP + P.

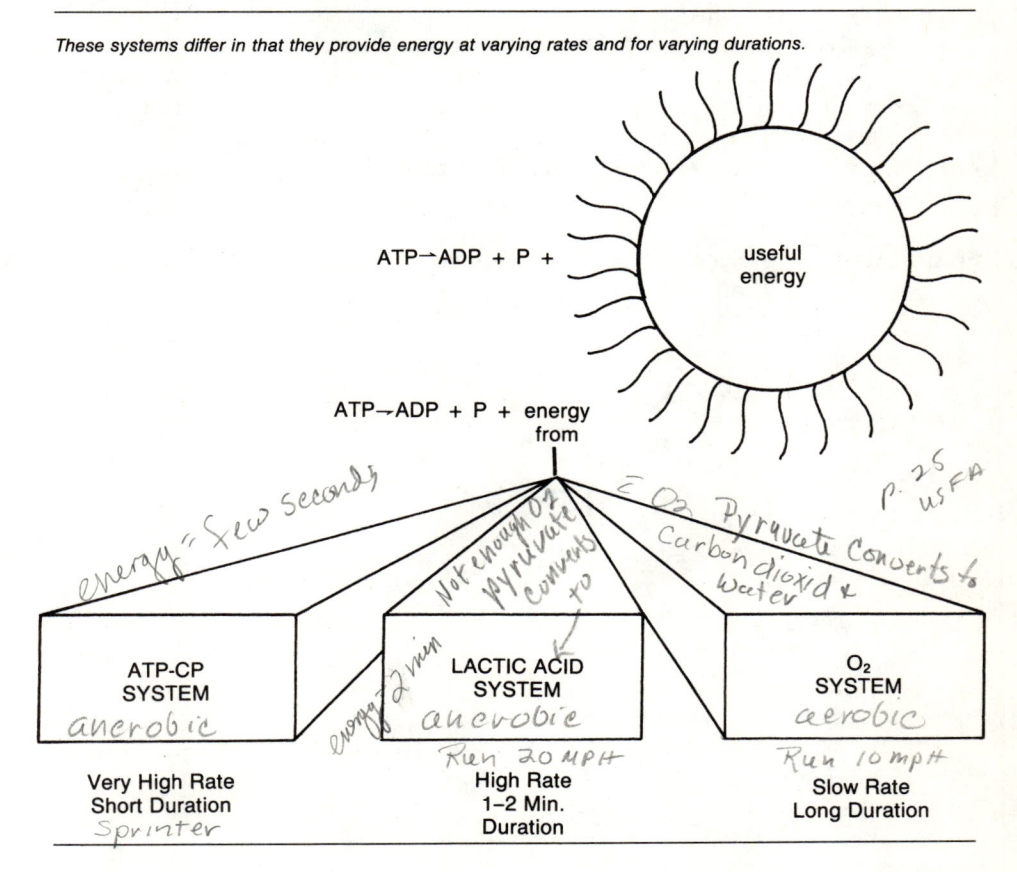

These systems differ in that they provide energy at varying rates and for varying durations.

ATP→ADP + P + [useful energy]

ATP→ADP + P + energy from

ATP-CP SYSTEM	LACTIC ACID SYSTEM	O₂ SYSTEM
Very High Rate	High Rate	Slow Rate
Short Duration	1–2 Min. Duration	Long Duration

is that only a small quantity of CP can be stored in cells, enough to support work for just a few seconds. When the CP is depleted, the work must stop or slow down. This is why the sprinter can run at very high speeds for only a few seconds and why you can lift very heavy weights for only one or two repetitions. However, if the sprinter slows down or you decrease the weight, work may be continued. This is because the decrease in exercise intensity has allowed for a different energy pathway to have time to resynthesize ATP molecules at a lightly slower rate.

Lactic Acid System

As soon as ADP + P becomes present in the cell, a series of chemical reactions called glycolysis begins. Glycolysis means the breaking apart of glucose which is a sugar molecule. A byproduct of glycolysis is pyruvic

32 ESSENTIALS OF AEROBIC EXERCISE

acid. The chemical reactions involved in glycolysis take place very rapidly and allow for the resynthesis of two molecules of ATP for every molecule of glucose. The chemical reactions involving pyruvic acid and the Kreb's Cycle (figure A.14) are much slower and depend upon the presence of oxygen (O_2). Therefore, if the sprinter selects a speed which requires ATP at a faster rate than can be provided by the Kreb's Cycle, pyruvic acid can temporarily accept H+ and form lactic acid. This pyruvic-lactic acid reaction can take place more rapidly than the Kreb's Cycle can take up pyruvic acid, therefore glycolysis can continue to resynthesize two ATPs

Figure A.14 The glycolysis pathway provides pyruvic acid to the O_2 system.

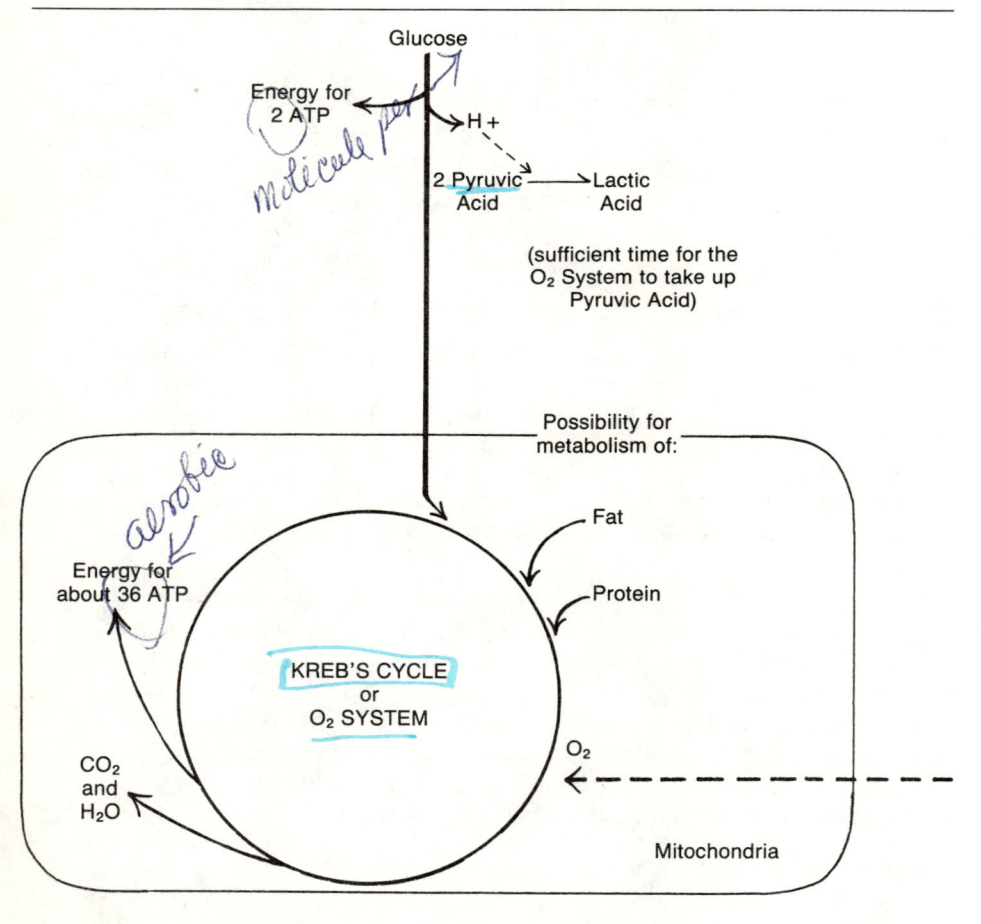

until lactic acid builds up too much. This build up of lactic acid can be experienced when you have tried to do exercises or run or perform any activity at a high rate of intensity. You have to stop because of the burning sensation in your muscles. This burning sensation is due to the build-up of lactic acid and other metabolic byproducts. The presence of excessive quantities of lactic acid simply creates an environment within the cells that makes it impossible for normal chemical reactions to take place. Since these reactions cannot persist, you cannot continue to do work because ATP cannot be made available rapidly enough. If you had selected a lower work intensity or a slower pace, you would have allowed for the recruitment of muscle cells that are well developed for the utilization of the O_2 system to resynthesize ATP. More details as to the functioning of the O_2 system will be provided in the next section.

O_2 System

The O_2 system represents that sequence of chemical reactions that take place inside the mitochondria. Mitochondria are small structures present in all cells. They contain the enzymes (proteins that stimulate various chemical reactions) necessary for the Kreb's Cycle to operate. For chemical reactions to continue to provide energy for the resynthesis of ATP, sufficient O_2 must be available to accept the H+s and result in the formation of carbon dioxide (CO_2) and water (H_2O). Fats and proteins can not enter the glycolysis pathway. We would never want to use protein as a fuel, but it is possible to do so in extreme starvation situations or when there is not enough carbohydrate (sugar or glucose) for glycolysis to result in the production of pyruvic acid for the Kreb's Cycle. This keeps us from dying under these situations. It also illustrates why low carbohydrate diets are inappropriate. They force the body to utilize some protein as well as fat to continue the energy metabolism processes.

On the other hand, if we are trying to lose fat weight, we can enhance the utilization of fat as a fuel by selecting activities that are of a low enough intensity for sufficient amounts of O_2 to be available for the Kreb's Cycle to function. If the activity is too intense, too much lactic acid is produced and the use of fat as a fuel for the Kreb's Cycle is sharply curtailed. One way of telling if the activity is of a low enough intensity is to check how long you can do the activity. If you cannot maintain the same pace for at least 15 minutes the activity is too intense. Preferably, to maximize fat utilization, you should be able to continue the activity for 30 minutes to an hour.

Anaerobic vs Aerobic

Up to this point, we have not used the terms anaerobic or aerobic to describe energy metabolism, but we could have. Anaerobic refers to those energy metabolism reactions which can occur without oxygen being present.

This means that we have two anaerobic pathways, the ATP-PC system and the lactic acid system. Even though they are both anaerobic, they play slightly different roles in our ability to engage in physical activities. The ATP-PC system provides the energy to almost instantaneously remake ATP from ADP + P, but because of a very limited ability to store PC, this system can support only a few seconds of explosive activity.

The conversion of pyruvic acid to lactic acid can also take place without oxygen being present, but as the lactic acid stockpiles, the chemical reactions which result in the releases of energy to remake ATP from ADP + P slow down. Consequently, the lactic acid system can be the dominant energy source for only a minute or two. If we are to continue activity for an extended time period, we must select a pace or an intensity that allows the circulatory system time to transport O_2 into the muscles and time for the mitochondria to take O_2 out of the blood and use it to accept the H+s. The chemical reactions involved in these *oxygen-dependent processes* are known as *aerobic metabolism* because of their *reliance upon* the *presence of oxygen*. The name *aerobics class* suggests that every activity in the class is aerobic and that really is not the case. The warm-up activities at the beginning of the class should be low intensity, and therefore aerobic. [IV: Warm-Up] Activities that are designed to develop muscular strength, e.g., using Nautilus equipment, are of a higher intensity, consequently they will be much more dependent upon anaerobic metabolism. Since muscular strength depends on the ATP-PC system, rest periods of 30 seconds to one minute should follow the high intensity exercises. This will allow time for the ATP-PC stores to be replenished. If development of the lactic acid system is a goal, as is necessary for the participants in many sports, fairly intense activities should be done for one to two minutes. Large muscle, low intensity movements should follow to help flush the lactic acid out of the muscles and speed the recovery processes.

The *build-up of lactic acid should not be a goal during the cardiovascular or "aerobics section"* of the class or routine. This is achieved by controlling the exercise intensity. Since each of us has a different cardiovascular system, capable of transporting different amounts of oxygen, and since we do not all have the same number of mitochondria in our muscles or the same efficiency for existing mitochondria, what is aerobic for one person may be quite anaerobic for another. Typically, target heart rate zones (explained in another chapter of this book) are employed to help people control the exercise intensity. If you are exercising at a heart rate that is in your target zone (assuming the zone is appropriate for you), you are aerobic. Even if your heart rate is below the zone, you are exercising aerobically. Remember *all* low intensity activities are aerobic. If your heart rate is in the target zone, this indicates that you are applying the *correct overload* to improve the body's ability to utilize aerobic metabolism. (See the chapter on Endurance Training for more information.) If your heart rate is above the target zone (we are still assuming that the zone is correct for you), this indicates that you are working at an exercise intensity that is requiring a greater and greater contribution of the lactic acid system to provide ATP at the rate that is necessary to sustain that pace or intensity. Consequently, the activity is becoming more and more anaerobic. Some people refer to the exercise intensity that results in a rapid build-up of lactic acid as the anaerobic threshold. In actuality, it is very difficult to identify one particular exercise intensity at which you suddenly cross the anaerobic threshold. However, it is true that as the activity becomes more and more intense for you, your brain will recruit muscles that are more and more reliant upon the lactic acid system as a source of ATP.

While the cardiovascular portion of the class may be either aerobic or anaerobic, depending upon the exercise intensity selected by the participant, to be most safe and effective it should be aerobic. **[VI.A: Aerobics]** You can help your students achieve this goal by encouraging them to restrict their motions, use less arm movement and slow the pace if they are over their target zones. Just the opposite adjustments may be made if the heart rate is below the target zone. Even though such low heart rates are still indicative of aerobic metabolism, they are not as effective in stimulating development of the heart and lungs.

Finally, the cool-down portion of the class should be aerobic in nature, involving controlled large muscle activities to help flush the lactic acid and other by-products from the muscles. **[VII: Post-Aerobic Cool Down]** (Some lactic acid is always produced, even during aerobic exercise. It is just not the *dominant* source of ATP during aerobic exercise.) The cool-down may be concluded with some relaxation activities, which again, because of their low intensity, are aerobic in nature. Any activity which requires only a few ATP per second is an aerobic activity. You do not have to be at your target heart rate to be aerobic.

Physiology Summary

Although there are many complex functions which must take place to enable us to participate in physical activity, the preceding material was limited to the consideration of energy metabolism as it applies to the design and implementation of fitness classes.

Sample Exercise Progression

1. Lie on your back with knees flexed and hands clasped behind the neck. With your feet flat on the floor, take a deep breath and relax.

Press the lower back against the floor and tighten your abdominal and buttock muscles. This should cause the lower portion of the pelvis to rotate forward and flatten your back against the floor. Hold this position for five seconds and then relax.
2. Lie on your back with knees flexed and your feet flat on the floor. Take a deep breath and relax. Now grasp one knee with both hands and pull the knee as close to your chest as possible. Return to the starting position and repeat with the alternate leg.
3. Lie on your back with knees bent and feet flat on the floor. Take a deep breath and relax before grasping both knees and pulling them as close to your chest as possible. Hold for three seconds, then return to the starting position.
4. Lie on your back with knees flexed and your feet flat on the floor. Take a deep breath and relax. Draw one knee to your chest, then extend the leg upward as far as possible. Return to the starting position, relax, and repeat the exercise with the alternate leg.
5. a. Lie on your stomach with hands clasped behind you. Pull your shoulders back and downward by pushing the hands down toward the feet. While pinching the shoulder blades together, lift your head from the floor. Take a deep breath and hold this position for two seconds. Now relax.
   b. Stand erect. With one hand, grasp the thumb of the other hand behind the back, then pull downward toward the floor. Stand up on your toes and look at the ceiling while exerting the downward pull with the hands. Hold momentarily and then relax. Repeat ten times at intervals of two hours during the day.

(The following exercises should not be done if the preceding exercises cannot be completed without pain.)

6. Lie on your back with one leg extended and the other flexed at the hip. Your arms should be at your sides. Take a deep breath and relax. Raise the extended leg as high as is comfortable and lower to the floor as slowly as possible. Repeat this procedure five times for each leg.
7. While lying on your back, flex your knees so that your feet are flat on the floor. Contract your abdominal muscles and lift your shoulders off the floor. Hold this position for three to five seconds. Your hands may be at your sides, folded across your chest, or clasped behind your head. If behind your head, do not pull on the head. A trunk-twisting action may also be added.

Commonly Asked Questions

Q: Why should straight leg sit-ups be avoided?
A. When a sit-up is begun with the hips and knees extended, tension is placed on the iliopsoas muscle so it becomes the major mover. If the sit-up is begun with the knees flexed, the rectus abdominis becomes the major mover. Consequently, flexing the knees helps to isolate the abdominal muscles and not the already overused iliopsoas.

Q. Can bones become stronger with exercise?
A. Exercise that is of an appropriate intensity for one's fitness level can result in the restructuring of the internal framework of the bones involved in the activity. In addition, the physical activity can stimulate the production of new bone cells and the increased deposition of calcium and other minerals, with the end result being a stronger bone.

Q. Bones become more fragile with aging. Can exercise stop this aging process?
A. Much of the decrease in bone density that is observed during aging is thought to be a result of decreased levels of physical activity associated with growing older. Consequently, because of the exercise effects mentioned in the previous question, regular physical activity can slow down the decreases in bone density typically seen in the aged. In other words, older individuals who exercise have more dense bones than people of the same age who do not exercise.

Q. What is a stress fracture?
A. A stress fracture is a decrease in the density of the bone at one or more points on the bone. Stress fractures are thought to be due to engaging in too much physical activity too soon. When a new activity is begun, existing bone is reabsorbed so that a new internal structure may be fabricated. Typically, the reabsorption of existing bone goes on for several days before the production of new bone catches up. If there is too rapid an increase in exercise intensity, the new bone production may never catch up and a stress fracture is the result.

Q. What is a ballistic exercise?
A. If an exercise is performed by utilizing momentum and/or gravity to rapidly move through the joint's range of movement, the exercise is said to be ballistic. These types of motions place unnecessary stress on the ligaments and tendons at the joints.

Q. Why should deep knee bends be avoided?
A. For many individuals, when the knees are flexed to more

degrees, as is required in doing deep knee bends, the ligaments that help to support the knee joint may be stretched. Good quadricep strength may be developed by doing "squat-type" exercises that only take the knee to 90 degrees of flexion.

Q. What is an aerobic activity or exercise?
A. Aerobic activities are those activities which are done at an intensity or pace which can be sustained for at least five to 10 minutes. They are large muscle, rhythmical activities that increase the heart rate and respiration so that oxygen may be delivered to the working muscles. In other words, exercises like walking, running, swimming, aerobic dance, etc. will be aerobic only if they are done at an intensity that allows the oxygen systems in the muscles to burn fats and carbohydrates to release the energy (ATP) necessary to do the activities.

Q. What is an anaerobic activity or exercise?
A. Any activity that is done at such a pace or intensity that the activity can only be continued for a few seconds up to a minute or two at most, is said to be an anaerobic activity. In order to provide the energy (ATPs) at the rate necessary to sustain intense exercise, the muscles have to utilize anaerobic (nonoxygen) energy-releasing processes.

Q. Is the Hurdler's Stretch a safe and effective exercise?
A. This exercise (a) is supposed to stretch the hamstring muscles of the extended leg and the groin muscles of the leg with the knee flexed. While the hamstring stretching phase is effective, the positioning of the leg with the flexed knee places undesirable stresses on the ligaments of the knee. Modifying the leg position as in (b) helps to prevent these knee stresses.

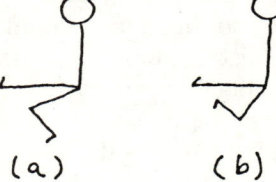

(a)   (b)

Q. What are the best types of activities for burning fat calories?
A. Only the O_2 system can utilize fat as a fuel. Therefore, an activity must be aerobic if significant numbers of fat calories are to be burned. In addition, the activity should be performed for at least 30 continuous minutes for the fat burning pathways to become fully operational.

When you "go for the burn" while doing an exercise, what does this 'ean?

A. The build-up of lactic acid in the muscles stimulates nerve endings, resulting in feelings of localized pain. This pain is similar to a burning sensation. Consequently, "going for the burn" means to do a high intensity exercise until build-up of lactic acid prevents further exercise.

References

Alter, J. *Surviving Exercise*. Boston: Houghton Mifflin, 1983.

Donnely, J. *Living Anatomy*. Champaign, IL: Human Kinetics Publishers, 1984.

Fox, E. and Mathews, D. *The Physiological Basis of Physical Education and Athletics*. New York: Saunders College Publishing, 1981.

Langley, L. and Telford, I. *Dynamic Anatomy and Physiology*, 5th Ed. Champaign, IL: Human Kinetics Publishers, 1980.

Sharkey, B. *Principles of Human Anatomy*. New York: Harper & Row, 1980.

Chapter 3

Medical Considerations of Aerobic Exercise

Arthur Siegel, M.D.

The purpose of this chapter is to review the cardiovascular aspects of aerobic exercise and fitness. Understanding the basic physiology of exercise and its benefits for the heart will enable instructors to guide students toward sound exercise programs for health enhancement. An overview of the potential complications and concerns related to heart disease and associated risk factors is discussed.

Exercise Conditioning and the Cardiovascular System

The basic concept of endurance fitness or aerobic capacity is based on the 20%-50% increase in work performance that an individual can achieve with maximum exercise participation. To understand this concept, it is necessary to review the physiology of exercise and the cardiovascular system, which is shown schematically in figure A.15. The top of the diagram shows the heart as a pump that circulates oxygenated blood to the body tissues including the exercising skeletal muscle mass. Deoxygenated blood is returned to the heart for circulation through the lungs where carbon dioxide produced by muscular work is exchanged and the blood is enriched with oxygen for redistribution to working tissues.

The central role of the cardiovascular system, consisting of the heart, arteries, capillaries, and veins (as shown in the central cogwheel in figure A.16) is as the conduit via which oxygen is brought from the air through the pulmonary system and delivered to the exercising tissue. The main source of energy for the life process in general and for exercise in particular is the oxidation of dietary substrates such as sugars and free fatty acids in the mitochondria of living cells. The flow of oxygen through the circulatory

Figure A.15 Schematic of the cardiovascular system

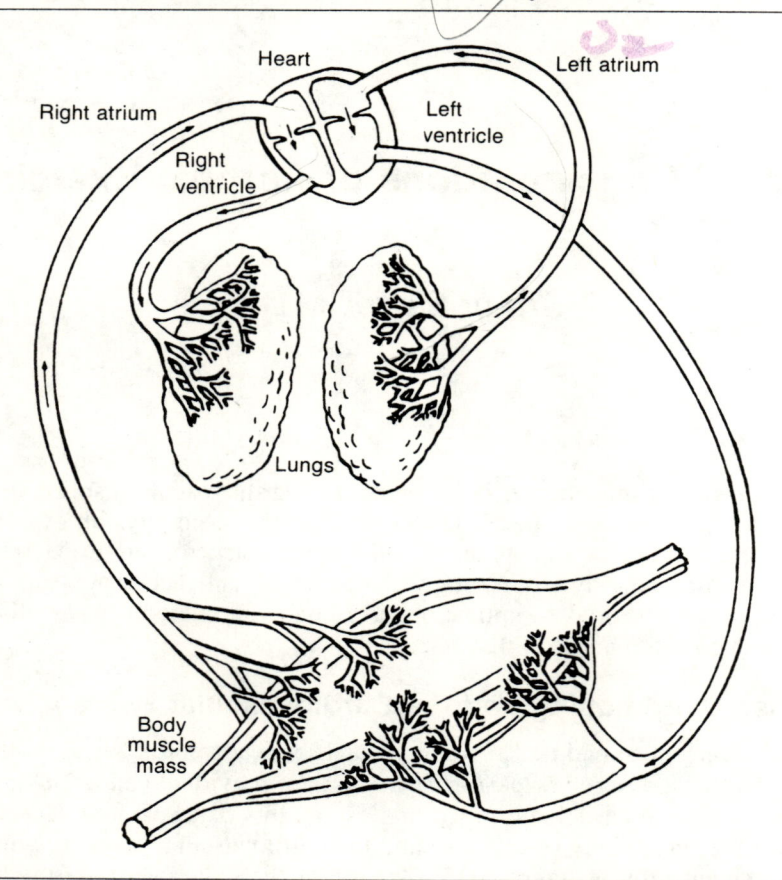

SOURCE: R.C. Cantu, Sports Medicine in Primary Care. The Collamore Press, D.C. Heath and Co., Lexington, MA, Toronto, 1982. (Reprinted with permission.)

system is from right to left in this diagram, whereas the production of carbon dioxide and its excretion runs from left to right (see figure A.15). During exercise, the quantity of oxygen consumed (VO_2) and the quantity of carbon dioxide produced (VCO_2) is determined by the amount of muscle activity. Conditioning involves improvement and efficiency of the heart as a pump and enhancement of the capacity of muscle to oxidize fuel substrates.

Figure A.17 illustrates the progressive decline in the maximum exercise performance or maximal oxygen (VO_2MAX) uptake with age. It also

MEDICAL CONSIDERATIONS OF AEROBIC EXERCISE 43

Figure A.16 Essential elements in gas exchange between the cell mitochondria and external environment

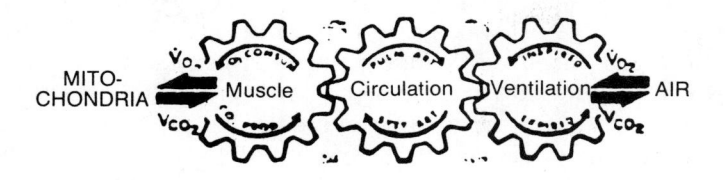

SOURCE: K. Wasserman, "Breathing During Exercise." New England Journal of Medicine, 1978:298:780. (Reprinted with permission.)

Figure A.17 Physical fitness classification

In the example shown (dot), the subject, aged 33, has a very low fitness level for his age group.

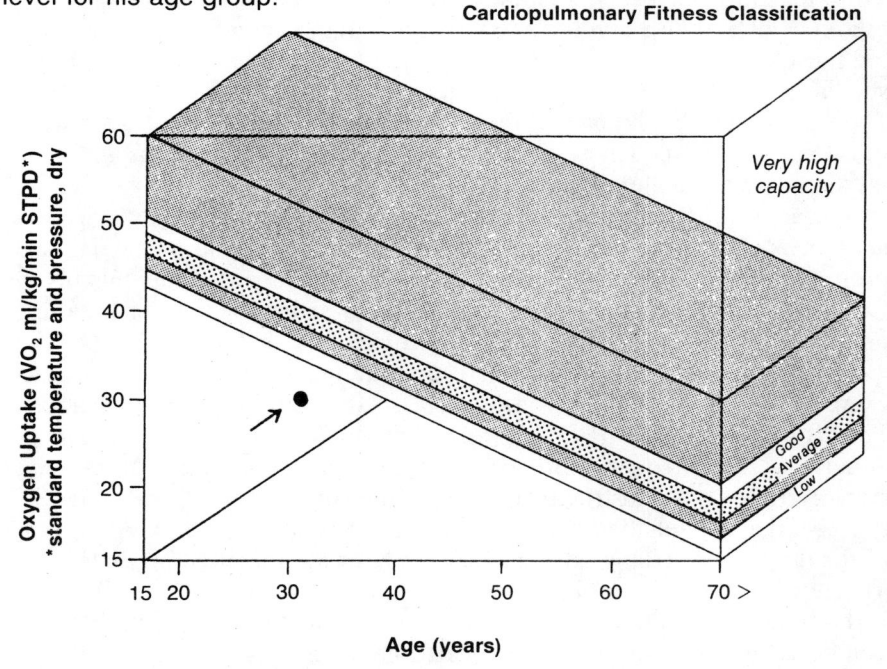

SOURCE: J.D. Cantwell, "Stress testing indicated in a variety of complaints," The Physician and Sports Medicine, 1977:February:70–74. (Reprinted with permission.)

illustrates the spectrum of low to very high cardiopulmonary fitness capacity existing for any individual at a given point in time. Regular aerobics training will move an individual up the oxygen uptake axis to a higher level of exercise performance. This is due to both cardiac and skeletal muscle adaptations to regular exercise. With the fitness effect, there is a greater amount of oxygen extracted from the blood per heartbeat. This is termed an increase or an improvement in the oxygen pulse. The exciting thing about this concept is that the principles of exercise physiology can be applied to the exercising individual by analysis of the resting and exercise-induced pulse rate.

The Exercising Individual

As discussed above, conditioning describes the improvement in exercise capacity with training through cardiovascular and skeletal muscle adaptations to physical work. This capacity is enhanced by activities involving the repetitive use of large muscle groups such as walking, jogging, dancing (aerobic!), swimming, cross-country skiing, or cycling. These types of exercise involve an increase in the oxygen binding capacity of the muscle cells together with an increase in the number of mitochondria, as shown in figure A.16, to assist the muscle in oxidizing fuels.

The rate of cardiopulmonary fitness development is dependent upon three exercise variables: frequency, duration, and intensity. Moderation and consistency are the hallmark concepts in the development of an exercise program, as the characteristics must be sufficiently intense to induce a training effect but avoid the hazards of overexertion and injury. Guidelines as proposed by the American College of Sports Medicine for the quantity and quality of exercise necessary to develop and maintain fitness in healthy adults prescribe 15–60 minutes of sustained exercise performed three to five times per week. These guidelines correspond to the frequency and duration of exercise during the optimal aerobics class as set out in the *Basic Exercise Standards and Guidelines* (BESG) of the Aerobics and Fitness Association of America. [I.A: Frequency of Workouts] [I.E: Training Effects] [VI: Aerobics] The central role of the instructor is guiding the student to a desirable level of exercise that will challenge his or her current fitness capacity. An optimal level for the healthy young adult is 70%–80% of the maximal predicted heart rate. This can be calculated by subtracting an individual's age from 220, the basal maximum attainable heart rate. For convenience, a table of percentages for maximum predicted heart rate at various ages is shown in table A.4. Exercise at this level of intensity will continue to enhance fitness for each individual and enable him or her to perform more vigorously and with more endurance. Please refer to BESG VI.H: Heart Rate for a review of the target heart rate concept.

Table A.4 Maximal heart rates predicted by age for normal untrained individuals with selected percentages of MHR

(Averages of 10 American & European Investigators, adapted from proceedings of National Workshop on Exercise)

AGE (Years):	25	30	35	40	45	50	55	60	65
MHR	190	186	182	181	179	175	171	168	164
90% MHR	171	167	164	163	161	158	154	151	148
85% MHR	162	158	155	154	152	149	145	143	139
80% MHR	152	149	146	145	143	140	137	134	131
75% MHR	143	140	137	136	134	131	128	126	123
70% MHR	133	130	127	127	125	123	120	118	115
65% MHR	124	121	118	118	116	114	111	109	107
60% MHR	114	112	109	109	107	105	103	101	98

SOURCE: *Jackson, F.W.: Performance and Interpretation in Exercise Testing Handbook. AMSCO Rehab Corporation, Division of American Sterilizer Company, 4950 Wilson Lane, Mechanicsburg, PA. 17055, 1974. (Reprinted with permission)*

The target heart rate should be looked at as the goal for a safe exercise intensity to produce aerobic fitness. Individuals can be instructed to take his or her pulse during exercise in order to ensure that this recommended zone is being attained. **[VI.H: Heart Rate]** Equally important is the postexercise pulse, which is an indication of the degree to which an individual can safely handle a given level of exercise intensity. The resting pulse should return to 60% of the peak exercise heart rate by 3–5 minutes after completion of a workout. Individuals should be urged to monitor this pulse, especially if any symptoms of fatigue or dizziness arise. If the pulse rate fails to return to this level (or below 100 beats per minute after 10 minutes), then the level of exercise intensity should be reduced. Students can also be instructed to take their early morning pulse before getting out of bed or thinking too much about the pressures of the day. A progressive training effect will lead to a progressive fall in this morning resting pulse unlike the pulse of individuals who may overtrain and show insufficient recovery. The morning pulse can act as a barometer for the individual to judge his or her training response; the postexercise pulse is an index of the ability to handle a specific workout.

A balanced exercising program involves rest and recovery as well as application of a safe amount of stress through incremental exercise intensity. Each workout should avoid pushing an individual to exhaustion (excessive anaerobic metabolism and blood lactate accumulation) just as the overall program should avoid progressive fatigue, which may lead to irritability, insomnia, and erosion of the positive psychological benefits of the exercise program.

Hazards of Exercise

Aerobic exercise involves the generation of internal heat through performance of muscular work. As the core temperature rises, an increased amount of cardiac output is delivered to the skin so heat can be dissipated in the form of sweating. Heat is lost principally through evaporation of sweat from the body surface, which cools the individual at the price of losing vital circulating fluids. Prolonged strenuous exercise invariably leads to dehydration, which may then lead to fatigue, confusion, lethargy, and persistent excessive body temperature. Advanced stages of heat exhaustion from exercise may lead to coma and even cardiac arrhythmias and sudden death. These rare and extreme hazards can be prevented by knowing ways to avoid dehydration and hyperthermia during exercise.

The first tenet of prevention is adequate hydration before exercise. This is best done by consuming 8–10 ounces of water 10–20 minutes before beginning a light workout. The warm-up phase of exercise allows the muscles and tendons to adapt to the biomechanics of exercise while the blood flow increases to exercising muscle. As body temperature rises, the sweating mechanism kicks into place with the perception of "second wind." **Prolonged exercise should involve breaks to consume additional water**. When appropriate, moisten the body surface by sponging or spraying to assist in the cooling process. Such cooling measures provide a form of "external sweating," which helps to dissipate heat without using internal fluid resources for evaporation.

Sweat is composed primarily of water lost from the tissues in a greater proportion than losses of sodium and chloride. This means that the body is under pressure to correct the imbalance. For this reason, salt substitutes are undesirable prior to strenuous exercise, and individuals should rely on the use of water alone to prevent heat injury or thermal stress.

Appropriate dress during exercise is another important consideration in the prevention of heat stress. This involves dressing in light and loose-fitting clothing during hot weather exercise, especially on humid days when the sweating mechanism is less efficient. In addition, exercising in full sun increases the risk of heat injury. Covering the head guards against the sun's radiant energy and will protect one from dehydration. Finally, individuals should avoid the use of saunas and hot tubs after exercise, which may compound the problem of fluid depletion.   [XII.C: Saunas and Hot Tubs]

Cardiovascular Complications of Exercise

In general, young healthy individuals require no medical clearance prior to undertaking an aerobic fitness program but would benefit from a general medical screening. Individuals at risk specifically for any cardiovascular disease, however, should have a prior medical clearance from a physician. Some of the major risk factors for development of coronary heart disease include hypertension, cigarette smoking, increased cholesterol levels, and a family history of heart disease. In addition, certain conditions such as mitral valve prolapse may run in families and be associated with serious arrhythmias and even with sudden cardiac death. Individuals with any of these factors in their family history should have a systematic medical evaluation prior to undertaking a vigorous exercise program.

The initiation of regular exercise is an opportunity to promote other positive health habits. Instructors should deliver a clear warning to students about the incompatibility of strenuous exercise and smoking. Once a regular exercise program has been established, the individual will be motivated to give up smoking.

Instructors should teach students that the warm-up and cool-down portions of exercise allow the heart and circulation a chance to accommodate and are important principles used in medical exercise rehabilitation programs to insure the safety of aerobic exercise. **[IV: Warm-Up] [VII: Post-Aerobic Cool Down]**

Another very important concept is that each individual should maintain a noncompetitive approach to his/her exercise program so that exercise intensity remains moderate and in a safe zone for target heart rate. **[II.D: Level of Participation] [II.E: Breathing]** Individuals who demonstrate any symptoms such as irregular heart rate, perceived palpitations, chest discomfort on exercise, or sudden breathlessness should be encouraged to seek medical consultation in order to exclude specific cardiovascular conditions. **[I.H: Danger Signs]** Heart patients often describe symptoms such as a dull ache or pressure in the chest. These complaints warrant referrals to a physician even if the individual does not describe these sensations as "pain." Extreme caution on the part of the exercise instructor is recommended in these situations.

Exercise instructors should also be aware of the potential cardiovascular complications of exercise including the rare cases of sudden death during sport. Studies in this area point to silent congenital heart abnormalities in the majority of cases of sudden collapse from heart arrhythmias during physical exertion. Such victims are young (aged 13–35) and often have a thickening of the heart muscle wall called hypertrophic cardiomyopathy. Individuals with a family history of sudden death during or even unrelated to exercise should have medical clearance prior to undertaking a progressive exercise program.

In contrast, victims of sudden death over the age of 40 usually suffer from atherosclerotic or coronary artery disease (CAD) as exemplified by the case of Jim Fixx. Such individuals have advanced CAD and may be asymptomatic or denying symptoms prior to collapse from heart fibrillation. The absence of a recent myocardial infarction suggests that these deaths are arrhythmia induced. This emphasizes the importance of appropriate screening in older patients, especially with risk factors for underlying heart disease. The warm-up and cool-down phases of an exercise session are safety factors against the onset of such arrhythmias. The risk for sudden death has been calculated as one episode per 400,000 person-hours of jogging, which is minimal compared to the overall benefits. Exercise testing should be considered by all, but especially when risk factors, hereditary factors or symptoms are identified.

Exercise-induced Conditions

As we breathe, our lungs serve to warm and humidify inspired air. This process involves heat exchange from the lung space to the outside air with condensation of moisture around the nose and throat. This accounts for the "runny nose" that all individuals experience when exercising vigorously in cold, dry weather.

Exercise-induced asthma

This process of heat exchange in susceptible individuals can lead to coughing and wheezing—the definition of exercise-induced asthma. Such individuals may have a background of allergies or be unaware of any respiratory symptoms except during exercise. Cold weather can also provoke coughing and the sensation of tightness in the central chest area.

Exercise-induced asthma is similar to the broncho-constriction experienced in "allergic" asthmatic bronchitis. Exercise-induced asthma is triggered, however, by the temperature and water exchange mechanisms described above and does not depend upon an allergic sensitivity. Symptoms may remain stable and then improve, only to worsen during the postexercise period. Once again, symptoms may be chest heaviness with cough and, in severe cases, wheezing.

Exercise-induced asthma can be blocked and even prevented by pre-exercise treatment with aerosol medication. While several over-the-counter preparations are available, the most effective bronchodilators must be prescribed by a physician. Individuals can also diminish symptoms by warming inspired air, such as exercising with a surgical face mask in very cold weather. While this technique does not lend itself to the class setting, students may use these tips in other sports activities, such as cross-country skiing.

Persons susceptible to exercise-induced asthma should be examined, treated, and encouraged to participate in full exercise activity for the benefit of physical conditioning. Lung function is maintained and preserved through such a program.

Exercise-induced anaphylaxis

Instructors should be aware of a rare but medically significant condition known as exercise-induced anaphylaxis. Some individuals may, during exercise, experience sudden facial swelling or a sense of tightness in the throat with difficulty in breathing. This reaction is similar to the type of reaction that can occur after a bee sting or penicillin exposure in a highly allergic individual. This condition requires emergency medical attention (epinephrine should be administered immediately). Patients who have this unusual reaction should, in fact, carry a bee-sting kit containing this medication so that attacks can be quickly treated. Anyone who develops a sudden difficulty in breathing accompanied by facial swelling should be suspected of having exercise-induced anaphylaxis. Fortunately, no fatalities have yet been reported.

Exercise-induced hives

Instructors may note that some individuals develop a blotchy red rash, sometimes with itching, at the beginning of a workout. This is called exercise-induced hives, or urticaria, and results from histamine release in the skin due to rapid superficial temperature changes. The student should be assured that this condition is harmless. Low doses of antihistamines can be helpful in diminishing symptoms as long as the side effects of drowsiness are not more bothersome.

Basic mastery of the concepts of exercise physiology and the role of the cardiovascular system will better prepare the instructor to inform students. This in turn will enrich their understanding of the body's adaptation to regular exercise and the specific changes involved in promoting fitness. See References for more information on cardiovascular and other medical aspects of exercise which will enable instructors to provide sound advice, guidance, and reassurance to their students.

References

American College of Sports Medicine. "The Recommended Quantity and Quality of Exercise for Developing and Maintaining Fitness in Healthy Adults." *Medicine, Science and Sports*. October 1978:vii.

Banner, A. et al. "Relation of Respiratory Water Loss to Coughing after Exercise." *New England Journal of Medicine*. 1984:311:883-886.

Cantu, R., Ed. *Sports Medicine in Primary Care*. Lexington, MA: Heath, 1982.

Cooper, K. *The Aerobics Way*. New York: Evans, 1977.

McFadden, E. "Exercise-Induced Asthma." *American Journal of Medicine*. 1980:68:4.

Siegel, A. "Exercise-Induced Anaphylaxis." *Physician and Sportsmedicine.* 1980:8(1):55-64.

Siscovick, D. et al. "The Incidence of Primary Cardiac Arrest during Vigorous Exercise." *New England Journal of Medicine.* 1984:311:874-877.

Strauss, R., Ed. *Sports Medicine.* Philadelphia: Saunders, 1984.

Thompson, P. and Mitchell, J. "Exercise and Sudden Cardiac Death." *New England Journal of Medicine.* 1984:311:914-915.

Chapter 4

Applied Physiologic Principles of Aerobic Exercise

Joanne Smith, MS

There is little doubt that engaging in regular physical activity in moderation while following safety guidelines provides numerous objective and subjective benefits. Participation in a group exercise activity helps provide the incentive and social support that encourages compliance with a regular exercise routine. The success attributed to a group exercise program will depend largely on the instructor's ability to provide an exciting, safe, and physiologically appropriate progression of exercise combinations for all program participants.

The purpose of this chapter is to apply physiologic principles to aerobic exercise, so that instructors will be aware of the positive outcomes and possible problem areas associated with aerobic exercise. The ability to conduct classes utilizing safe and effective conditioning techniques is a skill that will take considerable effort and planning on the exercise leader's part. With this challenge before us, the following topics of discussion are presented in this chapter:

- screening class participants
- participant orientation
- meeting the cardiovascular system's needs
- target heart rate, its nature and significance
- recognizing exertional intolerance
- special considerations

Screening Class Participants

Before beginning any strenuous exercise program, it is important to know if the participants have any medical problems that might be aggravated by vigorous exercise or preclude a successful outcome. Ideally, all persons planning to be in an aerobic exercise program should have a medical examination that includes an exercise stress test. This examination assists the participant to identify any preexisting conditions (e.g., anemia, heart disease, arthritis) that might hamper a positive outcome to the aerobic program.

Studies confirm that exercise carries with it a small but definite risk of cardiovascular complications, including sudden death. While not everyone is required to have an exercise stress test prior to enrolling in an exercise program, AFAA recommends that the following guidelines be followed for all participants.   [III.A: **Medical Clearance**]

- All participants who have not been exercising regularly should have a medical examination, unless they are under 30 years of age and have had a satisfactory check-up within the past year.
- If the participant is between 30 and 34 years of age, the medical examination should be within the last three months and should include a resting EKG.
- For participants 35 years and older, a medical examination and testing before an exercise program should include an exercise stress test. This will allow the physician to identify the presence of any possible contraindications to exercise; as the person's response to increasingly difficult levels of work is monitored on the electrocardiograph.
- Anyone, no matter what age, with a preexisting medical condition should be screened by his or her physician prior to beginning an exercise program.

To assist the instructor in becoming more familiar with the health backgrounds of new participants, a sample of the author's "Participant Health Information Form" (table A.5) is included at the end of the chapter. Revisions of the basic form should be made to make the information more suitable to each instructor's personal class needs. It is essential that instructors have an awareness of the capabilities and limitations of each and every participant in an exercise program for which the instructor is responsible. While the population of participants we generally work with will be low-fit but otherwise healthy adults, it is possible that within this population there are some class members who have medical limitations. Requiring each new class participant to complete a health information form and follow the new participant guidelines listed above can enable the instructor to provide a safe and effective class for each member.

Participant orientation

When new students join an instructor's exercise program, it is quite possible that they will understand very little about fitness itself, and

Table A.5 Participant health information form

NAME: _____ AGE: _____
ADDRESS: _____ HEIGHT: _____
_____ WEIGHT: _____
PHONE: _____

* * * * *

The information that is requested is necessary in order to provide each participant with a safe and appropriate exercise experience. All information will be kept confidential.

1. Do you have your physician's approval to participate in vigorous aerobic exercise activities?
   _____Yes   _____No
2. Date of most recent medical examination: _____
3. Name of physician who completed the examination: _____
   _____
        (town/city)   (state)
4. Please attach statement of physician's permission for you to participate in this activity (where required by instructor).
5. Date of most recent resting electrocardiogram: _____ Physician:_____
6. Date of most recent exercise stress test: _____ Physician:_____

(Please refer to attached list of AFAA guidelines to determine what medical screening is required of you, specifically, prior to engaging in this activity).

* * * * *

If you have been or are presently being treated for any of the following conditions, please indicate by checking the appropriate space(s). Also check any of the other appropriate spaces and provide the information that is asked. If you have any medical limitations that require program modification, I will work with you individually in order to provide you with a safe and enjoyable exercise experience.

____Heart Disease
____High Blood Pressure
 (Medication:_____)
     (include dosage)
____Diabetes: ____Type I ____Type II
____Epilepsy
____Arthritis, Bursitis
____Allergies: ____medications/drugs
    ____environmental
____Migraine Headaches
____Orthopedic Problems
 (Please specify: _____
 _____
 _____)
____have recently been hospitalized
 (please specify reason:_____
 _____)

____presently pregnant
 (____ months)
____recently gave birth
 (date: _____)
____presently a smoker
____have asthma
____have recently had surgery
 (Please specify:_____
 _____
 _____)
____have bad knees
____have other joint problems
 (please specify:_____
 _____)
____have flat feet

Estimated resting heart rate_____

Signature: _____
Date of Completion of this Form: _____

NOTE: *It is important that instructor is made aware of any changes in the information on the health record that may occur during the time period of our program.*

© Joanne L. Smith 1/10/85

probably lack appreciation for the importance of making exercise a regular part of their life patterns. Providing them with information in a new member orientation session about program structure, goals, and methods of attaining these goals in the program, and the importance of working at their own levels of ability and within their limitations, can be a strong determinant for their success and compliance with the program. Some important recommendations for new members prior to a new exercise program are: [**I.A: Frequency of Workouts**]   [**III: Preclass Procedure**]

1. Attending exercise sessions on a *regular* basis (AFAA recommends three to five one-hour sessions per week) is necessary to realize improvements in overall fitness, particularly improvements in maximal oxygen consumption. Attending one or two aerobic exercise sessions per week without supplementary aerobic training in another activity will be inadequate for effective improvement in aerobic fitness. Sporadic attendance is unsafe and ineffective in developing those components of fitness that most people are hoping to achieve, i.e., increased cardiovascular fitness, improved muscle tone, increased flexibility and agility, and an sense of improved well-being.
2. If a person wishes to maintain the "training effect" received from participation in an exercise program, such exercise must be continued on a regular basis. Fitness cannot be stored for later use! In fact, research indicates that as rapidly as two weeks after ceasing to exercise, a significant amount of detraining takes place. If a person stops exercising long enough, pretraining fitness levels will return. After approximately 2½–8 weeks without exercising, a return to pretraining fitness levels occurs. Four to 12 weeks of detraining has been shown to result in a 50% reduction in improvement in cardiorespiratory fitness.
3. On the other end of the spectrum, however, is the realization that overparticipation in strenuous exercise can result in orthopedic or cardiovascular complications that most probably would not have developed had the participant approached the exercise routine in a sensible and progressive fashion. Being either a "weekend athlete" who leads a relatively sedentary life five days a week and engages in vigorous aerobic activity on the weekends, or an "overdoer" who believes "the more and harder I train, the more fit I will become" are undesirable approaches to becoming fit.   [**I: Basic Principles, Definitions, and Recommendations**]
4. Participants must learn to listen to their bodies and ask themselves how they feel both during and following an exercise session. The saying "there's no gain without pain" is an inappropriate and unwise attitude to foster in anyone's approach to becoming fit. There is no

need for pain or discomfort the day following exercise participation. Being somewhat "stiff" or "tight" after an exercise session has different implications than being in real pain or so uncomfortable that daily activities must be altered.

Hints to instructors

Continually encourage program participants to reflect on the importance of a complete, personalized self-help health improvement program. In addition, be aware of the frequency with which each member attends your classes. A check-in list is helpful for keeping track of those who are attending any particular session. This attendance record may be important for legal purposes too, should anyone ever need documentation of his or her presence in your class on any specific day or time of day.

Discourage students from attending classes when they don't feel well. If they are feeling just slightly "under the weather," encourage them to work at a lower level of intensity and to not push themselves too hard. The instructor must never attempt to medically diagnose the reasons a participant is below par. Let the participant make decisions based on his or her own inclinations whether it is wise to participate when not feeling quite well. Suggest that the student seek medical advice for evaluation of the condition.

Meeting the cardiovascular system's needs

As the reader probably knows by now, there are many benefits of adequate and appropriate warm up prior to the aerobic phase of an exercise session. [IV: Warm up] To review briefly, some of the benefits are:

- An increased blood flow, hence oxygen delivery, to the working muscles.
- An increased core temperature produces increased muscular efficiency. Muscles contract more rapidly and forcefully when they are warmed up.
- A decreased potential for injuries to muscles, tendons, and ligaments due to their increased elasticity; this increased elasticity results from increased blood saturation within the muscles as well as increased core temperature within the working muscles.

As important as warming up is to the muscles, so it is also to the cardiovascular system. Blood pressure (BP) responses were significantly improved when the subjects warmed up prior to the strenuous work. Cardiovascularly, warming up is especially important because it helps avoid the build-up of lactic acid and excess oxygen debt and helps decrease one's potential for an ischemic response or cardiac arrhythmia.

In addition to understanding the importance of appropriate warm-up exercise, instructors must understand the difference between aerobic and anaerobic training and the implications of anaerobic training for certain

56 ESSENTIALS OF AEROBIC EXERCISE

populations of people. Persons with elevated resting blood pressures, for example, have a markedly different BP response to aerobic versus anaerobic work. Certain anaerobic workouts tend to result in more highly elevated heart rates and blood pressures (both systolic and diastolic) than comparable levels of aerobic exercise stresses. Participants with documented hypertension, therefore, are advised to not engage in certain types of anaerobic work (e.g., isometrics, heavy weightlifting); however, careful, controlled anaerobic activities such as tennis may be pursued by the hypertensive on recommendation from a physician. Any prospective class member who has a history of hypertension (high blood pressure) should have an exercise stress test and a physician's approval prior to engaging in an aerobic exercise program.   [III.A: Medical Clearance]   The exercise stress test, while not foolproof, can help determine whether or not a person can safely participate in aerobic exercise with or without medical supervision. The stress test, as discussed in the chapter on fitness testing, can also be helpful in developing an appropriate exercise prescription for the hypertensive person, indicating the safe target heart rate range for exercise.

It is important to continually stress proper breathing patterns during the various stages of the exercise session, particularly during movements in which the tendency might be to hold one's breath. Breath-holding during exercise elevates both the heart rate and BP rapidly and can result not only in a faster accumulation of lactic acid but also place the participant in a compromising situation cardiovascularly. Research has shown that many cardiac arrhythmias develop during or following breath-holding periods, since the heart is placed under increased stresses when the breath is held as the person "strains" to execute the maneuver (e.g., during push-ups).

Remember, too, as you reflect on physiology, that the initial four to six minutes of any aerobic exercise is not truly aerobic because the circulation is not able to respond to the increased need for blood and oxygen in the working muscles as fast as needed. During this period of oxygen deficiency, energy production is mainly anaerobic. Following this brief period of anaerobic work, *steady-state* is reached. This is when work can be maintained for a long period with aerobic energy production. During steady-state, class members should be certain to work within their target heart rate ranges. They should know what these ranges are and be comfortable in locating and counting their pulse according to the instructor's directions.   [VI.H: Heart Rate]

The "cool-down" period of an exercise session provides a transition between vigorous aerobic work and the calisthenics and stretching session. Breathing during this cool-down period should be relaxed, with the rate and depth of breathing dictated by one's physiologic reflexes.   [VII: Post-Aerobic Cool Down]   Prior to beginning calisthenics and stretching on the floor,

APPLIED PHYSIOLOGIC PRINCIPLES OF AEROBIC EXERCISE

AFAA recommends that the heart rate be monitored. It should not exceed 60% of maximum (220 minus the person's age times .6) five minutes after aerobic work. If the heart rate is higher, the person should walk slowly until the heart rate has lowered sufficiently to begin floor work.

Abrupt cessation of movement following vigorous aerobic exercise can cause pooling of the blood in the extremities, meaning accumulations of blood in the large muscles of the legs and less available to the heart and brain. This may cause a participant to become light-headed and, perhaps, even unconscious. Research has shown that cardiac arrhythmias can develop following exercise that did not necessarily occur during the aerobic work itself. Proper cool-down can help minimize the potential for clinically undesirable post-aerobic physiological conditions.

If one assumes a supine position on the floor immediately after vigorous aerobic work, there is an increased venous return to the heart that can put an added strain on the heart during the post-aerobic period. *Be sure to walk for two to three minutes after strenuous aerobic work to allow the heart rate to return to near-resting level (within 60% of age-predicted maximum heart rate) prior to doing less strenuous calisthenics and stretching.*

A final heart rate should be taken as stretches are finished and class members prepare to leave. The recovery heart rate at this point should definitely be below 60% of maximal heart rate for the individual participant. If a class member's heart rate is not at this level at the end of the workout, the person was probably exercising too intensely and should work at a less vigorous intensity for the next few classes, until he or she becomes more fit and better able to work at higher intensities. Cool-down stretches should be continued until one's heart rate has lowered to below 60% of maximal heart rate. **[XII: Final Heart Rate]**

Hot showers, saunas, and hot tubs

Hot showers, saunas, and hot tubs should be avoided following vigorous exercise because the heat causes the blood vessels to dilate. This, along with the tendency of blood to pool in the extremities, causes the heart and brain to receive inadequate amounts of blood and, therefore, oxygen. The person may faint or possibly experience more serious medical conditions. **[XII.C: Saunas and Hot Tubs]**

Target heart rate—its nature and significance

To improve the efficiency of one's cardiorespiratory system, it is necessary to exercise at an intensity that will stress the cardiorespiratory system adequately to realize at what is known as a "training effect." Researchers differ as to exactly what percent of the maximal heart rate one must exercise to achieve this training effect, but AFAA recommends that instructors have their classes work within 70%–80% of maximal heart rate. [**VI.H: Target Heart Rate**] Using the equation 220 minus one's age and multiplying that answer by .7 and .8 will provide the appropriate heart rate range for each participant to work within during the aerobic phase of the exercise session. Subtracting one's age from 220 gives the theoretical maximum at which anyone's heart can beat at that specific age. People *should not* exercise at this heart rate because it may represent a rate at which undue fatigue and possible injury can occur.

Some people refer to a single number when referring to target heart rate. For a 20-year-old person, the target heart rate for aerobic training would be 160 beats per minute. Others refer to a target heart rate *range* which has a lower and upper rate within which a person should work aerobically to realize a training effect over a period of weeks. Improved aerobic conditioning enables a person to perform similar work tasks more efficiently with a lower heart rate, less production of fatigue products, and the ability to continue the exercise intensity for longer periods of time. As a result of aerobic conditioning, the heart, lungs, and circulatory system become more efficient, processing and delivering oxygen more rapidly and efficiently to every part of the body.

One of the most important responsibilities of an exercise instructor is to guide class participants to work within their capabilities and limitations. Along this line, taking the time to instruct class members as to proper and accurate location of pulse and monitoring of heart rate is essential. Determining the heart rate during the aerobic phase of a workout provides a gauge as to whether the person is working below, within, or above the appropriate heart rate range for his or her age. Knowing the heart rate during an aerobic workout gives the participant information relative to the proper intensity for realizing a training effect over a period of time. AFAA recommends taking the heart rate five minutes after the beginning of active aerobic work. If monitoring the heart rate is not feasible at this point, AFAA recommends that the instructor find some time during the aerobic phase for the students to monitor their heart rates.

Monitoring heart rate involves the monitoring of the *pulse*. A pulse results from alternate expansion and relaxation of the arterial wall and from the beating of the heart. An impulse felt over an artery lying near the surface of the skin is created when the heart ejects blood into the aorta. Its impact on the elastic arterial walls creates a pressure wave ("pulse wave") that continues along the arteries. This impact is the pulse. All arteries have a pulse, but it is most easily felt at the point where the blood vessel approaches the surface of the body.

Arterial pulsations are counted for a specified period of time, either 6, 10, or 15 seconds. AFAA recommends counting the pulse for 10 seconds and multiplying the number of beats counted by six to determine the one-minute heart rate.

APPLIED PHYSIOLOGIC PRINCIPLES OF AEROBIC EXERCISE 59

The heart rate rapidly decelerates when vigorous aerobic work is interrupted by a slowing or cessation of movement to monitor heart rate. The deceleration that occurs within 6–15 seconds is so significant that counting the heart rate for 15 seconds and multiplying by four results in considerable underestimation of the actual exercising heart rate. Table A.6 shows target heart rates for three levels of workout corresponding to the age of the individual. Both one minute and ten second counts are listed.

Recognizing exertional intolerance

More than 500,000 cases of sudden death occur annually, with the victims often ranging in age from 40 to 65. Since an incident might occur in an aerobics class, an exercise instructor must be competent in CPR skills.

Table A.6 Target Heart Rates

Age	80%	70%	60%	Age	80%	70%	60%
15	164/27	144/24	123/21	47	138/23	121/20	104/17
16	163/27	143/24	122/21	48	138/23	120/20	103/17
17	162/27	142/24	122/21	49	137/23	120/20	103/17
18	162/27	141/24	121/20	50	136/23	119/20	102/17
19	161/27	141/24	121/20	51	135/23	118/20	101/17
20	160/27	140/23	120/20	52	134/22	118/20	101/17
21	159/27	139/23	119/20	53	134/22	117/20	100/17
22	158/26	139/23	119/20	54	133/22	116/19	100/17
23	158/26	138/23	118/20	55	132/22	116/19	99/17
24	157/26	137/23	118/20	56	131/22	115/19	98/16
25	156/26	137/23	117/20	57	130/22	114/19	98/16
26	155/26	136/23	116/19	58	130/22	113/19	97/16
27	154/26	135/23	116/19	59	129/22	113/19	97/16
28	154/26	134/22	115/19	60	128/21	112/19	96/16
29	153/26	134/22	115/19	61	127/21	111/19	95/16
30	152/25	133/22	114/19	62	126/21	111/19	95/16
31	151/25	132/22	113/19	63	126/21	110/18	94/16
32	150/25	132/22	113/19	64	125/21	109/18	94/16
33	150/25	131/22	112/19	65	124/21	108/18	93/16
34	149/25	130/22	112/19	66	123/21	108/18	92/15
35	148/25	130/22	111/19	67	122/20	107/18	92/15
36	147/25	129/22	110/18	68	122/20	106/18	91/15
37	146/24	128/21	110/18	69	121/20	106/18	91/15
38	146/24	127/21	109/18	70	120/20	105/18	90/15
39	145/24	127/21	109/18	71	119/20	104/17	89/15
40	144/24	126/21	108/18	72	118/20	104/17	89/15
41	143/24	125/21	107/18	73	118/20	103/17	88/15
42	142/24	124/21	107/18	74	117/20	102/17	88/15
43	142/24	124/21	106/18	75	116/19	102/17	87/15
44	141/24	123/21	106/18	76	115/19	101/17	86/14
45	140/23	123/21	105/18	77	114/19	100/17	86/14
46	139/23	122/20	104/17	78	114/19	99/17	85/14

NOTE: *All percentages include heart rate for 1 minute followed by number of beats to count for 10 seconds. Equation: 220 minus one's age times percent was used to arrive at above heart rates.*

© *Joanne L. Smith 1985*

Should a sudden death emergency occur during a class session, it is imperative that the instructor follow predetermined emergency protocol for obtaining immediate medical help. It is ultimately the instructor's responsibility to administer CPR until that medical assistance arrives.

Coronary artery disease (CAD) is the main cause if such death occurs within 24 hours of the onset of symptoms. Since people with CAD can have inherited tendencies to the disease, it is important that those with strong family histories of heart disease see a physician and have an exercise stress test prior to enrolling in a strenuous exercise program. More importantly, persons experiencing frequent chest pains on exertion that disappear at rest, or those who suspect, for any reason, that they might have a cardiac problem, must cease exercise and report these symptoms to their physician.

The following signs and symptoms are danger signals that indicate the necessity to stop exercising and to consult a physician either immediately or as soon as possible, but definitely before continuing in the exercise program. [I.H: Danger Signs]

- nausea or vomiting
- inappropriate shortness of breath, labored breathing, or appearance of chest pain
- mental confusion; disorientation
- unusual or severe fatigue
- dizziness or feelings of faintness; actual syncope (unconsciousness)
- musculoskeletal pain or extreme discomfort, particularly in the legs
- staggering or persistent unsteadiness
- appearance of signs of vasoconstriction, i.e., pale or clammy skin

Instructors should continuously be aware of all participant's responses during exercise sessions, particularly scanning those members who are new to the program. If any of the signs or symptoms of exertional intolerance become apparent, the instructor should urge the person to have a medical examination as soon as possible. In addition, the intensity and duration of exercise for that person should be reduced until the person can tolerate greater intensities of exercise stress without becoming symptomatic. The suggested care for someone who exhibits any signs of exertional intolerance is to stop the person from exercising immediately, make that person sit or lie down as warranted, and seek medical assistance as necessary.

Special considerations

Hypoglycemia There are many symptoms of hypoglycemia and frequently, symptoms that seem to indicate hypoglycemia are actually indicative of some other medical condition. However, if a class member complains of numbness that occurs several hours after eating, along with accompanying symptoms of chilling, hunger, trembling, headache, dizziness, weakness or fainting, this may indicate that the person has hypoglycemia and needs to seek medical advice before continuing with the exercise program. While numbness in the extremities can be a sign of hypoglycemia or other serious medical problems, a person complaining of this condition should be advised to seek medical evaluation prior to beginning or continuing an exercise program.

Diabetes   It is quite likely that one or more participants in your exercise program are diabetics. Exercise-induced hypoglycemia is a well-recognized complication in insulin-treated diabetes. While diabetics are aware of signs of hypoglycemia, the instructor should be aware which participants, if any, are more likely to develop this condition and what immediate care can be given until medical assistance arrives. The time of day in which the diabetic takes insulin, the type and time of meals, and the intensity and duration of the exercise session are all factors that can affect the diabetic's potential for becoming hypoglycemic. Under the physician's supervision, the tendency toward exercise-induced hypoglycemia can be minimized.

Since there is a close relationship between diabetes and heart disease, a diabetic person should have an exercise stress test and a complete cardiovascular evaluation prior to enrolling in an aerobic exercise program. This is essential if the person is 35 years of age or older. A diabetic participant under the direct care of his or her physician should be able to participate successfully in an aerobics program. The impact of the exercise on the individual's physiologic status must be consistently monitored by his or her physician.

Medications   Although the participants in an aerobics class may not be fit, they may be basically healthy young and middle-aged adults. Still, it is possible that within this population there are some class members who are taking medications for various reasons. Any participant who is being medically treated for hypertension, diabetes, thyroid problems or the like should be well aware of the medication he or she is taking and how that medication affects resting and exercise heart rate. If the person is taking a drug which alters exercise heart rate, then determining target heart rate range using the standard formula will be less accurate. The participant should undergo an exercise stress test while remaining on the medication to determine the heart rate response at varying levels of work intensities. Many anti-hypertensive drugs have a slowing effect on the heart and therefore may lead a person to think he or she is not working up to target when, in fact, he or she may actually be working hard enough even though the heart rate doesn't demonstrate this. It is important that the participant work closely with the physician in becoming familiar with the appropriate exercise prescription for his or her present medical status. Anyone using a heart-rate altering medication cannot appropriately determine target heart rate range using the equation for participants who are not limited by medical conditions. Heart rate for persons using heart-rate altering medication can be monitored by using ratings of perceived exertion (RPE). RPE utilizes one's perceptions of how one feels at any specific point in a workout as a relatively accurate indication of actual work intensity.

Anaphylactic reactions to exercise   Anaphylactic reactions are severe allergic attacks that may result in death if not treated. The symptoms can be one or more of the following: skin rashes, fainting, bronchial constriction, nausea, diarrhea, and severe headaches. Some participants may suffer chest tightness and wheezing with exercise signifying development of exercise-induced bronchospasm.

Side-stitch   Many people ask, "What exactly is a side-stitch?" It can best be described as sudden, sharp pains experienced in the upper part of the abdomen during exercise. These pains are a form of muscle cramp, probably of the diaphragm, the large flat muscle that controls breathing.

A common cause of the side-stitch, especially in novice athletes and beginning exercisers, is thought to be gas distending the colon. The colon makes up the last three feet of the intestinal tract and acts as a muscular tube which moves stool toward the rectum. As food gets digested, gas is formed throughout the entire intestinal tract. Exercise speeds up intestinal contractions and pushes gas toward the rectum. If the flow of gas is retarded, the colon becomes stretched like a balloon, resulting in what we know as a stitch, usually in the upper right part of the abdomen.

Other causes are eating just before exercise and sensitivity to certain food substances, often milk or wheat. When exercising on a full stomach, blood that is needed in the digestive tract to digest the meal is going to the working muscles, creating an inadequate blood supply to the intestinal tract for the digestion. Intolerances to some food substances occur when a person lacks the chemical enzymes in the intestinal tract to break down either sugar in milk (galactose) or protein in wheat (glutin). When those who are susceptible eat one of these foods, they may develop cramping or diarrhea. Some food-sensitive people develop such symptoms only when they exercise vigorously within 24 hours of eating the above foods.

To cure a stitch: slow down and push your fingers deep into the site of the pain, usually just below the bottom right rib. Bend forward and exhale, pursing your lips. The stitch should soon disappear and exercise can then be resumed. When someone gets a stitch, it usually isn't necessary to see a doctor.

Preventing injuries   It is true that an "ounce of prevention is worth a pound of cure!" Instructors should provide a safe program for all participants at all times! If someone should happen to be injured during a class, be sure to know the proper procedures for handling the injured person, including emergency phone numbers to call and appropriate temporary care until medical assistance arrives, if it is necessary. In the event of suspected strains or sprains, use the RICE method of treatment until medical assistance can be sought. RICE, which stands for **R**est, **I**ce, **C**ompression, and **E**levation should be the immediate course of action to help minimize swelling and discomfort. Remember, too, that most injuries occur due to fatigue or lack of common sense. Be sure your class members always work within their individual ability levels. No one should try to perform at a level that is potentially unsafe to joints, ligaments, muscles, and the cardiovascular system. It is imperative that all exercise instructors provide a proper progression of movements, including intensity and duration considerations, that will allow participants to warm-up appropriately, safely engage in the aerobic phase after having been appropriately warmed up, and then cool back down again. [AFAA: Standards and Guidelines]

Environmental considerations   During hot, humid weather, encourage class members to dress comfortably in clothing that "breathes," e.g., cotton. Air circulation and frequent water breaks are important also. Never prevent participants from taking cool water as they need it.

Summary

Regular physical activity is necessary in order to sustain the effects of exercise training. In addition, regular physical activity may serve as an incentive for improving all-around health including cessation of smoking, weight control, stress reduction, nutritional balance and similar life-style improvements. The potential risks of participation in an exercise program can be greatly reduced by following a safe, wisely-constructed exercise program based on research principles of appropriate exercise. The instructor of a group exercise program assumes considerable responsibility not only for providing a safe physical environment for exercise but also for conducting classes according to those practices and procedures that have been identified as being scientifically sound.

Vigorous exercise *does* present some medical risks, especially for those persons having undiagnosed heart disease and those engaged in activities that are too strenuous for their present level of conditioning. Instructors must screen participants carefully and monitor their performance abilities as they participate in the exercise program. Watch for signs of inadequate adjustment to the stresses of the exercise program. Take the responsibility for educating class participants concerning the importance of approaching exercise with common sence—starting slowly, progressing gradually, and paying attention to any warning signs or symptoms, no matter how fit they seem to be. Any time a participant experiences pain or unusual discomfort during or following exercise, the instructor must never try to analyze or diagnose the reason for the discomfort but should advise the participant to seek medical advice before continuing the exercise program.

Instructors must realize the important role they are assuming as exercise leaders. Continuing education in exercise physiology, kinesiology, and other related fields, as well as keeping abreast of related literature will help to ensure that participants are receiving the highest quality exercise program the instructor is capable of offering.

Commonly Asked Questions

Q. Will a person become fit more quickly if he or she works out at a heart rate slightly higher than his or her determined heart rate range?

A. No! In addition, working at greater than 80% of maximal heart rate sets the person up for a variety of potentially serious medical conditions. Orthopedic problems and cardiac dysrhythmias are much more common when someone exercises at an intensity greater than 85% of maximal heart rate. For a safety margin, AFAA recommends working no higher than 80% of maximal heart rate to minimize the potential for cardiac and orthopedic complications.

Class members with special needs (e.g., pregnant women, or anyone with a history of cardiopulmonary problems) should consult their physicians regarding their individual range. In any case, it is recommended that new members work at the lower end of their HR range for the first 8–10 weeks of their new program.

Q. When counting beats to monitor one's heart rate, how should one start?

A. Instructors should train their students to locate the pulse quickly once the cue is given to monitor the heart rate. It is highly recommended that participants become accustomed to monitoring their HRs while walking slowly, so that blood doesn't pool in the lower extremities during this period. Instructions should be clear and precise for the onset and cessation of the 10-second count. Typical verbal cues to monitor the pulse might be: "Continue walking slowly, locate your pulse, ready—COUNT!" A 10-second pause follows, then "STOP!"

When taking exercising HRs, instructors should be sure to use a consistent pattern of verbal cues to signal the initiation and cessation of pulse counting. Give a quick signal loud enough for everyone to hear. Use a stop watch or an accurate wristwatch with a second hand for determining the onset and cessation of the ten-second count.

The two big advantages of heart rate monitoring are first, that the procedure allows each participant to work at the appropriate level of intensity for his or her needs. Also, HR monitoring has a built-in progression because as a person becomes more fit, the heart rate response to a given workload will be less, and the person will have to work somewhat harder, on a progressive basis, in order to elevate the heart rate to within the target zone.

Q. What anatomical site should be used for monitoring heart rate?
A. The radial artery (wrist) is the most commonly used site for palpating the pulse. Correct location of the radial pulse is on the thumb side of the wrist between the bony prominence (the styloid process of the radius) and the forearm tendon (the flexor carpi radialis).

Q. Why is it some people can easily locate a radial pulse and others cannot?
A. There are several factors related to one's ease or difficulty in locating a radial pulse. Among them, the size of the artery, the strength of the actual arterial pulsations, the amount of subcutaneous fat around the radial artery, the amount of pressure used in feeling for the pulse, the location of the fingertips on the wrist, and the part of the fingertips used are the most important ones. It is helpful to palpate the artery with gentle pressure using several fingers for greater accuracy. Using more than one finger provides a greater, more sensitive surface to palpate the pulse wave.

If a student is continuously unsuccessful in locating a radial pulse during exercise, the person can be taught to palpate the carotid pulse. Anatomically, this site is located at the carotid artery on the side of the neck, about halfway between the sternal notch and the earlobe, and can be found by gently placing the fingertips on the side of the throat in a position directly in line with the outside corner of the eye on that same side. While some people consider palpation at the carotid artery to be easier than at the radial artery, there are some cautions that exercise instructors should be aware of concerning palpation at the carotid artery. Fingertip placement at the carotid artery should be *gentle* and on only **one side of the neck**, since excessive pressure or simultaneous pressure on both sides of the neck can elicit an extreme vagal response (stimulating the vagus nerve of the parasympathetic nervous system), slowing the heart rate. Some people have such a sensitive carotid artery that the heart can actually be slowed down to a point which causes the person to become unconscious. In very extreme cases, cardiac standstill could possibly occur.

Q. Does chest pain always indicate the presence of heart disease?
A. No. In addition to heart disease, there are many other causes of chest pain, including indigestion, drinking carbonated beverages, swallowing

air when eating rapidly, smoking, and chewing gum. A constricting substernal chest pain that develops during exertion and is relieved by rest may be angina pectoris. This pain, commonly associated with heart disease, will sometimes spread to the left shoulder and down to the elbow or wrist and occasionally to the right arm or the jaw. If a participant complains of these symptoms during or following exercise in your class, advise him or her to stop exercising and seek medical attention as soon as possible and to have a thorough checkup before returning to any exercise program. If, during a class, someone complains of lasting, crushing chest pain that is *not* relieved by rest, seek medical assistance immediately! These symptoms may indicate a heart attack. In addition to the crushing chest pain, the person may be belching, retching, or vomiting, and/or may have extreme shortness of breath. These latter symptoms can occur in the absence of chest pain and still indicate the possibility of a heart attack occurring, which is an immediate medical, life-threatening emergency (see appendix C, *Medical Emergencies*).

References

American College of Sports Medicine. *The Recommended Quantity and Quality of Exercise for Developing and Maintaining Fitness in Health Adults*. (Position Statement) 1978.

American College of Sports Medicine. *Reference Guide for Workshop/Certification Programs in Preventive/Rehabilitative Exercise*.

Chow, R. and Wilmore, J. "The Regulation of Exercise Intensity by Ratings of Perceived Exertion." *Journal of Cardiac Rehabilitation*. 1984:4:9:382-387.

Ellested, M. et al. "Standards for Adult Exercise Testing Laboratories." *American Heart Association*. 421A-427A.

Gornick, C. et al. "Sudden Cardiac Arrest: Developing a Preventive Strategy." *Primary Cardiology*. 1984: 10:11:84-99.

Koivisto, V. and Felig, P. "Exercise in Diabetes: Clinical Implications." *Cardiovascular Reviews and Reports*. 1984: 5:4:399-404.

Painter, P. and Hanson, P. "Isometric Exercise: Implications for the Cardiac Patient." *Cardiovascular Reviews and Reports*. 1984: 5:3:261-279.

Ruderman, N. et al. "Exercise as a Therapeutic Tool in the Type I Diabetic." *Practical Cardiology*. 1984: 10:2:143-153.

Wenger, N., Ed. *Exercise and the Heart*. Philadelphia: Davis, 1985.

Zabetakis, P. "Exercise and Mild Hypertension." *Primary Cardiology*. 1984:10:8:47-63.

Chapter 5

Body Composition

John E. Thiel, M.Ed.

Obesity is associated with a wide variety of degenerative diseases that cause an increase in the premature deaths of millions of Americans. It is estimated that about 50 million men and 60 million women in the United States between the ages of 18 and 79 are "too fat" and need to reduce excess weight.

One of the major reasons that Americans have taken up aerobic exercise over the past two decades is to reduce risk factors associated with cardiovascular diseases and weight control.

An important first step in formulating an intelligent program of total fitness for yourself or participants in an aerobic exercise program is an accurate assessment of body composition. The use of the popular height-weight tables offers little information in telling us anything about the quality or composition of one's body weight.

In the chapter that follows we will discuss the magnitude of the problem of obesity in the United States and provide an understanding of the concepts of overweight, overfat, essential fat, and storage fat. Also included will be the underlying rationale for the evaluation of body composition in terms of lean body weight and fat body weight.

Sex differences in essential body fat, and the association of body fatness in women and menstrual irregularity will also be presented. A simple and accurate method for the measurement of body composition by skinfold techniques will be discussed. Average percent fat values and associated values for overfatness and desirable percent fat for men and women of various age ranges will be presented as a means of increasing one's understanding of body composition.

Obesity in America

Overweight and obesity are two of the most significant health hazards in the United States today. They are either directly or indirectly associated with a wide variety of diseases such as cardiovascular disease; hypertension (high blood pressure); impaired metabolism; diabetes; joint, bone, and gall bladder diseases; and pulmonary dysfunction. These diseases account for 15%–20% of the annual United States mortality. It is estimated that in the developed countries, approximately 35% of the adult population is obese with evidence that obesity is on the increase.

The problems associated with obesity in the United States are enormous. To illustrate their magnitude, it was estimated that in 1973 around $10 billion dollars were invested in the diet industry. Of this amount, it was estimated that $14.9 million was spent on Weight Watchers International, another $220 million on health spas and reducing salons, $54 million on "over-the-counter" diet pills, $100 million on exercise equipment, and another $1 billion spent in the diet food market.

Since the mid-1970s, it has not been unusual to see at least one diet book on the bestseller lists in the United States at any one time.

Some authorities look at the economic costs of obesity in a very different manner. Taking skinfold fat data from the 1975 National Health Survey, a group of researchers estimated that about 50 million men and 60 million women between the ages of 18 and 79 (out of an adult population data base of 146.8 million) were "too fat." This excessive "overfatness" was calculated to be about 377 million Kg or 831 million pounds of excess fat in men and 667 million Kg or 1470 million pounds of excess fat in women, for a total of 1044 million Kg or 2.3 billion pounds for the total adult excess fat in the United States. If the energy saved by dieting to achieve desirable weight and body fat in these men and women were converted into fossil fuel, it would be equal to the total electrical demands of the cities of Boston, Chicago, San Francisco, and Washington, DC for a full year. The energy savings accrued from the weight loss and maintenance of desirable weight would be equal to 1.3 billion gallons of gasoline, or enough gasoline to fuel 900,000 average US autos at 12,000 miles per year and at 14 miles per gallon.

Evidence shows that physical inactivity may be the major cause of obesity in the United States—even more significant than overeating.

Overweight or overfat?

In order to understand what is meant by body composition, it is first important to define the terms of overweight and overfat. *Overweight* refers only to an individual's body weight which exceeds some known average standard. This standard is based on sex, height and frame size. The standardized height-weight charts first formulated in the early 1900s by the Society of Actuaries and Association of Life Insurance Medical Directors of America were recorded with shoes (one and two inch heels for men and women, respectively) and a four to nine pound allowance for clothing. Over time, these tables were revised for weight range provisions for small, medium and large frame sizes and one inch increments in height.

The problems of using standardized height-weight tables for determining an individual's desirable or ideal weight were best illustrated in a study in the early 1940s, when Dr. Albert Behnke, a Navy medical physician and pioneer in the field of body composition assessment, found 17 of 25 professional football players to be grossly overweight when compared to insurance companies' height-weight tables and "unfit" for military service. A careful assessment of each "rejected" player's body composition revealed that 11 of the 17 players had very high specific gravities, indicating low levels of body fat weight and high levels of lean muscle and bone mass.

The height-weight tables provide little information about the quality of one's body weight. It is possible to be overweight, such as the football players in the example above, but to have normal or below normal levels of body fat. It is also possible to be "overfat" and yet be within the normal weight range for height and frame size. It is important to point out that there is still no accurate method to categorize exact bone-frame size. The use of a height-weight table can **only** tell you if you are overweight or underweight and nothing about the amount of body fat that may be stored on the body. Since Dr. Behnke's work, several other studies have confirmed that standard height-weight tables do not provide accurate estimates of desirable or ideal weight and do not take into consideration the composition of the body.

Body Composition

Generally speaking, body composition refers to the types and amount of tissues that make up the body. The four major component parts of the human body are muscle mass, bone mass, fat mass, and organ mass. The last component includes the skin and various other non-muscle organs of the body. The most widely accepted model of body composition is the two-component scale which divides the body weight into lean body weight and fat weight. The lean body weight component consists of 40%–50% muscle mass, 16%–18% bone mass, and 29%–34% body organ mass. This component represents the active energy-producing tissues of the body. The second component of fat weight refers to the essential fat and inactive storage fat tissue that serves as a long-term energy reservoir.

Essential fat and storage fat

The total amount of fat weight in the human body can be categorized under two areas or sites depending upon its function. The first site where a small amount of fat is stored is in the bone marrow, heart, liver, lungs, intestines, spleen, kidneys, cell membranes, nerve tissue and certain tissues in the spinal cord and brain. This fat is commonly termed *essential fat*. This fat is required for normal physiological function of the various organs. In men and women, this essential fat accounts for about 3% of the total body weight. However, in females the essential fat also includes what is known as "sex-specific" or "sex-characteristic" fat. This "sex-specific" essential fat usually accounts for an additional 9%-12% of body weight in a woman. Its development is related to normal sex-hormone control. The mammary glands and the pelvic region are the primary areas of storage of this fat. In one recent study it was found that the weight of the breasts only accounts for about 4% of this "sex-specific" fat in a group of women who varied in percent body fat between 14% and 35%. The majority of this "sex-specific" fat is probably located in the hip, thigh and pelvic regions and is under sex hormone-related influence.

The second major site of the body fat is the fat that accumulates in the subcutaneous tissue between the muscle and skin. This is called the "storage" body fat. This storage fat or adipose tissue serves several bodily functions. First, it serves as a shock absorber to cushion and protect bones, muscles, and internal organs from injury. Storage fat also functions as an insulator against hot and cold environments. It can help maintain a somewhat constant core body temperature while at rest. However, it should be pointed out that excessive storage fat acts as a hindrance in regulating body temperature while exercising. During exercise the body has a decreased ability to transfer heat to the periphery, which is generated as a result of an increased muscle metabolism, through excessive amounts of stored adipose tissue. In addition to interfering with heat transfer through the subcutaneous layer, excess body fat directly adds to the metabolic cost of aerobic activities in which the body weight must be moved. The overfat person in an aerobic exercise class is at a distinct disadvantage in terms of heat regulation and physical performance.

The major function of storage fat is for energy. It is the largest reservoir of stored energy. During sustained-endurance aerobic activity, the primary fuel for energy comes from the breakdown of the storage body fat into simple fatty acids. The distribution of storage fat in males and females is very similar. The average amount of stored body fat in young men is around 12%, 15% in females.

Lean Body Weight

Lean Body Weight (LBW) refers to the physiological lower limit in which an individual cannot reduce his body weight without impairing health. To calculate LBW, subtract weight of storage fat from total body weight.

technique is based on Archimedes' principle, in which the density of the body can be calculated. Because of time, equipment, subject cooperation, and technical skill involved, this method is not recommended for non-laboratory settings or mass testing. Anthropometric measurements of skinfolds, body circumference and diameter measures are more practical for use in the health-exercise club setting. Numerous prediction equations have been developed to estimate body density, lean body weight, fat weight and percent body fat. These equations for anthropometric measurement correlate well with the underwater weighing techniques and have many advantages. The necessary equipment is inexpensive, requires very little space, and measurements can be obtained easily and quickly.

Measurement of body composition by skinfold techniques

A skinfold is a pinch of the skin plus the underlying fat taken at various sites over the body. The skinfold caliper provides a quantitative measurement of the amount of fat immediately below the skin. Approximately 50% of the body's total fat content is located in tissue just below the skin. The skinfold technique allows a reasonably valid estimate of the total body fat. The sum of several skinfolds provides a more representative sample of subcutaneous body fat and is more highly correlated with body density than just one or two sites. In recent years, the development of generalized rather than population-specific equations have been widely used.

The following nomogram for determining percent body fat was developed by Baun, et al., using the generalized equations reported by Jackson and Pollock (1979) and Jackson, et al. (1980). Ages range from 18 to 61 years and 18 to 55 years for males and females, respectively. This nomogram was designed to aid in making rather accurate determination of percent body fat. Please keep in mind that the major criticism in skinfold techniques is not the formula used to calculate body composition but the skill and experience of the person taking the measurements and the selection of proper sites. One should observe the following general guidelines for measuring skinfolds:

1. Pick up the subject's skinfold between your index finger and thumb. Be sure that you have two layers of skin and the underlying fat. Allow the skinfold to follow its natural stretch line as you lift it. If you doubt that you have a true fold, have the subject contract the muscle underneath it; you will be able to retain your grasp on the skin, if it is a true skinfold. Make all measurements of skinfolds on the right side of the body.
2. Apply the calipers perpendicular to the fold approximately 1 cm (¼-½ inch) from the thumb and index finger. It should be applied where the two surfaces of the fold are parallel. Do not apply the calipers where the fold is rounded near the top, or where it is broader near its base.

BODY COMPOSITION 73

Figure A.18   A nomogram for the estimate of percent body fat for Male and Female populations and the sum of three skinfolds

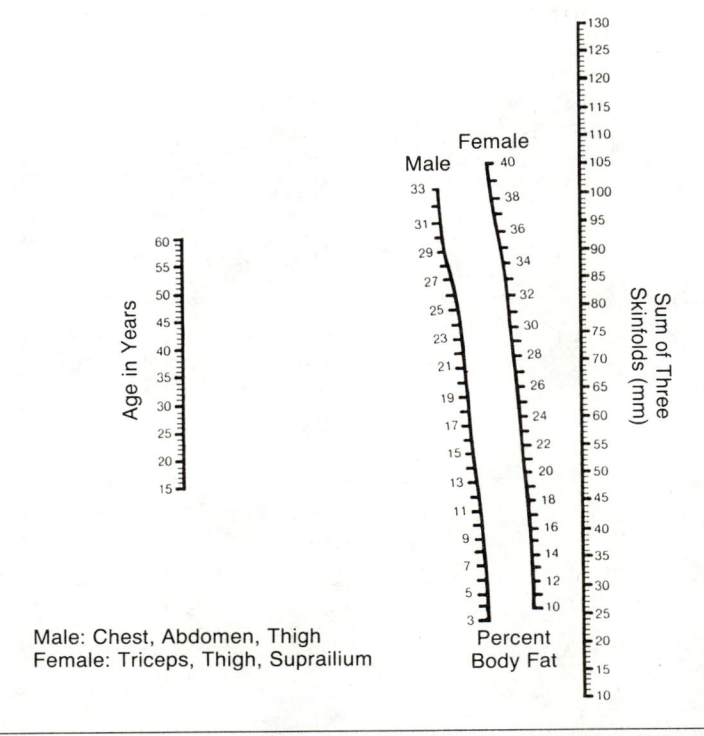

```
Age in Years        Male    Female     Percent      Sum of Three
                                       Body Fat     Skinfolds (mm)
```

Male: Chest, Abdomen, Thigh
Female: Triceps, Thigh, Suprailium

SOURCE: Baun, W. B., Baun, M. R., and Raven, P. B., A nomogram for the Estimate of Percent Body Fat from Generalized Equations. Research Qtr. for Exercise and Sport. (52, 380–384, 1981.) Modified and reprinted with permission.

3. While maintaining a grasp of the skinfold, allow the caliper grip to be released, so that the full tension is exerted on the skinfold. The dial is read to the nearest 0.5 mm (Lange) and 0.1 mm (Harpenden) approximately one to two seconds after the grip has been released.
4. A minimum of two measurements should be taken at each site. If the repeated measurement varies by more than 1 mm, keep repeating the measurement until two measures of the desired accuracy are obtained (maintain 5% accuracy; e.g., if the first measurement is 20 mm, the second measurement must be between 19 and 21 mm). Use as the recorded value, the average of the two or three measures which represent the skinfold fat site best.
5. The following six sites (male: chest, abdomen, and thigh; female: triceps, suprailium, and thigh) as indicated by their anatomical landmarks should be used (see figure A.19):

74 ESSENTIALS OF AEROBIC EXERCISE

Figure A.19 Anatomic location and position of skinfold caliper.

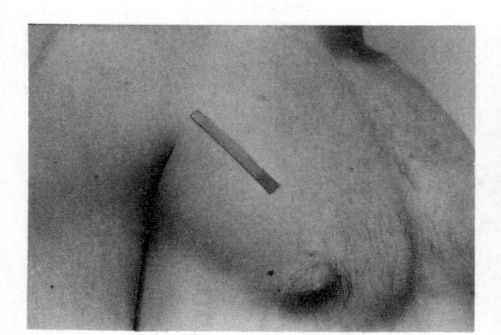

LOCATION　　　　　　　　　CALIPER POSITION

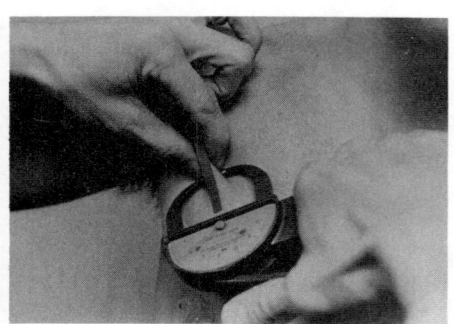

1A & 1B: Chest (men)

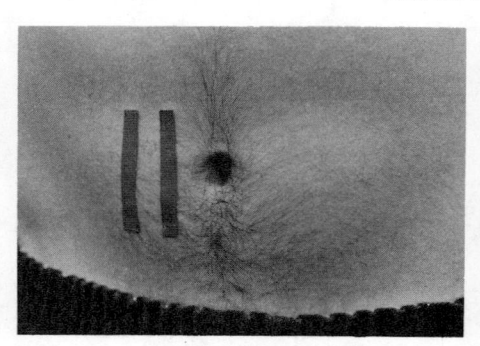

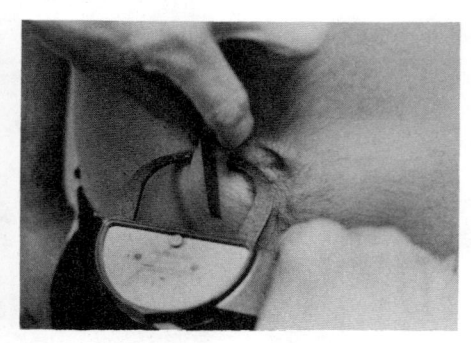

2A & 2B: Abdomen (men)

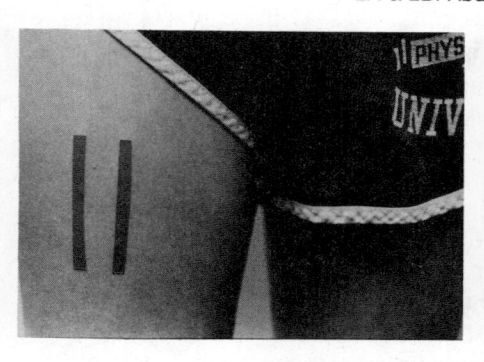

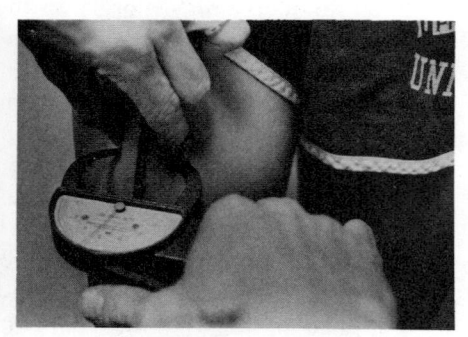

3A & 3B: Front of Thigh (men and women)

BODY COMPOSITION 75

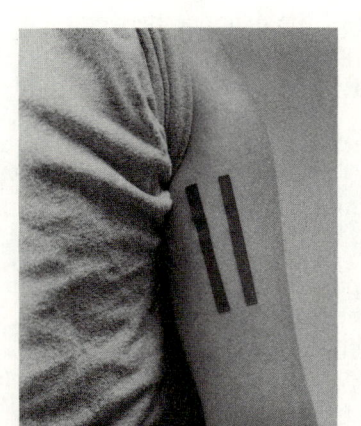

LOCATION   **CALIPER POSITION**

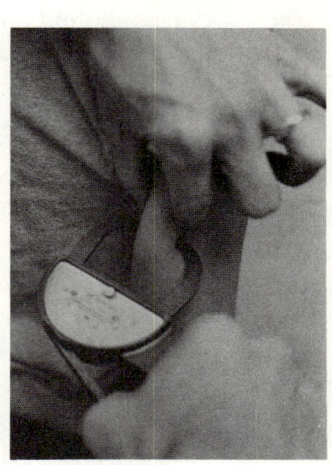

4A & 4B: Triceps (women)

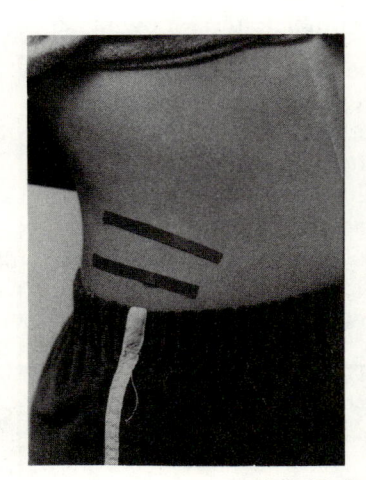

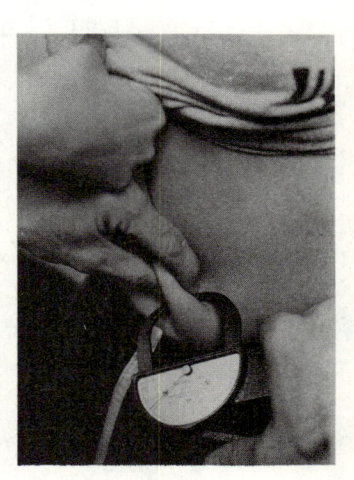

5A & 5B: Suprailium (women)

50% of body's total fat = in tissue just below skin

Male
a. **Chest:** A diagonal fold one-half of the distance between the anterior-axillary line and the nipple.
b. **Abdomen:** A vertical fold taken approximately 2 cm (1") laterally from the umbilicus.
c. **Thigh:** Vertical fold on the anterior aspects of the thigh midway between the hip and knee joints. The body weight should be placed on the opposite leg so that the thigh muscle is in a relaxed state.

Female
a. **Triceps:** A vertical fold on the posterior midline of the upper arm (over triceps muscle), halfway between the acromion and olecranon processes with the elbow extended and relaxed.
b. **Supraileum:** A diagonal fold above the crest of the ilium at the mid-axillary line.
c. **Thigh:** Same as in males above.

Calculation of percent fat
In order to calculate percent body fat, complete the following steps:

1. Take the values you reported for the three skinfolds (chest, abdominal, and thigh in males; triceps, suprailium and thigh in females) and add them together. Percent fat is then estimated by placing a straight-edged ruler (clear plastic works best) on the nomogram that connects the individual's age (left axis) with the sum of the three skinfolds (right axis) and reading the value from the appropriate percent fat scale with respect to sex. Record the percent body fat value.
2. Determine fat weight (FW) as follows:

FW = Percent fat (Step 1)/100 x body weight in lb (from scale)
---

3. Determine LBW by subtracting the fat weight from the total body weight.

LBW = Body weight (lb) − Fat weight (lb)

Average percent fat values for body composition
Values for average percent body fat in males and females of various age groups varies throughout the United States. There is a considerable number

of published studies available concerning the average body composition of men and women, young and old, physically active and inactive, but there are no systematic large scale evaluations of the body composition of representative samples from the general population that would justify the establishment of precise normative or "desirable" values of body composition. The table A.7 shows average values taken from published studies for men and women of various age groups. The ranges of percent body fat under the headings of "Excellent," "Very Good," "Average," "Fair," and "Poor" are hypothetical, based only on a review of the studies in athletic, normal, and obese populations.

A general observation based on the table above is that as men and women increase in age, the percentage of body fat tends to increase. It is difficult to say that the increase in body weight with age should be interpreted as being "desirable" or "normal." There are several reasons why adults gain more body fat with age. The primary reason is that there is generally an adaptation of a more sedentary life-style as one ages. Physical inactivity can cause an increase in storage fat accumulation and a reduction in muscle

Table A.7 Average values of percent body fat with optimum health/poor health scales and hypothetical ranges for desirable % body fat for males and females of various age groups.

Sex/Age Range	TOWARD OPTIMUM HEALTH ←		HEALTHY?	AWAY FROM OPTIMUM HEALTH →	
	Excellent "Lean"	Very good "Trim"	Average* "Healthy"	Fair "Plump"	Poor "Overfat"
MALE					
19 & Under	≤ 8.0	8.5–10.5	11.0–13.5	14.0–18.5	>19.0
20–29	≤10.0	10.5–12.0	12.5–15.0	15.5–19.5	>20.0
30–39	≤11.0	11.5–12.5	15.0–18.0	18.5–22.5	>23.0
40–49	≤12.0	12.5–15.0	18.0–22.0	22.5–26.5	>27.0
50 & Over	≤13.0	15.5–19.0	20.0–24.0	24.5–28.5	>29.0
FEMALE					
19 & Under	≤13.0	13.5–17.5	18.0–21.0	22.5–28.5	>29.0
20–29	≤15.0	15.5–20.0	23.0–27.0	27.5–31.5	>32.0
30–39	≤17.0	17.5–21.0	24.0–29.0	29.5–33.5	>34.0
40–49	≤19.0	21.0–24.0	27.0–32.0	32.5–36.5	>37.0
50 & Over	≤21.0	24.5–28.5	29.0–34.0	34.5–38.5	>39.0

*Average values taken from published studies. Boxed values represent a hypothetical "Desirable" percent fat for corresponding age range.

NOTE: It should be emphasized that the above concept of "desirable" percentages of body fat are based on hypothetical considerations. Very little actual published data other than the mean data taken from various carefully conducted age group studies are reported.

SOURCE: John Thiel, © 1985 (used with permission).

mass. Another reason for increases in body fat with age can be the reduction in bone density. An aging skeleton becomes demineralized and porous.

It is difficult to say that a 25% body fat value in a 50+-year-old male or a 34% body fat value in a 50+-year-old female and absence of other risk factors is "unhealthy." The data to substantiate "normal" or ideal levels of body fatness associated with the aging process are not available at the present time.

Desirable Body Weight

Excessive amounts of body fat are undesirable for optimum health and fitness. It is difficult to say what would be an "ideal" or "desirable" body weight for every individual. Desirable values will vary from person to person for a variety of reasons such as age, genetic factors, personal health, fitness-related goals, and psychological attitudes toward body image.

To determine desirable body weight once actual percent body fat is known, select a desired body fat level (use the "Hypothetical values for desirable percentages of body fat" from the table above) or consider what might be "desirable" based on

- weight at age 21 (if subject didn't have a weight problem then), or
- subject's weight at any age before he or she experienced an undesirable weight gain.

Standards for overfatness have been somewhat arbitrarily set at approximately 5% above reported average values of young men and women. Although the average value for percent body fat increases with age, this does not imply that men and women should get fatter as they get older. To calculate desirable body weight, use the formula illustrated below.

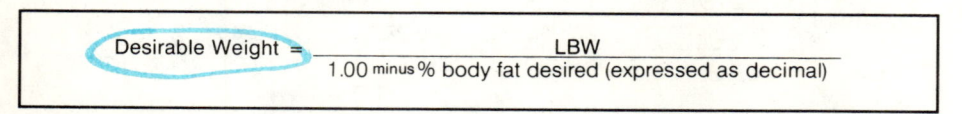

$$\text{Desirable Weight} = \frac{\text{LBW}}{1.00 \text{ minus } \% \text{ body fat desired (expressed as decimal)}}$$

It is recommended that a desirable weight range be established for an individual instead of an absolute value for the desirable weight. A weight range of plus or minus one percent of desirable weight might be considered.

Summary

Overweight and obesity are associated with a wide variety of diseases such as cardiovascular disease, high blood pressure, and diabetes that account for 15%–20% of the annual United States mortality. It is estimated that approximately 35% of the adult populations in developed countries are obese.

Commonly Asked Questions

Q. What is the best way to lose excessive body fat?

A. Research has shown that a combination of diet and exercise is the most effective way to lose weight safely. It can produce a weight loss of about 1½–2 lb per week. If weight loss is achieved this way, most of the loss is fat because exercise not only helps prevent the loss of lean tissue, it can cause a gain in lean tissue that lowers your percent of body fat even more than the weight loss would indicate.

Q. What recommendations should an instructor take when an excessively overweight person begins to exercise in an aerobic exercise program?

A. Several considerations should be taken when working with an obese individual in your exercise class. In order to assure a safe progression in physical activity, it is advisable to begin an overweight individual at 50%–60% of their target heart rate for the first several weeks. Specific routines or exercises that require quick and strenuous movements such as running and jumping should be avoided. Minimize movements that can cause possible injury to ankles, knees, hips, and lower back. You should encourage only walking in movement routines and allow the person to perform every other repetition when doing sets of various exercises.

Q. Is amenorrhea (disruption of the normal menstrual cycle) caused by a too low body fat level?

A. It is very difficult to say what causes an increase in amenorrhea in physical activity in women. There is a complex interaction of physical, hormonal, psychological, nutritional, and environmental factors on menstrual function. Several studies have shown an association of low body fat levels and amenorrhea. One particular study suggests that a body weight level below 17% fat triggers hormonal and metabolic disturbances that affect the normal menstrual cycle. It should be pointed out that there are many women athletes in all sports who are below the 17% body fat level and have normal menstrual cycles.

Q. What is the "desirable" percentage of body fat in older men and women?

A. Optimum body fat levels cannot be stated in precise percentages for any one individual. Desirable or ideal levels vary from person to person and are influenced by a variety of factors. Based on young healthy adults and athletes, it appears that it would be ideal to maintain a body fat level at 15% or less for men and 25% or less for women throughout one's adult life.

References

Baun, W. et al. "A Nomogram for the Estimate of Percent Body Fat." *Generalized Equations Research Quarterly for Exercise and Sport.* 1981:52:380–384.

Bonen, A. and Keizer, H. "Athletic Menstrual Cycle Irregularity: Endocrine Response to Exercise and Training." *Physician and Sportsmedicine.* 1984:12(August):78–90.

Katch, F. and McArdle, W. *Nutrition, Weight Control and Exercise,* 2nd Ed. Philadelphia: Lea and Febiger, 1984.

Lohmom, T. "Body Composition Methodology in Sports Medicine." *Physician and Sportsmedicine.* 1982:10(December):47–58.

Mayhew, J. "Body Composition." *Journal of Physical Education, Recreation and Dance.* 1981:September:38–40.

McArdle, W. et al. *Exercise Physiology—Energy, Nutrition, and Human Performance.* Philadelphia: Lea and Febiger, 1981.

Pollock, M. et al. *Exercise in Health and Disease—Evaluation and Prescription for Prevention and Rehabilitation.* Philadelphia: Saunders Co., 1984.

Weltman, A. and Stamford, B. "Fat: Understanding the Enemy." *Physician and Sportsmedicine.* 1982:10(March):159.

Chapter 6

General Nutritional Needs

Laura Pawlak, RD, Ph.D.

Life requires balance for growth, development, and survival. Thus, the human body relies on food as fuel for existence and then utilizes these nutrients within the diet for the positive growth, maintenance and work requirements of daily living. The amount of food fuel required for bodily energy and growth needs varies daily but the basic principle of balance must be retained for optimum health:

| Food-Fuel | | Energy-Growth |
| Intake | △ | Output |

Nutrients: The Food Fuels

Nutrients are chemicals necessary for the proper functioning of the body. There are seven nutrients essential for life:

- protein
- carbohydrates
- fats
- vitamins
- minerals
- fiber
- water

Although fiber is not absorbed and therefore cannot be considered a nutrient by definition, its vital role in the diet warrants inclusion in the category of nutrients

Water

Function   Water, the most abundant body constituent, is also the most basic of nutrient needs. It performs three functions that are essential to life:

- It contributes to the structure and form of the body.
- It provides the liquid environment for cell processes.
- It aids in regulation of body temperature.

Balance: intake vs excretion   Intake is accomplished through three routes:

- water within solid foods (fruit/vegetable group)
- liquids consumed (water, milk, other beverages)
- water generated within the cell through oxidation during normal metabolic processes

Water from foods and liquids is absorbed via the stomach, the rate depending on the temperature of the water. Although water can be absorbed throughout the small intestine, water absorption occurs mainly in the large intestine.

Intake of this nutrient should balance the output of water daily from:

- urine excretion
- stool excretion
- respiration losses through lungs
- losses from skin evaporation and sweat

Requirement   The multitude of factors determining water loss precludes a set minimal water requirement. Water losses through the skin and lungs can increase three to ten times during strenuous physical activity, especially when combined with exposure to high elevations or hot, dry climates. Water needs for the physically stressed person will be discussed in Chapter 8. However, the standard of 1 ml/calorie for adults is adequate under non-sweating conditions. Stated in simpler terms, for each 1,000 calories consumed, one needs about one quart of water intake primarily from fluids and water-containing foods.

Protein

Function and structure   Proteins make up the basic structure of all living cells and are essential for formation and maintenance of the organism. They are known as the building materials of the body. The individual building units are called amino acids. The quality of the protein as a building material is classified as complete or incomplete, depending on the type of amino acids and their percentage in the specific protein food. Therefore, the quality of the protein source can only be discussed in terms of the quality of the constituent amino acids.

GENERAL NUTRITIONAL NEEDS 83

Amino acids are categorized as essential or nonessential. The nine identified essential amino acids that cannot be manufactured by the human body are therefore "essential" for life, growth and development and only available through outside food sources. Complete proteins are those that contain all essential amino acids in sufficient quantity and proper ratio to support life's maintenance, growth, and development needs. Proteins unable to fulfill this definition are categorized as incomplete.

Sources Proteins of animal origin, (meat, poultry, fish, milk, cheese and eggs) are complete. The quality standard for a complete protein containing the best ratio and quantity of essential amino acids is the egg albumin (egg white), although all the proteins stated are excellent. Incomplete proteins, those deficient in one or more essential amino acids, are of plant origin (grains, legumes, seeds and nuts).

Digestion and absorption Although digestion begins in the stomach, the very long protein structure is only slightly decreased in size within this organ. Total digestion and absorption of the protein into its basic amino acid composition occurs within the small intestine. The amino acids then proceed via the blood system primarily to the liver for use as needed in building bodily structure. Proteins eaten beyond daily needs are digested and absorbed completely. However, upon entrance to the liver, they are metabolized as an energy source at the rate of four calories per gram.

Requirements There is no set protein requirement for all persons since need varies with the following three factors:

- **Tissue growth and maintenance:** Age-related growth spurts, pregnancy, lactation, and tissue repair due to injury significantly increase protein needs. Although an individual with above average muscle mass requires more protein per day to maintain the tissue, requirements set for adults should more than adequately protect these persons.
- **Illness and disease:** Physical trauma dramatically increases our protein requirements since protein is needed for repair and, in addition, is often wasted as an energy source during these periods.
- **Diet:** True evaluation of the amount of protein required by the body is based on the quality of the protein source and its digestibility by the gastrointestinal tract. Since all essential amino acids must be provided in sufficient quantities for construction of needed proteins by the body, a diet emphasizing complete proteins (animal protein) as the food source provides acceptable levels of essential amino acids at a lower intake than a diet consisting primarily of plant sources of protein (incomplete protein).

84 ESSENTIALS OF AEROBIC EXERCISE

Within a meal, a combination of complete and incomplete protein is comparable to a meal of only complete protein since the amino acid inadequacies of the incomplete protein foods are compensated by the amount an number of essential amino acids in the complete source.

Those persons choosing to eliminate all animal proteins from their diet must plan each meal carefully to achieve combinations of necessary amounts of the essential amino acids. The following diagram (figure A.20) illustrates food combinations that create the proper balance of essential amino acids for body needs.

Figure A.20 Complementation of proteins

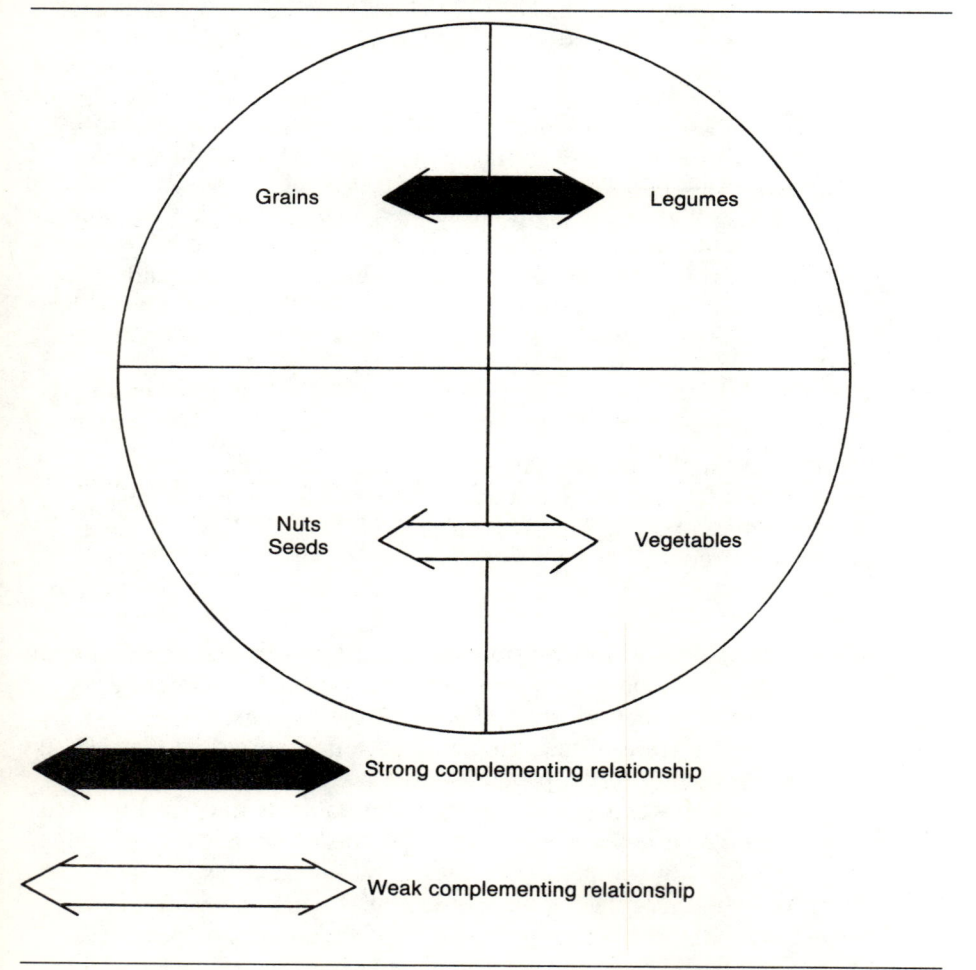

Assuming a variety of animal and plant proteins in the daily diet, a standard of 0.8 gm per kilogram of body weight is recommended for the healthy, nonstressed adult, e.g., for a person of approximately 150 pounds about 1½ ounces of pure protein of high quality is needed per day. Let us remember, however, that protein is part of a mixture of nutrients in foods and by weight is only half or less of low fat meat and dairy products.

In most cases, the American diet contains two to three times the standard of protein recommended for adults with the excess intake being an extremely expensive source of energy that could be supplied by carbohydrate foods.

Carbohydrates

Functions and structure   The power for body work can simply and rapidly be derived from carbohydrate food sources. Instant muscle and other organ energy needs can be met by carbohydrates even in the absence of sufficient oxygen for short periods of time. Its presence in the diet is important to avoid the misuse of protein as an energy source.

The carbohydrates are classified by their structure and divided into the following three groups:

- **Monosacharides**, called the simple sugars, are the smallest individual units of carbohydrate important in human nutrition (e.g., glucose, fructose, galactose).
- **Disaccharides** are sugars composed of two monosaccharides (e.g., table sugar [sucrose] = glucose and fructose; milk sugar [lactose] = glucose and galactose).
- **Polysaccharides** are composed of many monosaccharide units, with chemical binding between each unit which may or may not be digested as an energy source. For example, starch from plant food and glycogen from muscle digests into usable monosaccharides. In contrast, fiber, though a polysaccharide, is not digestible by the human body.

Digestion and absorption   Little digestion of carbohydrates occurs in the mouth. Stomach enzymes have no effect on them. Total digestion to monosaccharides is accomplished by the enzymes in the small intestine. These simple sugars are then absorbed into the blood stream and distributed to organs as needed for energy usage through the action of insulin, a hormone secreted by the pancreas.

Sources   Carbohydrates, of varying structure, are part of plant foods such as legumes, nuts, grains, vegetables, and fruits. They provide four calories of energy per gram weight.

Requirement   Current health standards recommend that approximately 55%–60% of our daily caloric intake be consumed as carbohydrate.

Carbohydrates isolated from foods, called refined sugars, should be limited to approximately 10% of the total carbohydrate intake since these sources are greatly deficient in nutrient value. The total calorie intake is determined by individual need.

Fiber

Function and structure   Dietary fiber is an item defined as the sum of indigestible carbohydrate and carbohydrate-like components of food, including cellulose, lignin, hemicellulose, pentosans, gums and pectins. Although there is no metabolic requirement for dietary fiber, its physiological significance warrants discussion in spite of the fact that it cannot be categorized as a nutrient due to its indigestibility.

Each type of fiber has a distinctive role as it is transported through the gastrointestinal tract; but in general, fiber functions as:

- a bulk agent, easing elimination and decreasing appetite
- a chelating agent, decreasing the absorption of cholesterol and, in excess, vital minerals from the diet
- an agent that decreases the rate of absorption of glucose from meals

Digestion   Although defined as indigestible carbohydrate, some forms of fiber can be metabolized by bacteria in the large intestine and thus are considered poor bulking agents.

Sources   Fruits, vegetables, whole grains, seeds, nuts, and legumes contain mixtures of fibers.

Requirements   Although no requirement has been set for fiber intake, it is recommended that the American diet be drastically changed from the current approximation of 10-20 gm of fiber per day to 50 gm of dietary fiber. The fiber should be obtained in natural foods; it is not recommended that isolated fiber be consumed.

Fats

Function and structure   Fat combines with other nutrients to form important structural compounds, among which are blood lipids, steroids, cell membranes, bile and vitamin D. Fat also aids in regulating body temperature since it insulates the body against rapid heat loss. Fat adds palatability and satiety to a diet and adds to the synthesis of vitamins by the body.

All fats are insoluble in water and are often called lipids. Lipids have the same structural elements as carbohydrates but are linked together very differently. When metabolized as an energy source, fats are then able to produce more energy, i.e., nine calories per gram of fat metabolized.

Lipids in foods can be divided into two types of basic components:

GENERAL NUTRITIONAL NEEDS 87

- animal fats—saturated fatty acid and cholesterol
- plant fats—unsaturated fatty acids

The plant fats are primarily mono- or polyunsaturated, with safflower, sunflower and corn oil having the greatest percent of polyunsaturated fat components.

Digestion and absorption Digestion occurs primarily in the small intestine through the action of enzymes that break the complex fat molecule apart into simpler absorbable components and bile salts acting as emulsifiers in the digestive process. Small fatty acids are absorbed directly into the bloodstream while the longer chain fatty acids and cholesterol, due to their lack of solubility in water, must filter first into the lymph fluid for reorganization. When combined with water-soluble carrier proteins, the lipids can then filter into the blood for transport to liver or adipose cells.

Sources Unless removed by processing, fat is found in greater or lesser quantities in plant and animal foods, the quality varying with the source.

Requirements As in protein nutrition, there are a few essential fatty acids that cannot be manufactured by the body and must be supplied by diet. However, there is no specific lipid requirement in the diet since the fat content of a balanced food intake provides adequate amounts of the essential fatty acids. The average American ingestion of fat, especially animal fats, far outweighs the bodily needs.

Vitamins

Function, food sources and requirements The term "vitamin" is derived from the root word "vita," essential to life. Today vitamins are defined as a group of organic compounds other than protein, carbohydrate, and fat, that cannot be manufactured by the human body yet are required in minute amounts for specific body functions of growth, maintenance, reproduction and repair. Vitamins are broadly classified solely on their solubility as water or fat soluble since each one is unique in its construction, properties, functions and distribution. Tables A.8 and A.9 summarize the functions, food sources, and requirements of the vitamins established as essential for human life.

Digestion and absorption Vitamins require no digestive process and are absorbed intact into the bloodstream. They are better absorbed when obtained through natural food sources than in tablet form. The fat soluble vitamins can be stored in the liver when excess is ingested; thus the potential exists for toxic effects from "mega" ingestion (more commonly by supplementation than through food sources). The water-soluble vitamins, when absorbed in excess of needs, are quickly excreted through the kidneys.

Table A.8 Water Soluble Vitamins: Functions, Sources, and Requirements

Vitamins*	Function	Food Sources	Adult Requirements
Thiamine (B$_1$)	Energy production	Pork, Organ Meats, Sausage, Eggs, Whole-grain or enriched breads and cereals, Green leafy vegetables, Nuts, Legumes	1.5 mg
Riboflavin (B$_2$)	Respiration of tissue cell; Normal cellular growth; Tissue maintenance of skin and mucus membranes	Organ meats, milk; Cheese, eggs, meat, whole-grain and enriched cereals, leafy greens	1.7 mg
Niacin (B$_3$)	Energy production and tissue respiration; Normal functioning of all cells	Liver, lean meat, fish, poultry, peanuts, enriched or whole-grain cereals	20 mg
Ascorbic Acid (C)	Formation of intercellular cement; Normal bones, teeth, skin	Citrus fruits, broccoli, cabbage, strawberries, tomatoes, greens	60 mg
B$_6$ (Pyridoxine)	Protein, carbohydrate, and fat metabolism	Muscle meats, liver, vegetables, and whole-grain cereals	2 mg
B$_{12}$	Participation in protein, fat, and carbohydrate metabolism, functioning of cells in bone marrow, nervous system, and gastrointestinal tract	Animal foods only: liver, kidney, muscle meat, milk, cheese, fish, eggs	6 mg
Folacin	Formation of red blood cells	Green leafy vegetables, liver, kidney, asparagus, lima beans	0.4 mg
Biotin	Formation of fatty acids; Energy production	Liver, kidney, egg yolk; Nuts, cauliflower, legumes, mushrooms	0.3 mg
Choline	Nerve function	Liver, kidney, meats, legumes, nuts, skim milk	—
Pantothenic Acid	Formation and breakdown of fatty acids	Liver, kidney, fresh vegetables, organ meats, whole-grain cereals, yeast, egg yolk (Pantothenic acid is widely distributed in foods)	10 mg

GENERAL NUTRITIONAL NEEDS

Table A.9 Fat Soluble Vitamins: Functions, Sources, and Requirements

Vitamins*	Function (needed for)	Sources	Adult Requirements
A	Normal growth	Liver, egg yolk, kidney	5000 I.U.
	Normal vision	Whole milk, butter	
	Normal skin	Fortified margarine	
	Formation of enamel	Fortified skim milk, yellow and dark green vegetables	
D	Bone and teeth formation	Sunshine (absorbed through the skin), fortified milk	400 I.U.
E	Healthy red blood cells (still being studied for a direct link with E)	Whole-grain cereals, salad oil, shortening, margarine, fruits, vegetables	30 I.U.
K	Blood clotting	Green leafy vegetables, egg yolk, liver, cauliflower, tomatoes (Vitamin K is also produced by bacteria in the small intestines)	----

*Constant excesses of some vitamins can be harmful:
Overdoses of Vitamin A may cause dry, peeling skin, loss of hair, headache, loss of appetite, lumps on extremities, thickening of bones.
Overdoses of Vitamin D may cause calcification of soft tissue, blood vessels, kidney tubules.
Vitamin E is an antioxidant that inhibits oxidation of Vitamin A.
Overdoses of Vitamin K (in research with rats) have been found to cause rupturing of red blood cells.

Minerals

Function, food sources and requirements Minerals are inorganic elements (metals) essential to man as control agents in body reactions and cooperative factors in energy production, body building and maintenance activities. The essential minerals are categorized into two main groups according to the amount used by the body:

- the **major** minerals present in large amounts
- the **trace** minerals utilized in lesser quantities

Tables A.10 and A.11 summarize the functions, food sources, and requirements of these minerals.

Digestion and absorption Minerals require no digestion and are absorbed intact from the small intestine. Some minerals can be stored in the liver when ingestion exceeds need. It is therefore important to avoid intake above those values established as safe especially when oral supplements are consumed.

Preventive Health Formula "The Basic Four Food Groups"

How can one determine on a daily basis that all nutrient needs are met for optimum body function? The impracticality of considering each nutrient

90 ESSENTIALS OF AEROBIC EXERCISE

Table A.10 Major Minerals: Function, Sources, and Requirements

Mineral	Function (needed for)	Sources	Adult Requirements
Calcium	Formation of bone and teeth Clotting of blood Muscle function Nerve function	Milk and milk products, mustard, greens, kale, broccoli	800 mg *1000 – 1500*
Phosphorus	Energy production Nerve function Muscle function Bone and teeth structure	Cereals, meats, fish, legumes, eggs, milk, dairy products	1000 mg
Magnesium	Bone constituent Catalyst for chemical reactions in body; building of protein.	Brains, sweet breads, liver, egg yolk, dark leafy greens, nuts, whole-grain cereals, beans, coffee, tea, cocoa	400 mg
Potassium	Energy production	Citrus juices, bananas	—
Sulfur	Hair, skin, nails	Protein foods: meats, seafood, fish, poultry, eggs, cheese, legumes	—
Sodium	Muscle and nerve	Milk and milk products, meat, deep leafy greens, seafood salt	1–3 gm estimate
Chloride	Muscle and nerve functioning	Protein foods	—

need in meal planning is obvious. A "Daily Food Guide" was therefore designed by the US Department of Agriculture to provide a flexible framework for making food selections to meet the nutrient needs specified by the Recommended Dietary Allowances (RDA values). The Daily Food Guide is intended to be easy to use, easy to remember, adaptable, and to increase one's choice of achieving sound nutrition on a daily basis. The guide does not specify individual foods to be eaten, rather it combines foods which make similar nutritional contributions in four large groups:

1. Milk
2. Meat and other proteins
3. Fruits and vegetables
4. Grains

The Daily Food Guide is frequently called the *Basic Four*. Table A.12 further delineates the types of foods in each Food Group and the major nutrient contribution of each group to good health. The number of servings

Table A.11 Trace Minerals: Function, Sources, and Requirements

Mineral	Function	Sources	Adult Requirements
Iron	Normal red blood cells, muscle functioning	Liver, meat, organ meats, egg yolk, legumes, dried fruits, whole-grain cereals and breads, deep green leafy vegetables	18 mg
Copper	Formation of red blood cells, formation of bones	Liver, kidney, shellfish, oysters, nuts, raisins, legumes, chocolate	2 mg
Iodine	Normal growth and development, reproduction, lactation.	Iodized salt, seafood	150 mg
Cobalt	Formation of red blood cells	Widely available in food	—
Zinc	Liver, bone, skin, blood	Liver, eggs, oysters, meats, brains	15 mg
Fluoride	Bone structure Prevention of dental caries	Fluoridated water Gelatin, organ meats, seafood	—
Manganese	Normal bone growth and development, lipid metabolism, reproduction, nerve function	Nuts, legumes, whole grains	35–70 mg (estimate)
Molybdenum	Normal growth	Legumes, whole grains, organ meats	0.15–0.50 mg (estimate)
Selenium	Influences action of drugs, affects oxidation reaction	Meat, seafood, cereals	50–200 mg (estimate)
Chromium	Component of glucose tolerance factor in control of blood sugar	Yeast, beer, liver, whole grains, meat, cheese	50–200 mg (estimate)
Silicon	Bone formation	Not clearly defined	—
Arsenic Nickel Vanadium	Not clearly defined	Not clearly defined	—
Cadmium Lead Tin	Questioned role in human nutrition		—

recommended for a minimum balanced nutrient intake each day are listed in table A.13.

Because of the growing trend toward vegetarianism, especially among today's young adults, I have included a Basic Four Food Group Guide that states the number of servings recommended for the two large classes of vegetarians (see table A.14).

Table A.12 The Basic Four Food Groups:
A Simplified Method for Adequate Nutrient Intake

Group	Major Nutrient Contribution

Milk
1 cup milk, yogurt,
OR Calcium Equivalent:
  1½ oz. cheddar cheese
  1 cup pudding
  1¾ cup ice cream
  2 cups cottage cheese
	Calcium
	Protein
	Riboflavin

Meat
2 ounces cooked, lean meat, fish or poultry
OR Protein Equivalent:
  2 eggs
  2 slices (ounces) cheddar cheese
  1 cup dried beans, peas
  4 T. peanut butter
	Protein
	Iron
	B_1, B_3, B_6, B_{12}, Copper,
	Phosphorus, Magnesium, Chloride, Sulfur

Fruit-Vegetable ½ cup cooked or juice 1 cup raw Portion commonly served as medium apple, banana	Vitamin A Vitamin C Folic Acid Potassium Magnesium
Grain 1 slice bread 1 cup cold cereal ½ cup cooked cereal ½ cup pasta, grits	B_1, B_3 Vitamin E Phosphorus Iron

Table A.13 Minimum daily requirements

Basic Food Groups	Minimum Requirements (no. of servings)		
	Child	Teen	Adult
Milk*—1 cup/svg.	3	4	2
Meat—3 oz/svg. (or protein alternatives)	2	2	2
Fruits/Vegetables—½ cup/svg.	4	4	4
Bread—1 slice/svg. Cereal—½ cup/svg.	4	4	4

*In light of current research, the number of servings from the milk group for an adult should be increased to three per day for adequate calcium intake. The current Recommended Daily Allowance of 800 mg. for calcium will soon be raised to a minimum level of 1000 mg. per day for adults, with a possible need of up to 1500 mg. for some women.

Table A.14 Vegetarian: minimum daily requirements

Basic Food Groups	Minimum Requirements Lacto/Ovo Vegetarian	Strict Vegetarian
Milk	3	0
Eggs (optional 4/week maximum)		0
Fruits	1–4	1–4
Vegetables	3	6
Grains		3–5
Breads	6	4
Nuts/Seeds		1
Legumes		2
Possible Nutrient Deficiencies	Iron, B_{12}	Iron, B_{12}, Vitamin D, Riboflavin, Calcium.

The more restrictive the diet, the more difficult it becomes to reach balanced nutrition. Adequate nutrient intake is possible for vegetarians, but the strict vegetarian must take care when preparing each meal to ensure that the correct quantity and type of essential amino acids are provided for immediate protein needs. The method for combining food proteins so that their amino acid strengths and weaknesses balance out was shown previously in figure A.20. Use this "complementary" principle to ensure a mixture of protein foods of good value.

Goal Weight Determination

The next question then is, "What size person do you want to be?" What goal weight is best for long term health? The Metropolitan Life Insurance Company has actively researched those weights considered "ideal" since the 1940s. The newest table of weight for height is based on the industry's largest survey of weight vs longevity (conducted in 1979 with approximately four million individuals over the previous 22 years). The standard (see table A.15) divides each height per sex into three groups depending on frame size. Frame size can be determined using the formula stated in table A.16. However, no consideration is given to those physically fit persons with a high percentage of muscle tissue, and thus less body fat. Body composition, body fat, and lean muscle determination were discussed in the last chapter. Per equal volume, muscle tissue is far heavier than adipose tissue and becomes a significant variable when establishing ideal weight.

Cooper, in his latest book *The Aerobics Program for Total Well-Being*, 1983, bases ideal weight on the principle that a set of maximum *athletic*

Table A.15 New Height and Weight Tables

Men

Height	Small frame	Med. frame	Lg. frame
5'2"	128–134	131–141	138–150
5'3"	130–136	133–143	140–153
5'4"	132–138	135–145	142–156
5'5"	134–140	137–148	144–160
5'6"	136–142	139–151	146–164
5'7"	138–145	142–154	149–168
5'8"	140–148	145–157	152–172
5'9"	142–151	148–160	155–176
5'10"	144–154	151–163	158–180
5'11"	146–157	154–166	161–184
6'0"	149–160	157–170	164–188
6'1"	152–164	160–174	168–192
6'2"	155–168	164–178	172–197
6'3"	158–172	167–182	176–202
6'4"	162–176	171–187	181–207

Weight at ages 25–59 in shoes and 5 pounds of indoor clothing.

Women

Height	Small frame	Med. frame	Lg. frame
4'10"	102–111	109–121	118–131
4'11"	103–113	111–123	120–134
5'0"	104–115	113–126	122–137
5'1"	106–118	115–129	125–140
5'2"	108–121	118–132	128–143
5'3"	111–124	121–135	131–147
5'4"	114–127	124–138	134–151
5'5"	117–130	127–141	137–155
5'6"	120–133	130–144	140–159
5'7"	123–136	133–147	143–163
5'8"	126–139	136–150	146–167
5'9"	129–142	139–153	149–170
5'10"	132–145	142–156	152–173
5'11"	135–148	145–159	155–176
6'0"	138–151	148–162	158–179

Weight at ages 29–59 in shoes and 3 pounds of indoor clothing.

SOURCE: 1979 Build Study, Society of Actuaries and Association of Life Insurance Medical Directors of America, 1980.

Table A.16 Determining Body Frame Size

Frame Size	Wrist	Height
Small	5½" or less	5'2"–or under
	6" or less	5'3"–5'4"
	6¼" or less	5'5"–5'11"
Medium	5½"–5¾"	5'2"–or under
	6"–6¼"	5'3"–5'4"
	6¼"–6½"	5'5"–5'11"
Large	5¾" or more	5'2"–or under
	6¼" or more	5'3"–5'4"
	6½" or more	5'5"–5'11"

body fat should be 15%–19% for men and 18%–22% for women. Under this principle, the formulas are stated as follows:

- **Men:** current height in inches x 4 − 128 = ideal weight
- **Women:** current height in inches x 3.5 − 108 = ideal weight

These formulas need adjustment only for the large framed person by adding 10% to the final number to equalize the added skeletal mass.

Summary

Nutrition is the sum total of the processes by which the living organism receives and utilizes the materials necessary for survival, growth, and repair of tissues. These vital materials called nutrients are: proteins, carbohydrates, fats, vitamins, minerals, water, and fiber. This chapter discusses the function, major food sources, and requirements of each nutrient.

The Basic Four Food Group Guideline is explained as a minimal insurance for adequate intake of all nutrients on a daily basis. Adaptations of the guideline for vegetarians are included.

Commonly Asked Questions

Q. If my daily food plan does not meet the requirements of the Basic Four Food Groups, what type of supplement should I take?
A. I recommend a multiple vitamin/multiple mineral table containing approximately 100% of *all* the RDA needs including iron. Most vitamin/mineral supplements will not contain calcium in any appreciable amount, so one must also consider a calcium supplement if daily consumption of foods from the milk and dairy product family is less than three servings per day. Remember, we are still studying the nutrients in food, and still discovering new elements essential to human life. No pill or combination of oral supplements can completely substitute for balanced meals.

Q. Is it true that as an adult I no longer need to drink milk?
A. There is nothing sacred about milk but dairy foods are important as a primary source of calcium in the diet. Yogurt and cheese are certainly appropriate substitutes. The important principle to remember is that adult requirements are two or more servings per day or a calcium supplement equivalent to the RDA of 1,000 mg of calcium per day.

Q. Is it safe to consume foods containing sugar substitutes?
A. Both saccharin and aspartamine (Equal/Nutrasweet) are available on the market. At this time, it is questionable whether saccharin, a non-caloric, non-nutritive sweetener, will continue to be available due to past animal studies showing toxicity. Aspartamine, a natural dipeptide, is stated to be safe for human use with no adverse effects. Because of the nature of this dipeptide, it breaks apart into the constituent amino acids (aspartic acid and phenylalanine) upon heating and losses its sweet taste. Only those with a rare disease, known as phenylketonuria, are unable to consume aspartamine safely.

References

Deutsch, R. *Realities of Nutrition*. Palo Alto, CA: Bull Publishing Co.
Doyle, R. *The Vegetarian Handbook*. New York: Crown.

General Foods Corporation. *The Set Point Diet*. White Plains, NY.
National Academy of Sciences. *Recommended Dietary Allowances,* 9th Ed. Washington, DC: 1980.
Pemberton, C. *Getting In Shape*. Berkeley, CA: Creative Arts Book Co.
The Nutrition Foundation, Inc. *Present Knowledge in Nutrition*, 5th Ed. Washington, DC: 1984.
William, S. *Essentials of Nutrition and Diet Therapy,* 3rd Ed. St. Louis: Mosby, 1982

> LBW = Total weight (from scale) - Fat weight
> (determined by body composition assessment)

LBW includes the essential fat that is required for normal physiological functions. Recall from earlier discussion that essential fat is approximately 3% of the total body weight of males and 12% of females. These values represent the lower limits of body fatness, and any usage of these reserves may impair normal bodily function or the ability to exercise. Percent body fat values lower than 3% in men and lower than 10%-12% in females have been observed in elite athletes, but are very rare. Most reported percent fat values that are lower than these limits are physiologically impossible.

Lean Body Weight in women

The lower limit of fatness for women in good health appears to be about 10%-20% of body weight. The concept of the lowest lean weight in women that incorporates about 10%-12% essential fat in adipose tissue is equal to the lean body weight in men that have approximately 3% essential fat.

Low body fat and menstrual irregularity (amenorrhea)

The theory that women with a low percentage of body fat experience amenorrhea (disruption of the normal menstrual cycle) has been postulated by several researchers. One researcher suggested that a body weight at around 17% fat is the critical fat threshold and reducing below this weight leads to hormonal and metabolic imbalances that can affect the normal menstrual cycle. It should be mentioned that there are many women athletes in all sports who are below the 17% body fat and have normal menstrual cycles. This lean-to-fat ratio appears to be important, but several other factors must be taken into consideration. The complex interaction between physical, hormonal, nutritional, environmental and psychological factors on menstrual function are difficult to study independently but can contribute significantly in the alteration of menstrual regularity. It has been shown in several studies that exercise-associated disturbances in menstrual function are reversible with changes in life-style activity. This is an area of great interest and concern for aerobic exercise instructors, particularly those of child bearing age. Concerned instructors should consult with their physicians if menstrual irregularity is perceived as a problem.

Measurement of Body Composition

The most acceptable method of assessing body composition is hydrostatic (underwater) weighing. In this method, the subject is weighed on dry land and again while submerged under water. The underwater weighing

Chapter 7

Developing Endurance

Patricia Eisenman, Ph.D.

The ability to jog a few feet, to execute a combination of steps in an aerobics class, to pedal a bicycle or to swim a few strokes represents the final coordination of countless physiological and neurological events. The precise combination of muscle fibers must be stimulated to provide the exact amount of force for the activity. Energy, in the form of ATP molecules, must be made available at the appropriate rate and the byproducts must be removed.

These are just a few of the events that need to transpire for us to participate in physical activity. While the human body may not be capable of perfectly executing all of these events, it does have the potential to improve, and that is what training is all about . . . for training is the process of improving abilities and capacities. Consequently, endurance training is the process of improving the ability to engage in a physical activity for an extended period of time. Not only must the nerves and muscles be capable of the coordination of the events just described, but they must be able to continuously repeat these physiological events. [I: **Basic Principles, Definitions and Recommendations**]

At this point you might well ask, "Why do I need to know about the complexities of physiology? Let's just get on with the rules for endurance training." While it is true that exercise scientists have identified a number of training principles, there is also an art to endurance training. And part of that art rests upon having an appreciation for the complexities of the training process. If you realize that the cells need time to use the amino acids in the food that you eat to produce the enzymes and mitochondria (see chapter on *Anatomy and Physiology*) necessary to develop ATP for long duration activities, you will be less likely to apply the training principles too rapidly.

If you realize that not everyone has exactly the same anatomical structures (again, refer to *Anatomy and Physiology*), the need to individualize and modify routines for certain students will make more sense. While this chapter will be devoted to presenting and explaining endurance training principles, it is important to realize that these principles are not like recipes in a cookbook. Rather, they are more like guidelines. They should provide you with direction, but if you are to be a truly effective fitness instructor, you should help students individualize the application of the training principles. In so doing, you will be applying the art and science of endurance training.

Training Principles

Four major endurance training principles will be presented in this chapter. They are

- specificity
- overload
- variability
- reversibility

An explanation of each of these and some application guidelines will be identified in the text following each topic.

Specificity

The training principle of specificity is based on the observation that the various tissues, organs and systems in the body are capable of improved functioning if that particular tissue, organ or system is placed in a situation in which it has to function. For example, the circulatory system is responsible for circulating blood containing oxygen and nutrients to the various cells of the body, including skeletal muscle cells. If the circulatory system is placed in a situation in which more oxygen and nutrients than normal are required, as is true in physical exercise, the circulatory system can respond by improving its ability to deliver oxygen and blood to the muscle cells that need it. This last phrase—to the muscle cells that need it—is a very important one. For with endurance training, improved circulation is most improved to those cells involved in the specific endurance activity. This is why the highly conditioned distance runner may not be able to complete the 20-30 minute cardiovascular section of an aerobics class. The runner's muscles are not specifically trained for aerobics movements.

The principle of specificity is important in that you can design training programs for very specific purposes, but it also requires that fitness instructors be quite knowledgeable about the effects of various types of training regimes. The material that is presented in table A.17 should be

Table A.17 Training Effects

CENTRAL: as a result of participating in intense aerobic training (the HR, heart rate, is at or close to the upper limit of the THRZ, target heart rate zone).

Site	Type of Effect
A. Heart	Improved ability to burn fat.
	May be an increase in number of capillaries.
	Improved ability to pump blood (hearts of some endurance athletes have an increased volume called cardiac hypertrophy, athletes who lift heavy weights sometimes have thicker heart walls—both types of hypertrophy are normal).
	Decreased Resting Heart Rate (RHR).
B. Lungs	Decreased residual volume (the amount of air left in the lungs after exhaling)
	Increased volume of air that can be taken in per breath so that trained individuals can take fewer breaths per minute (more efficient)
C. Blood Distribution	Redistribution of blood from the less active tissues, such as the digestive organs and kidneys, to those in greater need, such as the heart and working muscles. (When exercising in the heat, the skin—for cooling—becomes an area of need.)
D. Blood	Increased blood volume
E. Body Composition	Decreased percent of body fat

PERIPHERAL: as a result of long duration exercise at a heart rate toward the lower limit of the THRZ.

Site	Type of Effect
A. Muscle Fibers	Improved ability of the muscles to burn fats (especially in the muscles working during a specific type of aerobic activity). This improved ability is due to: —increased number of mitochondria —increases in O_2 system enzymes —increased number of muscle capillaries
B. Bones, Ligaments and Tendons	Improved functional abilities
C. Nervous System	Improved skill or efficiency at the activity

helpful in this regard. A variety of types or modes of activity may be utilized to burn calories and/or to develop cardiovascular fitness, but this does not mean that you will be able to perform all cardiovascular activities at the same intensity or for the same duration. Consequently, when students have been doing only one type of cardiovascular activity and wish to start another, care must be taken not to overstress the muscles, ligaments, tendons, and bones involved in the new activity. It is not uncommon to see highly trained aerobics students develop a stress fracture if they are overzealous in initiating a running program. Even if injuries are not sustained, students can become discouraged with their apparent ''lack of fitness" in the new activity if they are not aware of the specificity of training principles.

Even if an individual has been consistently participating in 10K (about 6.2 miles) races or fun runs and now wants to complete a marathon, the body has to be specifically trained to run for two hours or more. Exercise of this duration needs a highly developed circulatory system in addition to muscles which have been specifically trained to provide energy for long periods of time. Since the amount of carbohydrate (glucose) that can be stored is limited to about a two-hour supply for activity, endurance trained muscles become well suited to burning fat. To develop the enzymes and mitochondria to allow the energy production system to burn fats efficiently takes time and the completion of long runs every week or so.

The principle of specificity also applies to such things as altitude and temperature. A cross-country skiing trip to the mountains will place a new set of specific demands on your heart and lungs if you are not used to high altitude. The body can adapt by producing more red blood cells to transport oxygen, but this can take up to two weeks. Similarly, if you are used to doing your workouts in an air-conditioned room, your body has adapted to those conditions, and you will not be able to perform as well if the temperature rises. It will take several days for your body to adapt to exercising in the heat. When it does adapt, you will sweat sooner, produce more dilute sweat (less salt in it), and have improved blood flow patterns to cool you better. The point is, the body can adapt to the specific demands of exercise in the heat, if you give it time, drink plenty of fluid, preferably water, and do not overexercise. This admonishment to not overexercise is sometimes a bit confusing, especially since one of the major training principles is the overload principle. Hopefully, the next section will help you to see how it is possible to "overload" without overexercising.

Overload principle

The overload principle mandates that in order for a specific adaptation to take place, a demand must be placed on the function that is to be developed. [I.F: Overload Principle] On the other hand, if too much demand is placed on the function, an overuse injury is likely. Therefore, exercise scientists have conducted a number of studies to determine procedures for quantifying the amount of overload that is necessary for endurance training. These studies indicate that an appropriate degree of "overload" may be achieved by manipulating the intensity, frequency, and duration of the activity as well as the type of activity.

Since endurance activities require that the cardiovascular system provide a constant supply of oxygen and nutrients, the heart has to increase its pumping rate to accommodate the increased need for blood. Consequently, in healthy individuals, heart rate or pulse rate is a good indicator of how hard the cardiovascular system is working. [VI.H: Heart Rate] The higher the heart rate, the more intense or demanding the activity is for an individual. Early researchers noted that if the heart rate was not above a critical or threshold value, the cardiovascular system would not improve in its ability to function. On the other hand, if the heart rate was too high, further aerobic improvement was not realized and the likelihood of injury was increased. These observations led to the concept of a Target Heart Rate Zone (THRZ) that was most appropriate for cardiovascular training. The lower limit of the THRZ, known as the aerobic threshold, implies that there is not enough overload for improvement of the aerobic energy-releasing pathway unless the heart rate is above this value. If one exceeds the upper limit of the THRZ, the activity is so intense that anaerobic chemical reactions (anaerobic glycolysis, which produces fatiguing lactic acid) rather than aerobic reactions are becoming the dominant source of energy. Further research has noted that the THRZ varies somewhat for different individuals. It is somewhat lower for the individual who does not have a very well trained cardiovascular system. On the other hand, the individual who is in the excellent cardiovascular fitness category needs to apply more "overload" to realize further improvement. Consequently, the training THRZ for this individual is at the higher end of the spectrum. The training THRZs for those individuals who are in the "fair" and "good" fitness categories are intermediate to the zones for those in the poor and excellent fitness categories.

There are techniques to determine individualized heart rate zones. One of the better procedures utilizes the Karvonen Heart Rate Reserve method for calculating a THRZ. Karvonen was one of the original researchers to note that there was a minimal threshold for training the cardiovascular system. In the formulas seen in table A.18, the Heart Rate Reserve (HRR) or the

Table A.18 Target Heart Rate Zone Formulas for Individuals of Varying Cardiovascular Fitness

1. Individuals in the POOR FITNESS CATEGORY:
   THRZ = RHR* + 60–70% (MHR** – RHR)

2. Individuals in the FAIR FITNESS CATEGORY:
   THRZ = RHR + 70–80% (MHR – RHR)

3. Individuals in the GOOD FITNESS CATEGORY:
   THRZ = RHR + 80–85% (MHR – RHR)

4. Individuals in the EXCELLENT FITNESS CATEGORY:
   THRZ = RHR + 85–90% (MHR – RHR)

*RHR = Resting Heart Rate
**MHR = Maximal Heart Rate

difference between the resting heart rate and the maximal heart rate is used to determine the THRZ for healthy individuals. If an individual has completed a maximal fitness test and actually knows his or her maximal heart rate value, this value is utilized in the formula. More frequently the maximal heart rate is not known. In those cases, maximal heart rate may be predicted by subtracting the individual's age in years from 220. **[VI.H: Heart Rate]** Resting heart rate is determined by taking the pulse rate for one minute. It is best to do this before getting out of bed in the morning. This is the true resting pulse rate (from now on pulse rate will be assumed to be equal to heart rate). Pulse rates may be counted by placing any finger (but not the thumb because it has a pulse of its own) over any artery. The two most commonly used arteries are the carotid in the neck and the radial artery at the wrist. If you choose to utilize the carotid artery, place two fingers over the carotid artery on one side of the neck and apply pressure lightly. If too much pressure is applied, it is possible to occlude blood flow to the brain and/or trigger a reflex response in the baroreceptors located in the neck, which will cause the heart rate to slow down or skip a beat. If light pressure is applied, none of these possibilities should occur. *Do not press hard or place thumb on opposite side of neck at the same time, as the blood flow could be impeded.* **[VI.H: Heart Rate]**

The decision as to which of the formulas to select depends upon a knowledge of the individual's cardiovascular fitness. This is obtained by administering a cardiovascular fitness test. (See Part B, Chapter 1, *Fitness Testing and Prescription*.) Although less accurate than an actual fitness test, the Physical Activity Index in table A.19 could be employed to approximate a fitness category so that a THRZ formula could be selected.

Perhaps the best way to describe the calculations necessary is to utilize an illustration, so let's take a look at table A.20. Alexis works in an office from 8:00 A.M. to 4:30 P.M. and then goes home to a growing family. She does not have a regular physical activity program, therefore she has circled 1 for the "Intensity" value on the Physical Activity Index. Since she frequently goes to the mall and takes the kids to the zoo, etc., she has selected 3 from the "Duration" category and a 3 from the "Frequency" category. Her activity index is found by multiplying her score for each category. Her resultant score places her in the poor fitness category, so she will use the first THRZ formula. To complete this formula, she took her resting pulse and found it to be 84. She does not know her maximal heart rate, but since she is 38 years old, by subtracting 38 from 220, she predicts that her maximal heart rate is about 182.

Now she has all the necessary information and when she finishes the calculations (table A.20) she has determined that her individualized THRZ is 143 to 153. This means that during the cardiovascular development

Table A.19 A Physical Activity Index as an Indicator of Fitness

Directions: The Physical Activity Index in calculated by multiplying your score for each category (Score = Intenxity × Duration × Frequency). Then find the fitness category which corresponds to your final score.

	Score	Activity
Intensity	5	Sustained heavy breathing and perspiration
	4	Intermittent heavy breathing and perspiration (as in tennis)
	3	Moderately heavy (as in recreational sports and cycling)
	2	Moderate (as in volleyball, softball)
	1	Light (as in fishing, walking)
Duration	4	Over 30 minutes
	3	20 to 30 minutes
	2	10 to 20 minutes
	1	Under 10 minutes
Frequency	5	Daily or almost daily
	4	3 to 5 times a week
	3	1 to 2 times a week
	2	A few times a month
	1	Less than once a month

Evaluation and Fitness Category

Score	Evaluation	Fitness Category
100	Very active lifestyle	High
60 to 80	Active and healthy	Very good
40 to 59	Acceptable (could be better)	Fair
Under 40	Not good enough	Poor

activities that she does, she should periodically check her pulse rate and see if it is in her THRZ. Because it is difficult to take a pulse rate while you are exercising, except if you are on a stationary bicycle, it is best to slow the body's movements so that a count may be taken. When activity is stopped or slowed, the heart rate begins to rapidly decrease. Consequently, it is recommended that a 10 second pulse rate be taken during exercise while full minute checks are best for determining resting heart rate values. Remember that the first pulse that you feel is counted as "zero" and the second as "one," etc.

If Alexis counts incorrectly and gets only 14 pulse beats when she should have counted 15 in the 6 second period, she will mistakenly assume that she is working below her THRZ at a heart rate of 140 beats per minute when in fact she is at the top of her zone at 150 beats per minute. Consequently, she may increase the intensity of the exercise and exceed her THRZ. For a healthy person this does not necessarily pose an immediate problem, but over several days it could mean that Alexis overexercises. Thus, it is worthwhile to take some time and make sure that students know how to take correct exercise pulse checks.

Table A.20 Sample Calculations for Alexis.

Physical Activity Index

	Score	Activity
Intensity	5	Sustained heavy breathing and perspiration
	4	Intermittent heavy breathing and perspiration (as in tennis)
	3	Moderately heavy (as in recreational sports and cycling)
	2	Moderate (as in volleyball, softball)
	①	Light (as in fishing, walking)
Duration	4	Over 30 minutes
	③	20 to 30 minutes
	2	10 to 20 minutes
	1	Under 10 minutes
Frequency	5	Daily or almost daily
	4	3 to 5 times a week
	③	1 to 2 times a week
	2	A few times a month
	1	Less than once a month

1 x 3 x 3 = 9

Evaluation and Fitness Category

Score	Evaluation	Fitness Category
100	Very active lifestyle	High
60 to 80	Active and healthy	Very good
40 to 59	Acceptable (could be better)	Fair
(Under 40)	Not good enough	(Poor)

1. Alexis has a resting heart rate (RHR) of 84 beats per minute.
2. She does not know her Maximal Heart Rate (MHR), but she is 38 years old, so by subtracting 38 from 220 she can predict that her MHR is 182.
3. The THRZ formula for individuals in the poor fitness category:
   $$THRZ = RHR + 60\text{-}70\% (MHR - RHR)$$

THRZ = 84 + .60(182 − 84)   THRZ = 84 + .70(182 − 84)
       84 + .60(98)   84 + .70(98)
       84 + 59   84 + 69
       143   153

182 − 84 = 98
98 × .60 = 58.80 = 59
98 × .70 = 68.60 = 69

Therefore, the Target Heart Rate Zone goes from a heart rate of 143 to an upper value of 153.

Even though there are less complicated target heart rate formulas, it is worth the time and effort to have your students utilize the Karvonen THRZ formulas. They emphasize that the target zone is a personalized one because the person has to enter his or her personal resting heart rate and maximal heart rate. In addition, the person's cardiovascular fitness level is taken into consideration. The concept of personalization should be taken still further by having your students recalculate their target heart rate zones every two to three weeks for the first months of increased physical activity.

Although the actual counting of pulse rate serves as a useful index for evaluating exercise intensity, stopping to take counts is tedious for some people and undesirable in some situations, like a 10K run. Under these circumstances, the rating of perceived exertion (RPE) can become a very useful tool for the fitness instructor.

"Rating of perceived exertion" (RPE) utilizes one's perceptions of how one feels at any specific point in a workout as a relatively accurate indication of actual work intensity at that same point. It is based on the theory that most people will naturally work within their appropriate THRZ without being told what that heart rate range should be. Working lower than THRZ seems too easy for the person and working above THRZ range puts that person at a level of work that cannot be endured for any great length of time.

The term "perceived exertion" refers to the total amount of exertion and physical fatigue that one perceives, combining all feelings of physical stress, effort, and fatigue. A person using the RPE method estimates, as accurately as possible, the total inner feeling of exertion, paying attention to breathing rate and intensity, feelings in the muscles and joints, the ease with which one can carry on a conversation, and the overall feeling of exertion. In most cases, if a person's heart rate is taken during the time when he or she is working at the subjectively described intensity, it is found that the heart rate will be within the THRZ. When used in stress testing, a person might be asked to think in terms of a scale that ranges from 6 to 20, and as the stress test proceeds and the person is asked at what level of intensity he or she perceives to be working, if the response is "12," the actual heart rate is at or very near 120. If the person says "16," his or her heart rate is most probably 160. At the lower intensity exercise levels, people seem to be less accurate in their ability to pace themselves than at the higher intensity levels.

Using RPE for exercise prescription is a very subjective way of assigning a workload for aerobic training. It works quite well for some people and very poorly or not at all for others. It does seem to be innate in most of us, however, to work within a level of intensity that is comfortable for us—which will most often be within our THRZ.

Advocates of the RPE method suggest that increasing one's awareness of physiologic stress can decrease one's dependence on external monitoring systems, i.e. watches. RPE might be used as the sole indicator of work intensity in situations in which a timepiece is unavailable, in competitive events, and for persons with impaired vision.

An advantage of using RPE to monitor exercise intensity for the healthy population is that it can be performed continuously. The THRZ method, when used alone, requires an elaborate monitoring system.

As you teach your students about the relationship between exercise intensity and target heart rates and have the students stop to take their pulse rates you can also encourage them to learn to read their own body signs. Use questions like, "How does your breathing feel when you are exercising in your THRZ?" "How do your legs feel when you are exercising over your target heart rate zone?" "Can you feel your heart beating in your chest when you are exercising below your THRZ?" There are some aerobics class enthusiasts who sing lyrics to themselves as they exercise. When they can no longer remember the lyrics, they know they are exercising too intensely. There are runners who do simple math problems in their heads. When they can no longer complete the calculations they know they are exercising too intensely. Each of these individuals is using a perceptual clue to evaluate the intensity of their exercise. Research results have demonstrated that there is a very good relationship between people's perceptual feelings and how hard the exercise is and what their actual heart rates are. This is a skill to be cultivated. Do not try to get your students to ignore the feedback from their bodies as they exercise. Granted, this may get them through one or two exercise sessions, but in the end, it is not an effective or a safe procedure.

You should now have an appreciation of how you can help your students apply the overload principle to cardiovascular fitness. You can help your students determine and individualize their THRZ and sensitize them to the concept of perceived exertion. Students can also use pulse rate and perceived exertion after they have stopped exercising. If their heart rates do not return to normal within one half hour after exercise, or if they feel spent or wiped out after exercise rather than relaxed and refreshed, the exercise was too intense. If such overly intense exercise sessions are the rule rather than the exception, injury is inevitable.

Exercise intensity is not the only factor which can bring about exercise-related injuries. The duration and frequency of the exercise are also important. Although numerous studies have indicated that to achieve a level of endurance or cardiovascular fitness that is compatible with good health, one should exercise so that the heart rate is in the THRZ for 20-30 minutes three to four times per week, not everyone can immediately tolerate this prescription. The less fit individual will not be able to exercise continuously for 20 minutes with the heart rate in the THRZ. Table A.21 summarizes the relationships between fitness level and the appropriate duration and frequency recommendations. Not only should you provide your students with an individualized THRZ, but you should also design programs which allow students in the lower fitness categories the opportunity to take longer to warm-up and do more developmental exercises so that they do not have to complete 20-30 minutes of cardiovascular activities.

Another alternative is to encourage those students in the lower fitness categories to walk and move in place after they have completed their

Table A.21 Frequency and Duration Prescriptions for Individuals in the Various Fitness Categories

Fitness Category	Frequency	Duration
Poor	Every other day	Start with about 10 min in your THRZ
Fair	Every other day	Start with about 10–15 min in your THRZ
Good	May like to try a couple of days in a row	Start with about 15 min in your THRZ
Excellent	May like to try 5–6 days per week	Try starting with 20 min in your THRZ

prescribed time exercising with their heart rate in the THRZ. So, if Clyde is in the poor fitness category, he might start out exercising for 10 minutes with a heart rate in his THRZ. Then he could drop his exercise intensity while the rest of the class continues for the remaining 10–20 minutes. Clyde can increase by one or two minutes the amount of time spent exercising in his THRZ. If he makes such increases every two to three weeks, he will be applying the gradual overload principle to his endurance training program. Again, the resting pulse rate values and Clyde's perception of exertion will serve as excellent evaluation tools. If the resting pulse rate values (remember they are taken first thing in the morning) are not coming down or at least staying the same, or if Clyde has continual feelings of fatigue, the training is inappropriate. Perhaps the THRZ is too high. Remember, it was based upon some predictions. Perhaps Clyde's maximal heart rate is not as high as the age-predicted value used in the THRZ formula, or perhaps Clyde increased the duration of his cardiovascular workout too rapidly. So, have Clyde try exercising at a lower intensity or have him reduce the number of minutes of work in the THRZ. The frequency of exercise may also be the problem. If he is exercising more than four days per week, or if there are no days off from exercise, a switch to exercising every other day may be necessary. Do not, however, have Clyde reduce his exercise program to less than three days per week. This number of days of training is essential for the physiological and neurological adaptations associated with endurance training to take place.

Other possible explanations for the lack of improvement in aerobic fitness despite participation in an exercise program are a lack of sleep and/or inadequate nutrition, or another illness or health problem such as previously undetected heart disease which may contraindicate vigorous physical activity.

It is also possible that the type of activity is the culprit. Certain movements or movement patterns in a class may be inappropriate for certain students. Or, perhaps it is the floor or surface or the shoes that are inappropriate. Stationary bicycles, swimming, cross-country ski machines and other non-weight bearing activities are sometimes good substitute aerobic activities. Theoretically, any large muscle, rhythmical activity may be employed to apply the "demand" to overload the cardiovascular system so that an endurance training effect takes place. In fact, recognition of this fact has resulted in the formulation of the third major training principle which will be discussed in the next section.

Variability

The principle of variability refers to the fact that if "demands" are placed on the body, the body adapts to these "demands," and no further improvement is realized until the "demands" are met. In training jargon, this lack of improvement in spite of continued training is sometimes referred to as a plateau. Recent research suggests that by varying the types of "demands" placed upon the body, such a plateau may be avoided.

In practical terms, the principle of variability translates into systematically altering the exercise demands by employing one or more of the strategies outlined in table A.22. In other words, endurance training, particularly for health benefits, is probably best accomplished by having some exercise sessions which are easier than others. This would be a major change for many class situations, because typically every class has the same components and is conducted at a similar intensity. Why not adopt a pattern of having one or two days a week designated as "hard" days, another couple of days as "easy" days and the remaining days of the week as "moderate" days? That way, your students could select accordingly. It would also be good for instructors, who are even more likely to be injured

Table A.22 Techniques for injecting variability into a training program

Technique	Description
Hard-Easy Days	Vary the exercise intensity with easier days following more intense days.
Use Different Types of Exercise	Vary activities with the seasons or alternate activities as in supplementing aerobics classes with sessions on the stationary bicycle.
Use Fartlek Days	Fartlek is the Swedish word for speed play. It means to vary the intensity within a workout (e.g., do 25 jumping jacks as fast as possible followed by jogging in place at ½ speed, and then do one minute of 2-foot hops at ¾ speed).
Stair-step Overloading	Increase the overload by increasing the intensity, frequency or duration of the activity every 2–3 weeks.
Supplemental Training	Utilize strength training to improve the strength of the specific muscles involved in your specific aerobic activities.
Play Supplements	Use "play" activities such as tennis, day hikes, cross-country skiing tours, bicycle trips, racquetball games, etc. to supplement your workouts.

than are participants. Many fitness instructors are also starting to alternate exercising on equipment (bicycles, rowing machines, etc.) with choreographed routines or calisthenic routines. This is a very effective strategy for applying the training principle of variability while maintaining specificity. In addition, it is probably an excellent way to minimize overuse injuries to specific parts of the body and prevent boredom.

Reversibility

The last of the major training principles to be discussed in this chapter is reversibility. This principle alludes to the fact that if one stops participating in a regular physical activity program, all of the positive adaptations which have occurred will be lost. You cannot store fitness. It must be maintained on a regular basis. Consequently it is important that fitness instructors design programs that allow participants to enhance their cardiovascular fitness in a safe and effective manner. If people can realize the positive psychological feelings associated with improved cardiovascular fitness, they are more likely to continue with such programs. Similarly, if participants remain injury free because their programs have been well designed, they are more likely to remain life-long participants. The possibility of all of these outcomes is greater if the four training principles of specificity, overload, variability and reversibility are applied by manipulating the intensity, frequency, duration and type of activity delivered by the fitness instructor. The material presented in this chapter should provide instructors with the background needed to begin to apply the endurance training principles to their class situations. Finally, the readings in the reference sections should provide sources for fitness instructors to learn even more about the subtleties of endurance training.

Commonly Asked Questions

Q. What is the difference between an endurance activity and a strength activity?
A. Strength refers to the ability to exert maximal muscular force. Since it is maximal, that amount of force may only be produced once or twice in a given workout. Endurance implies that the amount of force produced is submaximal and therefore can be repeated numerous times. In fact, with training, endurance activities can be continued for hours.

Q. What is specificity of training?
A. Specificity of training is the process of selecting training activities and exercises that utilize the functions and/or processes which one would like to improve. For example, to improve the ability of the muscles to

hop on one leg for extended periods of time, those particular muscles need to be involved in progressively longer periods of one-legged hopping.

Q. What is meant by the overload principle?
A. This training principle mandates that in order for a specific adaptation to take place, a demand greater than that normally encountered must be placed on the function that is to be developed. For example, muscular endurance is developed by gradually increasing the number of minutes of participation in physical activity.

Q. Why should target heart rate zones (THRZ) be utilized?
A. According to the overload principle, a demand needs to occur before an adaptation takes place. A THRZ represents an objective technique for approximating the correct overload for the cardiovascular system. If the heart rate is not above the lower limit of the zone, there is probably insufficient demand for improvement in cardiovascular fitness. If the heart rate is above the upper limit of the zone, there is too much reliance upon anaerobic systems and the likelihood of overuse injuries and fatigue is increased.

Q. What is the "talk test?"
A. If you are able to carry on a conversation with a companion while doing your endurance training activity, you are doing it aerobically. Consequently, the talk test can be utilized along with target heart rates as a way of controlling exercise intensity.

Q. How many times a week must one workout to be aerobically fit?
A. In order to be aerobically fit, one should exercise so that his or her heart rate is in his or her THRZ for 20 to 30 minutes for three to four days each week. These workouts should occur on alternate days. Although it is possible to adapt to working out five to seven days per week, this is *not* necessary for health-related fitness.

Q. What is involved in the training principle of variability?
A. Each and every workout session should *not* be exactly alike. Instead, some sessions should be of a slightly higher intensity, while others are of moderate intensity and still others are of a very light intensity. You can also vary the type of activity and include such activities as jogging, walking, rope skipping, aerobics dance movements, calisthenics, bicycling, and swimming. Such variety can help to prevent overuse injuries and boredom.

Q. Why are some exercise class participants able to exercise day after day with heart rates that are over their THRZ?

A. Remember that several predictions or estimations are used in the calculation of the THRZ. The age-predicted maximum heart rate (220 − age in years) is just an approximation. Some people have maximal heart rates that are somewhat higher than this age-prediction. Therefore, the upper limit of the calculated THRZ is a bit low for these individuals. This *does not* mean that THRZs are useless; they are excellent guide points. However, they are not absolute commandments. If an exerciser feels fine while exercising at a slightly higher target heart rate, and he or she recovers quickly after exercise, a slightly higher THRZ may be more appropriate. Conversely, some individuals have maximal heart rates that are lower than the age-predicted values, so they will find it difficult if not impossible to exercise in their calculated THRZ. A downward modification of the zone is appropriate for them. It should *always* be kept in mind that this formula applies to healthy individuals only.

Q. *Is heart rate the same thing as pulse rate?*
A. For the normal healthy heart, the heart rate and pulse rate will yield identical values. Each time the heart contracts, blood surges through the arteries. Because the arterial walls are elastic, this surge of blood is felt as a pulsing sensation in the finger or fingers that are taking the pulse. To be most accurate, the heart rate should be taken with a stethoscope or by placing the hand directly over the heart and feeling the heartbeats.

Q. *Is it dangerous to take pulse rates at the carotid artery?*
A. There has been some research which has indicated that if too much pressure is placed on the carotid artery, irregular heartbeats may result. It is also possible for excessive pressure to cause reflex slowing of the heart rate. If this occurs during an exercise heart rate check, the exerciser could underestimate the intensity of the exercise and mistakenly increase the exercise intensity too much. Both of the preceding situations can be avoided by emphasizing that the fingers be *lightly* placed over only one carotid.

Q. *What is the reversibility training principle?*
A. This principle stipulates that if one stops regular participation in exercise, the adaptations in the cardiovascular system and other organs and tissues in the body will revert to the lower functional abilities which they had before the training was initiated.

References

Fox, E. and Mathews, D. *The Physiological Basis of Physical Education and Athletics.* New York: Saunders College Publishing, 1981.

Getchell, B. *Physical Fitness: A Way of Life.* New York: Wiley, 1983.
Marley, W. *Health and Physical Fitness: Taking Charge of Your Life.* New York: Saunders College Publishing, 1982.
Sharkey, B. *Physiology of Fitness,* 3rd Ed. Champaign, IL: Human Kinetics Publishers, 1984.

Chapter 8

Nutrition for Endurance and Training

Laura Pawlak, RD, Ph.D

It has become increasingly clear in recent years that knowledge of nutrition and exercise physiology has reached a level at which certain dietary recommendations can be stated to meet the particular needs of those persons involved in intense exercise one or more hours per day. Whether an individual exercises as part of a job requirement, for fitness maintenance, or athletic competition, the attainment and maintenance of optimum nutrition under daily physical training requires knowledge of special nutrient needs. A good diet cannot, in itself, guarantee fitness or competitive success, but a poor diet can ruin your chance of success.

Caloric Demands During Exercise

The demand for higher caloric intake due to energy expenditure in an exercise program can best be met by increasing the number of servings of food from the Basic Food Four Groups. The food recommendations for adults are *minimum* nutrient needs and contain approximately 1,200 calories. Energy expenditure in the training or performance stage of sport participation can elevate caloric needs from 300 to 3,000 calories per day. The body demands more than increased energy for optimum performance; nutrient dense foods, as found in the Basic Four Food Groups, assure *quality* caloric consumption.

Although protein, fat, and carbohydrates can provide calories, prevention of muscle fatigue requires that the supply of carbohydrates be adequate to prevent depletion of muscle glycogen, the storage form of carbohydrates.

Special attention should be given, therefore, to increasing the number of servings in those food groups that supply carbohydrates as well as the vitamins and minerals needed to complete the metabolic processes that convert glucose, the simplest carbohydrate, into energy. Emphasize increased portions from the bread and cereal and also the fruit and vegetable groups. Glucose, not immediately needed for work, will replace lost stores of glycogen in the liver and muscle for future activity.

Short spurts of intense exercise (anaerobic exercise) exclusively utilize glucose for energy while exercise of longer duration at low-to-moderate intensity (aerobic) burns approximately equal percentages of fat and glucose for the work. However, fat always burns in the "flame" of carbohydrate; as carbohydrate availability decreases, fatigue increases.

Total storage of glycogen in the body is normally about 1,800 calories. The trained body that consumes a high carbohydrate diet (approximately 55% of calories each day) will generally have greater glycogen stores. Hard physical workouts, especially those repeated two or more times per day, can result in total muscle fatigue since glycogen depletion has far exceeded replenishment. A diet as high in carbohydrate as 500–600 grams per day can replace exhausted muscle glycogen losses in 24 hours. A review of table A.23 shows the grams of carbohydrate in *one serving* of each food group. Note that the meat group, with the exception of dry beans and peas, is a very poor source of carbohydrates.

The snacking pattern of physically active persons can be a useful tool for increasing carbohydrate intake. Choose snacks wisely; avoid those that are rich in fat or added sugars (white, brown, or powdered sugar, molasses, honey, corn syrup). Nutrient rich snacks for all occasions are suggested as follows:

- *lunch pail treats*: fig bars, dried fruit, apples, bananas, raisins, dates, bagels, muffins, carrots, crackers
- *half-time boosters*: juicy fruit (e.g., apples, plums, oranges, peaches, pears, and fruit juices)
- *vending machines*: milk, fruit, juice, yogurt, trail mix, cheese/crackers

Table A.23 Basic Food Groups/Nutrition in one serving

Food Group	Serving Size	Cho (grams)	Nutrients Protein (grams)	Fat (grams)
Milk	1 cup	12	8	10–0
Meat	2 ounces	0	14	6–20
Fruit	½ cup	10	0	0
Vegetables	½ cup	0–5	0–2	0
Grains	½ cup	15	2	0
Fats	1 tsp.	0	0	5

Those engaged in more than two hours of continuous, strenuous workouts should consider the use of glucose or fructose drinks to prevent low blood sugar. As the stores of glycogen are depleted, the muscle draws on blood sugar to replenish its energy need. The liver glycogen can assist muscle needs by releasing glucose into the blood but supplies are quickly depleted. The resultant low blood sugar level can lead to dizziness, nausea, confusion, and partial blackout. For best absorption, these beverages should contain no more than 2½% sweetener and consumption should begin in the first hour of the exercise, at a rate of ½–1 cup every 15–20 minutes.

Protein Needs

Protein requirements are identical for the untrained and trained athletic person. Exercise can increase muscle mass, often at the expense of fat loss; however, the protein recommendation of 0.8–1.0 gram per kilogram of body weight is more than adequate for adults. Excess protein intake results in its utilization by the body as an energy source. Regardless of the portion of calories devoted to carbohydrates in the diet, one must supply the body with its .8 gm of protein for optimum health.

Fat, a Hidden Foe

It is important for the athletic person to be able to distinguish between food choices that are good sources of carbohydrate and those that are primarily composed of fat. Aerobic exercise burns fat as a major fuel but even lean marathon runners are well equipped to supply that fat from bodily storage areas.

Drinking for Endurance

Proper hydration before, during, and after exercise is essential for optimum performance. Heat generated in the body core during physical work must be dissipated into the surrounding environment when the temperature of the performance is maximized. However, prolonged exercise in an extremely humid environment or in nonbreathable clothing will cause body core temperature to elevate and lead to early fatigue since the evaporative process is hindered. Table A.24 may be helpful for detecting dehydration.

Responding to thirst is an unreliable guide to needs during the profuse sweating stage of performance. Weight measured immediately before and after strenuous exercise is an accurate determination of losses and replacement needs. Remember, one pint of fluid consumed replaces each pound of weight loss. A convenient guide to fluid requirements follows:

Table A.24 A Guide to the Detection and Treatment of Dehydration

Weight Loss (% of body wt)	Symptoms	Treatment
3%	Impaired performance	Increase fluid consumption.
5%	Heat Cramps Thirst Chills Clammy skin Rapid pulse Nausea	Increase cold fluids by ½ cup/15 minutes. Remove as much clothing as possible. STOP exercise, increase fluids, sit in a cool environment; perform static stretch of involved muscle groups.
6–10%	Heat Exhaustion Sweat Dizziness Headache Shortness of breath Rapid pulse Dry mouth Fatigue	STOP EXERCISE; cool environment; drink 2 cups water per pound loss; ice bag on head; cold shower.
Greater than 10%	Heat Stroke* Swollen tongue No sweat or urine High body temperature Hallucinations, aggression Visual changes Unsteady walk	Life threatening emergency medical care; ice bag on back and front of head; cold shower; alcohol over body. Utilize any available action to reduce body temperature.

NOTE: *Heat stroke can occur in susceptible individuals with less than 10% weight loss.*

- 2 hours before performance: 2½ cups or more
- 15 minutes before performance: 2 cups
- each 15–20 minutes during performance: ½–1 cup

Following performance, fluids should be taken as needed to reinstate weight. Plain cold water is the best fluid to drink. Absorption will be dramatically improved if the water is iced.

Electrolyte Losses—Sodium, Potassium, Calcium, Magnesium

It is difficult to generalize the electrolyte losses of the athlete who sweats profusely since a multitude of variables must be considered:

- acclimatization
- adrenal cortical activity
- temperature
- humidity

However, it should be noted that replacement need not be immediate. This eliminates the controversial argument regarding the requirement for "salted" fluids during the exercise session.

Table A.25 Good Iron Sources

Food Group	Foods
Milk	None
Meat	Liver, dry beans, peas, tofu, red meat, eggs.
Fruit/Veg	Prune juice, prunes, figs, raisins, watermelon
Bread/Cereal	Cold cereals: Most, Product 19, Total.
	Hot cereals: Cream of Wheat, Malt-O-Meal, Wheat Hearts.

Long-term electrolyte deficiencies should not occur if a variety of foods from all four groups—foods innately high in nutrient density—is a part of the training program.

Special Vitamin, Mineral Considerations

Conversion of carbohydrate particles into energy molecules requires the cooperative effect of B vitamins in increased amounts. However, it is unclear whether the current recommended doses of the B-complex vitamins as well as vitamin C and E and iron are ample for daily stress exercise needs.

It is shown that adherence to a well-balanced diet with servings increased amply to sustain ideal weight provides more than sufficient levels of vitamins for body maintenance and exercise demands. Emphasis must be placed on good eating habits, however. A recommendation of iron supplementation on a temporary basis may also be warranted for those females who sweat profusely on a regular basis and experience excessive monthly menstrual losses.

To Load or Not To Load

Carbohydrate loading is a dietary procedure utilizing a high carbohydrate diet (80% carbohydrate) and a set seven day exercise pattern to maximize muscle glycogen storage. Recent research has shown two equally effective techniques (designated A and B) in accomplishing this goal.

Table A.26 Carbohydrate Loading Techniques

Technnique	Phase	
A	I	Days 1–3: normal balanced diet with normal training exercise pattern.
	II	Days 4–6: carbohydrate loading (300–500 gm) with light exercise pattern.
		Day 7: Pre-event meal and event.
B	I	Days 1–3: low carbohydrate diet (100 gm) with normal training pattern.
	II	Days 4–6: carbohydrate loading (300–500 gm) with light exercise.
		Day 7: Pre-event meal and event.

Technique A is preferred to technique B since it avoids the metabolic stress resulting from severely restricted carbohydrate intake during exercise. It is not recommended that carbohydrate intake be increased through foods of low nutrient density (i.e., sugar, honey, sodas, marshmallow, hard candy). Choose a variety of foods from the fruit group as well as the many high complex carbohydrate foods of the bread and cereal group (listed below) during the loading phase while decreasing the intake of foods from the meat and fat groups for caloric balance. This manipulation can result in a two-fold increase in glycogen storage; however, repeated use of the technique (more than twice a year) decreases its effectiveness dramatically.

Bread and cereal group foods   Breads (all types), crackers (all types), cereals (hot/cold), biscuits, muffins, cornbread, popovers, pancakes, waffles, peas, lima beans, corn, popcorn, dried peas, beans, rice, spaghetti, noodles, potatoes, parsnips.

The loading technique is of no advantage in short-term, high intensity competition of less than four minutes for which the normal glycogen stores of 1,500 calories are adequate.

Active persons in all sports can benefit from maximized glycogen stores. A shortened version of carbohydrate loading, called *loaf-load* can increase glycogen stores enough in the physically active individual to make competition in most sports possible (table A.27).

Last Chance Meal: The Pre-Event Meal Plan

What you eat, when you eat, and how much you eat will dramatically affect your performance in any physical activity. A light meal must be consumed a minimum of two hours before exercise, or as early as three to four hours preceding activity if convenient. Food eaten after this will not be digested when exercise begins. Digestion will continue slowly, or not at all, during exercise since the available blood supply is shunted to the working muscles.

Guidelines
1. Increase the number of foods from the fruit, vegetable, and grain groups but be sure they are low in fiber, by
   a. Choosing juice, not fruit.
   b. Choosing starchy vegetables or vegetable juice, not crunchy, watery vegetables.
   c. Avoiding excessive intake of whole grain cereals and breads. Increased bulk (fiber) delays stomach-emptying time, thus prolonging the diversion of the blood away from the muscle.
2. Decrease the fat content of the meal by
   a. Avoiding margarine, butter, and other foods from the fat group.

Table A.27 Loaf-Load Regime

Day	Training	Diet
3	Moderate	Carbohydrate-loading diet
2	Moderate	Carbohydrate-loading diet
1	Rest	Carbohydrate-loading diet
0	Competition	Pre-competition meal

Table A.28 Pre-Game Meal

Skim milk	1 cup
Lean meat (or equivalent protein)	1 oz.
Fruit juice	½ cup
Bread or substitute	2 svgs or more
Fat spread	1 tsp
Beverages	1–2 cups

    b. Watching out for the hidden sources of fat in foods from the protein group. You need protein in the meal, but choose wisely.

    A fatty meal also delays emptying time in the stomach.

3. Avoid simple sugars by avoiding commercial jellies, jams, honeys, molasses, white and brown sugar.

    Concentrated sugars and exercise will cause disruption of the normal balance of glucose in the blood. The "energy high" doesn't last, while the resulting recoil to a very low blood sugar level is devastating to the body's stability and performance.

If you generally experience heat cramps during or following demanding endurance events, provide copious amounts of water several days preceding the period of heat stress.

In addition to proper timing, quality and quantity of food, psychologic well-being is the primary consideration of the athlete. Many athletes have superstitious beliefs regarding the role of food for peak performance and, regardless of logic or scientific facts, should eat what is comfortable and mentally reinforcing.

Your most critical fuel need (water) can be partially fulfilled before the event by *hyperhydration*. Consume as much water as possible half an hour prior to the match. One to two quarts, if tolerated, is recommended.
Become adjusted to the feeling of fluid in the gastrointestinal tract by using this technique regularly.

Summary

Prolonged physical exercise (endurance activity or training) requires a more finely tuned diet to satisfy the far greater bodily demands of maximum performance. Increased caloric intake for the exercise should be wisely chosen from nutrient-dense foods high in carbohydrates since protein and fat requirements are unaltered during strenuous activity. Dehydration is a major limiting factor in performance; one-half to one cup of water is recommended each 15 minutes of exercise. Additional electrolyte, vitamin or mineral supplements are generally not required if a balanced diet is consumed.

Carbohydrate-loading techniques are presented that may be valuable in delaying the onset of fatigue in long-term events. Guidelines for a properly-timed, nutritionally adequate pre-event meal are provided.

Commonly Asked Questions

Q. Is there any evidence that protein requirements for physically active persons should be increased? And if so, under what circumstances?

A. Most nitrogen balance studies suggest that there is no increase in protein requirement during the entire training period. However, during the first few days of training, athletes may actually be in a slight negative nitrogen balance. After this, nitrogen balance is once again achieved. This information suggests that increased protein might be useful during the first few days of training, if, in fact, the small negative nitrogen balance at the beginning of training is undersirable. A negative nitrogen balance also occurs in recovery from intensive exercise, such as marathons, comparable to the negative nitrogen balance normally seen in individuals under psychologic stress.

Q. Is a fructose-containing beverage more beneficial for maximum performance than one containing sucrose or glucose?

A. To date, no studies on *human* subjects have supported a superiority of fructose over glucose or sucrose as measured by performance. During competition, many athletes subjectively report that fructose feedings aided their performances. However, controlled laboratory studies have not always substantiated such claims.

A study at Ball State University looked at muscle and liver glycogen repletion in the rat, using fructose versus glucose. The results showed that fructose increased glycogen repletion in the liver and glucose increased glycogen repletion in the muscle. Therefore, beneficial effects of fructose ingestion during exercise may not be detectable. However, during recovery, repletion of liver glycogen may be enhanced. Other studies in rats have shown that there is greater muscle glycogen repletion per gram of fructose feeding than for glucose feeding.

Q. Are there any differences in glycogen storage after a person eats simple (glucose) versus complex (starch) carbohydrates?
A. In the first 24 hours, there is generally little difference. After 48 hours, there is greater storage after complex-starch consumption. Generally, the more carbohydrate eaten (from any source), the greater the glycogen storage possible.

Q. Will sports drinks hurt your performance?
A. Because they must stay in the stomach until diluted, sports drinks could possibly hurt the athlete's performance. The longer a fluid stays in the stomach, the longer it takes for the water to get where it is needed. In the meantime, the athlete can become overheated. As mentioned earlier, if athletes use sports drinks, they should be diluted at least 50%—one half cup sports drink plus one half cup plain water.

Q. Does the supplementation of vitamins and minerals over the recommended daily doses result in better performance?
A. Based on current research, vitamin and mineral supplementation appears to be ineffective in improving the performance of a well-nourished person. However, a number of controlled experiments are in progress to investigate the effects of additional B-complex, vitamin C and E, and iron on persons involved in daily aerobic exercise. The rule stands: a well-balanced diet elevated in calories to meet increased energy needs will cover added nutrient needs; an unbalanced, inadequate diet is not redeemed by supplementation.

References

The American Alliance for Health, Physical Ed., Recreation & Dance. *Nutrition For Athletes—A Handbook for Coaches*. Reston, VA.

American Dietetic Association. "Nutrition and Physical Fitness, A Statement." *Journal of the American Dietetic Association*. May, 1980(76):437.

Coleman, E. *Eating For Endurance*. Riverside, CA: Rubidoux Printing Co., 1980.

Costill, D. et al. "Muscle and Liver Glycogen Resynthesis Following Oral Glucose and Fructose Feeding of Rats." *Biochemistry of Exercise: Proceedings of the Fifth International Symposium on the Biochemistry of Exercise*. Champaign, IL: Human Kinetics Publishers Inc., 1983.

Getchell, B. *Being Fit: A Personal Guide*. New York: Wiley, 1982.

Katch, F. and McArdle, W. *Nutrition, Weight Control and Exercise*, 2nd Ed. Philadelphia: Lea and Febiger.
National Dairy Council. *Food Power: A Coach's Guide to Improving Performance.* Rosemont, IL: 1984.
Serfass, R. "Nutrition for the Athlete Update." *Contemporary Nutrition.* April 1982 (7)6:10
Sharkey, B. *Physiology of Fitness,* 2nd Ed., Champaign, IL:1984.
Williams, M. *Nutrition for Fitness and Sport.* Dubuque, IA: William C. Brown, 1982.

Chapter 9

Strength Training

Donald Chu, Ph.D.

Strength is a term used to describe the maximum force that can be applied to an object or that can be registered by an individual.

There are many forms of strength. The first is *absolute* strength. How much force can be developed regardless of sex, age, weight, or any other factor? Since the world of athletics often works on absolutes, we are very aware of the most weight lifted, home run hit farthest, fastest sprint time, or highest jump made by individual performers.

Then there is a *relative* strength. When force development is compared to a particular standard, such as body weight, we often find a very different picture. The biggest athletes may not be the strongest when compared to a specific variable. When men are directly compared to females, they appear to be 30%–40% stronger. However, when these values are expressed relative to body size and lean body weight, females have been shown to be slightly stronger than their male counterparts.

Age is also a factor in relative strength. Until males and females reach puberty, there is virtually no difference in strength capability. Once past puberty, however, the production of testosterone in the male accounts for larger muscle mass and an associated increase in strength.

Strength is also relative to the task being performed. Certainly those individuals using wrist and ankle weights are attempting to develop strength while performing aerobic dance activities. The absolute strength developed, although useful and adequate for the aerobiciser, will in no way approach that of a dedicated Olympic weight lifter.

Strength Development

It is a widely recognized fact that strength development occurs when an individual works against external resistance at some degree. The concept of *overload* is well implanted in our minds. **[I.F: Overload Principle]** Lift more weight and you get stronger. Practically, however, we know that this is not an endless succession.

At this point it is necessary to postulate a method of describing how the human system reacts to the stress of training for strength. The General Adaptation Syndrome (GAS) seems well suited to describe the effects of exercise and training.

In simplified form, the GAS suggests that an individual attempting to develop strength passes through three distinct phases:

Phase 1 The individual reacts to the stimulus of initial training. This phase is characterized by soreness and stiffness during the first few days of a new training program. A temporary drop in the level of performance often occurs.

Phase 2 The individual's body undergoes a number of physiological and biomechanical changes relating to efficiency, and the effect is enhanced performance. This phase continues with only minor fluctuations as long as the body is allowed the luxury of recovery and variability in exercise. If timed properly, "peaking" for ultimate performance is possible. If, however, the variables of exercise are not manipulated properly, and strength training takes place without rhyme or reason, then the third phase of GAS occurs.

Phase 3 Stress from training and/or other aspects of an individual's life becomes so great that exhaustion occurs. The body can no longer make the adaptations to continue benefiting from exercise and "overtraining" occurs. The body may fail in the sense of producing a poor performance or incurring an injury.

Organization of Strength Development

Strength training programs are dependent upon the following variables with regard to exercise:

- frequency
- duration
- intensity
- variation
- specificity

These variables must combine to create a format of training. This discussion deals primarily with the development of absolute strength. It considers the idea that a model plan for developing strength has been presented by researchers in muscle physiology and strength development.
[I: Basic Principles, Definitions and Recommendations]

Stone and Garhammer have presented their model program as being comprised of four parts:

1. Hypertrophy
2. Basic strength
3. Strength-power
4. Active rest

Hypertrophy

Hypertrophy is the development of size in a muscle with corresponding reduction to improve the tensile strength characteristics. Best developed by using a system of training with weights and lifting of a high volume (total number of repetitions) and low intensity (average weight of the object being lifted); e.g., three to five sets of 10 reps with 70% of the individual's one repetition maximum (RM).

Basic strength

The second phase is known as *basic strength* and characterized by training with a moderate volume of repetitions and a high intensity (lifting heavier weights); e.g., three sets of five reps with 80%–90% of one RM.

Strength-power

Strength-power is the third phase. It includes the use of a low volume of repetitions and very high intensity (maximum weights), e.g., three to five sets of two to three repetitions with maximum weight.

Active rest

Active rest is designed to allow the body to physiologically recover and prepare itself for a repeat of the model. It utilizes very low volume and very low intensity. It often involves participation in a different sport and using weight minimally.

The above model utilizes the concept of *periodization*. This is the art of cycling certain types of exercise systems to enhance strength-power development and reduce overtraining. The cycles or phases of the model may be designed to be four to six weeks in length. Athletes at the elite levels use this sort of training to reach "peaks" in conditioning (post phase 3) and prepare for their ultimate performance. Research by several authors has produced the following interesting results at the conclusion of each phase:

- significant gains in short-term (aerobic) endurance (phase 1)
- positive changes in body composition—decreased percent fat and increased lean body mass (phase 1)
- the model produced superior gains in leg, hip, and upper body strength (phase 2)

- superior gains in leg and hip power as measured by a battery of tests considering strength development as a function of time (phase 3)

This model of strength training has replaced the traditional thinking on methods of lifting weights. It is utilized by knowledgeable strength coaches and athletes throughout Russia, Europe, and the United States. The system has a sound physiologic basis and gives the athlete a program that brings the body to new levels of strength and power gain.

Strength development for performance must be specific. Exercises and weight training activities should relate to the demands of the athletic task. In a general fitness setting, the individual should consider weight exercises that involve all the large muscle groups. Exercise should take place on alternate days. If a daily workout is desired, the upper body should be exercised, then the lower body on the alternating days.

These considerations apply even when light weights are attached to the arms or legs. Attaching weights in this way will be effective in increasing strength up to a point. Once the body has adapted to the additional resistive torque provided by the use of such weights, another variable must come into play if strength gains are to be made. Increasing repetitions will generally lead to increased muscular endurance but do little for actual absolute strength gains.

Summary

In summary, we often view the strength of an individual as a physical characteristic based on some absolute figure. Unfortunately, the "more is better" concept is what prevails in our thinking. In reality, strength is a very difficult quality to pin down. If it is compared to an individual's size, age, sex, or other variable, we find that the notion of "strong" takes on new meaning.

Regardless of how resistance is applied to the body, the muscular system must adapt to this stress in a predictable way. The General Adaptation Syndrome is important when considering the effects of resistance training on the human body.

The "periodization" concept is a model for strength training. It has been investigated and found to be effective in maximizing strength grains when training with external resistances, namely weights.

Finally, the theory of specificity applies in all resistance training. Using ankle and wrist weights may do little to affect one's bench press, but it can contribute much toward caloric burn, muscle definition, and local muscle endurance.

References

Clarke, D. "Adaptations in Strength and Muscular Endurance Resulting from Exercise." *Exercise and Sports Sciences Review.* New York: Academic Press, 1973.

Fox, E. *Sports Physiology.* Philadelphia: Saunders, 1979.

Garhammer, J. "Periodization of Strength Training for Athletes." *Track Technique.* 1979:73:2398-2399.

Stone, M. et al. "A Hypothetical Model for Strength Training." *Journal of Sports Medicine and Physical Fitness.* 1981:21:336, 342-351.

Stone, M. et al. "Theoretical Model of Strength Training." *National Strength Coaches Association Journal.* 1982:4:36-39.

Chapter 10

Developing Flexibility

Donald Chu, Ph.D.

Flexibility is that component of fitness which is, perhaps, best understood by the majority of participants. *Stretching* involves increasing the extensibility of the muscles, tendons and ligaments. However, we would be remiss if we did not state that stretching beyond normal range of motion, particularly ligamentous tissue, is a negative aspect. All joint areas have a "normal" range through which they should move. Beyond this point, hypermobility of joints occurs, and the results can be an increased tendency toward injury.

It is of interest to point out that ligaments and tendons are tissues with low elasticity. These tissues are resistant to stretching and are designed to stabilize joints and provide strong bonds between muscle and bone. They will stretch, however, and once stretched, they do *not* return to their shorter, previous states.

Muscle tissue, with its great contractile properties, has the additional and unique ability to lengthen greatly under certain conditions. The Golgi Tendon Organs (GTOs) are sensory receptors which provide the muscle with certain information and are located at the musculo-tendon junctures. The purpose of the GTOs is protection. When a muscle is subjected to sustained stretch, it receives sensory information as to the force and duration of the stretching action. Given enough information, the receptors trigger an inhibiting response which causes the muscle to relax and, therefore, achieve greater length than it originally possessed. If a joint area such as the knee or elbow refuses to "stretch" out, it is possible the cause is related to other soft tissues of the joint (ligaments, joint capsule, etc.) and not the muscles surrounding the joint.

Flexibility does have a relationship to the sex and age of the participants. Research shows that females are generally more flexible than males. As we age, the problems of lack of circulation, collagen fiber breakdown, and reduced activity levels all help to reduce the body's flexibility. Thus, it becomes important to maintain range of motion and muscle extensibility as close to the normal range as possible.

As much as aerobic participants intuitively know about "stretching," there are often some myths or confusion about increasing flexibility.

Warm-Up

Stretching to increase flexibility is not warming-up. **[IV: Warm-Up]** The activity of "warming-up" indicates the elevation of muscle core temperature. Stretching, as an activity, has never been shown to accomplish an increase in core temperature. Warming-up should consist of 8–10 minutes of low intensity activity such as riding a stationary bicycle or calisthenics. Toning exercises which are done in a stationary position are excellent forms of warm-up. It is interesting to note that the greatest gains in flexibility occur after a period of warm-up. Flexibility is specific, and stretching the muscles of the lower extremities has no relationship to flexibility of the upper body. Therefore, muscles in all areas of the body should be attended to. Also, rhythmic exercise should be performed as part of the warm-up routine to prepare muscles for their all-out use during aerobic routines. Keep in mind that these movements are precursors to more strenuous activities.

Guideline for Stretching

Research shows that static stretching is just as effective as ballistic (bouncing) stretching in terms of increasing muscle range. **[IV.C: Stretching]** Static stretching has been judged to be a safe and effective means of accomplishing increased range of motion.

- Static stretching is performed by aligning the body properly so that stretch occurs along a longitudinal line with the direction of the muscle. This allows the GTOs to be stimulated as soon as possible, building in the inhibitive or relaxation response.
- Movement into a stretching pattern should be slow and easy, and when the end of the range of motion is reached, this position should be held for 10–20 seconds. This length of time is necessary to affect the GTOs.

- When stretching the muscles of the lower leg, particularly the hamstrings, adductors and rotators of the hip, keep the lumbar section of the spine extended and pivot from the hips.
- When inhaling, try to let the stomach go out, and when exhaling, pull the stomach in toward the spine. This is known as diaphragmatic breathing and helps to focus one's concentration on relaxation.
- Keep in mind that you should not bounce, but "reach and hold" on all movements.
- Some days you may be "looser" than others. Remember, flexibility varies with time of day, temperature, and stress levels.
- Make note of the fact that one side of your body is looser than the other. This is often due to greater use and consequent asymmetrical development as seen in some tennis and baseball players.
- Make sure you are aware of dynamic imbalances that may exist. Joggers often are subject to weak and tight hamstrings while their quadriceps and calves may be overstretched. This is due in part to the nature of their activity and the focus they tend to adopt in their training. Another example of an imbalance that may develop is the preoccupation with flexion exercises for the trunk as a way of reducing back problems. The human body is a cylinder, and no one side or area can be ignored without creating an imbalance.
- There are several theories as to the origin of muscle soreness. One that is plausible relates the onset of soreness to fatigue. As muscle fatigue occurs, incomplete relaxation takes place, leading to muscle contraction (spasm). Static stretching has been shown to reduce muscle soreness when performed pre- and postactivity.
- "Cooling down" from activity is an important aspect of high level performance. **[VII: Post-Aerobic Cool Down]** This involves the use of progressively slower paced rhythmic activities to restore normal heart rate and allow for recovery of the individual's metabolism. The final step in this process is the use of large muscle stretching to decrease the adverse effects of exercise such as muscle soreness and to better prepare one for the next day's activity.

Summary

Flexibility as it relates to stretching soft tissue such as muscles and tendons is a necessary component of fitness. Flexibility is best accomplished through static stretching techniques. It is specific to the area being stretched and one should consider the body as a dynamic system which operates best when all areas are developed and maintained. It should be noted that there are very tangible benefits to utilizing flexibility activities as part of a cooling down process, as well as the traditional warm-up on pre-activity stretching.

References

deVries, H. *Physiology of Exercise for Physical Education and Athletics*, 2nd Ed. Dubuque, IA: William C. Brown, 1974.

Jensen, C. and Fisher, A. *Scientific Basis of Athletic Conditioning*, 2nd Ed. Philadelphia: Lea and Febiger, 1979.

Wilmone, J. *Training for Sport and Activity*, 2nd Ed. Boston: Allyn and Bacon, 1982.

Chapter 11

Neuromuscular Power and Plyometrics

Donald Chu, Ph.D.

Power is the least understood component of fitness. Power, by definition, is the ability to apply strength rapidly. It is often expressed as the ability to develop force over a certain distance as rapidly as possible. It is the time factor that is crucial. Force must be developed in a very short period of time to classify as power. For example, track and field sprinters are powerful athletes, and as they run they exert tremendous forces against the ground. The paradox becomes apparent in high-speed film analyses of these athletes. Although they exert extremely large amounts of force against the ground, the actual amount of time they spend on the ground is very short. This example demonstrates the all important concept that powerful movements are large amounts of force developed in short periods of time.

Plyometrics

The term currently being applied to exercise systems designed to develop neuromuscular power is *plyometrics*. A plyometric exercise is an exercise in which the athlete utilizes the force of gravity to store energy within the muscular framework of the body. The storing of energy is then followed by an immediate reaction of equal but opposite magnitude, utilizing the natural elastic components of the muscles to produce a kinetic energy system.

For example, when an athlete steps from a box of 24–26 inches in height and drops to the ground, the athlete's body is accelerated over the distance by the force of gravity. Upon landing, the nervous system of the muscles senses a rapid eccentric contraction. It has been well established that the faster a muscle is lengthened, the greater the concentric force developed. The result is a movement that is more powerful in nature than one that could be developed from a ''standing'' start.

The essence of plyometrics, then, is to develop the nervous system so that it will react with maximal speed to the lengthening of muscle and in turn develop the ability of the muscle to shorten rapidly with maximal force.

It follows that the overload principle is the tenet of exercise to apply in this case. The Europeans found that by repeatedly dropping from specific heights they could stress a muscle spindle system and create a positive change in performance. The great Russian jump coach, Veroshanski, was one of the first to publish drills and exercises for developing the "total neuromuscular system." Veroshanski published specific recommended heights for one and two foot landings and labeled these exercises "in-depth" jumps. This Russian coach followed several guidelines in the establishment of training programs utilizing these exercises, and a revolution began.

Explosive-reactive power was the goal. The goal can only be accomplished by treating each exercise attempt as a maximal effort. The neuromuscular system utilizing the "stretch-reflex" principle demands that each effort require the utmost in concentration and physical effort.

In his early work, Veroshanski described his in-depth jumps as a straight line drop from heights of .75 and 1.10 meters. This drop requires that the athlete step off a box (not jump) and upon making contact with the ground, move his body directly upward as rapidly as possible. The essence of the movement is that it be "touch and go." The athlete must be mentally ready to reverse the dropping motion at the instant he or she feels the ground contact.

The time that lapses from ground contact to reversal of movement is known as the "amortization" phase. It is desirable that this time be minimal to a point within reason. The athlete must undergo some split second of neurological processing prior to accomplishing take-off. This is a process that can be developed and improved. Hence, the rationale for plyometric training is at hand.

It is noteworthy that not all sport movements are directly upward. Many are composed of horizontal as well as vertical force. Thus, another form of plyometric exercise developed named *bounding*. Bounds are an exercise form in which the athlete directs himself over the ground in both single, double, or alternating leg movement patterns. Since the athlete is covering ground, and the height from which he drops is controlled by angles of take-off projection and landing, the exercise and its inherent "amortization phase" becomes more complex.

Hopping activities are really a sub component of bounds. Hopping activities are both single- and double-legged in take-off and landing activities. Hops are generally shorter in attempted distance than bounds.

Use

This leads to a clarification of the usefulness of these activities, the *why, where,* and *when* of plyometrics. If the nature of the exercise is directed toward improving a specific skill such as single or double leg take-offs vertically for such sports as basketball, volleyball, and jumping events for heights, then those movement patterns should be approximated as closely as possible by the plyometric exercise, in this case, in-depth jumps.

If the need is for horizontal force development, the plyometric exercise should favor movement in a linear direction. The development of lateral movement power is one of the most overlooked areas of training by all athletes. A simple recognition of the forces necessary to stabilize the hips in a one-legged stance (e.g., running, one-foot jumping, cutting) should be enough to generate some thought into planning and development of this aspect of the conditioning program.

Acceleration

Plyometrics have often been credited with the development of acceleration and absolute speed in running. This can be accomplished only if planned for, with careful consideration of the exercises used. If acceleration is a desirable skill for improvement, then short (distance), intense plyometrics of high frequency (leg cycle or turn-over) would be the exercises of choice. It is generally accepted that leg cycle or turn-over is a most difficult trait to improve. Acknowledging that it is capable of small improvements, one must realize that leg frequency must be closely associated with force developed against the ground. Acceleration in running is the art of overcoming the inertia of one's own body at an ever-increasing rate. Pushing back against the running surface and more rapid leg movement are both crucial to success in this activity.

Absolute speed

Sustaining peak speed once it is attained is considered to be that characteristic known as *absolute speed*. The worst enemy of the runner is *deceleration,* or dropping below the peak speed of movement attained at the end of acceleration. This becomes an area of skill requiring the maintenance of leg frequency and maximum push against the ground. Attacking the problem of sustained speed generally requires plyometric drills that project the athlete linearly at angles specific to running and for high numbers of efforts or repetitions. Thus, bounding often encompasses distances close to or even beyond 100 meters. Distances beyond this may result in too much of a sustained effort, and fatigue will cause rapid deterioration in the skill level of the athlete.

Some sport activities such as volleyball, basketball and aerobic dance are plyometric in nature. Given the many jumping activities that occur in these sports, it might be difficult to see the value of training the body for single maximal explosive efforts. However, plyometric training also teaches a tremendous amount of body control and neuromuscular reactivity, and can certainly challenge the anaerobic conditioning threshold of the most avid fitness enthusiast.

Experts in the area of plyometrics are still few and far between. College track and field coaches are potential resources for further information in the area. Also, the National Strength Coaches Association has many informative articles on plyometrics in their journal.

Summary

In summary, plyometric training is an exercise system unto itself. It is based on a physiologic principle: namely, elastic components of muscle and neurological reflexes which support its rationale. It has a researched history, and although it is not a panacea for all power training ills, it has a valuable place in all conditioning programs. It is a system which provides the ultimate in flexibility and variety of training. Only the imagination of the user limits the system's variability and potential.

References

Chu, D. "Plyometrics: The Link Between Strength and Speed." *National Strength Coaches Association Journal*. 1983:4:20-21.

Chu, D. "Plyometric Exercise." *National Strength Coaches Journal*. 1984:5:56-61.

Grieve, D. "Stretching Active Muscles." *Track Technique*. 1970:42:1333-1335.

Starzynski, T. "Triple Jump Training." *Legkaya Athletika*. 1970:5:1436-1440.

Veroshanski, Y. "Specific Training for Power." *Legkaya Athletika*. 1976:5:9-11.

Wilt, F. and Ecker, T. *International Track and Field Coaching Encyclopedia*. West Nyack, NY: Parker Publishing Co., 1970.

Wilt, F. "From the Desk of Fred Wilt, Plyometric Exercise." *Track Technique*. 1970:64.

Chapter 12

Applied Sports Psychology

Barry Devine, Ph.D.

While several other countries around the world were quick to recognize the importance of sports psychology in the improvement of physical performance, the United States has been slower to emphasize this relationship. The mental approach to physical performance is much more important than most aerobic exercise instructors realize. Mental processes need to be developed just as we develop physical skills, and this always takes time. The instructor needs to know when to activate or relax thought processes in preparation for and during a class, and which processes are suitable for particular circumstances.

This chapter is directed toward the aerobic exercise instructor and emphasizes the application of sports psychology in the sequence of responsibilities the instructor undertakes in teaching classes. The preparation prior to leading the class is considered, especially in relation to preparing to lead subsequent classes on the same day. Next, the psychologic tools needed to ensure that the instruction itself is as meaningful as possible and in keeping with the potential of the instructor are addressed. Finally, the chapter will explore the concluding phase of the instruction, including what takes place after the class, especially if it is to be followed by another class on the same day.

Questions to be Answered in the Text

- How should the instructor deal with his or her anxiety before a class begins?
- How can the instructor prepare mentally for a class?
- How can the instructor sustain his or her motivation over weeks of instruction?

- How can the instructor deal with setbacks due to less than acceptable performance?
- How can the instructor evaluate critically, yet positively?
- How can the instructor utilize automatic and/or adaptive behavior instruction?

Considerations Prior to Instruction

Anxiety

Leading an aerobic exercise class is certainly meaningful enough to produce a state of heightened arousal with anxiety and tension. This is particularly likely for the less-experienced instructor, for one teaching a new class or level, or when teaching at a new facility. This anxiety is present in some degree in even the most successful and experienced instructor. Anxiety is all part of the mechanism that makes many seasoned entertainers very sick prior to every appearance on stage. The arousal permits us to really concentrate and focus upon the tasks ahead and then provides us with a surge of energy to accomplish these tasks. Clearly, if these emotions get out of control, it can be a problem for the instructor. Normal arousal in preparation to lead a class is helpful; too much arousal is a distracting, negative influence.

To cope with anxiety, there are several sound methods available. It should be noted that individuals develop different tolerances to anxiety, and that some thrive on it more than others. While many differences in tolerance can be accounted for by maturity and experience, there are also differences based upon other factors. A program of relaxation responses is the key to minimizing anxiety prior to conducting classes. These relaxation responses utilize the same skills the instructor might be nurturing among the class participants as part of the cool-down. Benson's relaxation response (a simplified form of meditation), transcendental meditation, yoga, self-hypnosis, progressive muscle relaxation, and other techniques have all been found successful in enabling the "trained" individual to relax. These techniques all require some practice developing enough skill to make good use of them.

Simple deep breathing enhances physical relaxation. The deep breath tenses the body while a controlled, lengthy exhalation relaxes it. If an instructor has the luxury of a quiet place to relax between classes, the breathing practice, the playing of soft music (perhaps from the cool-down segment of your exercise session), and the opportunity to be quiet and to imagine a favorite peaceful location are all excellent tools to deal with pre-activity anxiety.

Mental preparation

Two of the most effective techniques for mentally preparing for physical performance are the use of imagery and mental rehearsal. By the use of imagery, we are able to construct the conditions of the class as we perceive them in the upcoming workout. This allows the exercise leader to clarify expectations and to foresee complications or other difficulties that might have to be addressed in order to ensure that the goals of the workout are attained.

The mental rehearsal allows the exercise leader to reinforce a method of technical approach (such as an exercise transition), by repeated mental practice of an action or a sequence of actions. In each case, the instructor should be relaxed and attempt to picture actions as vividly and as positively as possible.

Considerations During a Class

Movement and varied verbal cues normally flow freely during the exercise session, and there is usually little need for deliberate cognitive intervention on the part of the instructor. The mental focus should be on the minimal number of relevant cues. Relaxation techniques can be applied *during* a session if the arousal state is too high. The individual must learn to monitor what is going on and must work toward controlling emotions so that they do not negatively affect performance.

Automatic behavior takes over once one is able to control emotions without conscious action. However, on days when several classes are taught, accumulated fatigue effects may make it necessary to utilize adaptive behavior in order to control some emotions. For example, if the instructor falls behind the pace due to injury or fatigue, or is not completing the proper range of movement, it may be necessary to move to a different set of exercises, or to take a break, face the class, and observe its form and timing.

Before a class gets under way, the successful leader has already thought through the entire session, addressing the beginning, the middle and the end of the session. The beginning of a session is a critical time, and realizing this, the capable leader sequentially thinks through such details as room lighting, setting music and volume in place, distribution of pads or towels (if not provided by participants), location from which he or she will make announcements, exercise clothing to wear, words of greeting to participants and announcement of class level, solicitation of information from any first-time participants in class, cautionary information to be announced, etc. [III: **Pre-class Procedure**] The beginning segment is especially important, because the tone for the whole session is established at this time.

After the class gets under way and the warm-up/stretching phase is over, the session moves into the middle of the workout, during which most of the aerobic exercise is done. The thoughtful instructor has again planned the sequence of events to ensure that the timing and transitions are right, and to be sure that the correct level of energy is maintained. It is appropriate to remind ourselves that the success of classes meeting for aerobic exercise is due in great measure to the music utilized to set the tempo. As well as motivating participants, the music allows the instructor to monitor the continuity of his or her sequence at any time, without reference to clocks or notes.

The end of the workout begins as the class eases into a cool-down routine. Any thoughtful instructor will have seen to it that the music selected is appropriate, and will have reviewed the activities and announcements that need to be undertaken to finish the session. It is necessary to bring the session to an end (closure), psychologically speaking, even if individuals are invited to bring questions or problems to the instructor after class. Also, closure can be achieved by use of relaxation exercises at the end of the cool-down period.

Clearly, all the demands upon the aerobic exercise instructor require a great deal of personal motivation if competence is to grow. Ideally, the instructor should be motivated for internal or personal reasons to prove how good he or she can be by working hard. An instructor should take pride in his or her efforts and achievements and set high (but attainable) goals to pursue. The drive toward self-fulfillment and competence is intrinsic (internal) motivation. Motivation based upon threats of termination or desire for monetary reward is extrinsic (external) and not as effective in the long run.

Considerations After a Class

When an instructor has more than one class to teach on the same day, he or she should learn to relax completely for a time, then activate mental and emotional processes to get into the optimal readiness state for the next class. Sustaining arousal and intensity from one class to the next can drain one's energy.

From time to time, as a learning experience, one needs to use the results of leading classes. We can review, evaluate, and learn from our performance by using analysis evaluation and constructive criticism. Dwelling on the negative is not productive; if a performance was not as effective as it should have been, analysis can provide appropriate goals and indicate changes that will create improvement in the future. Remember that improvement is a tangible measure of success. When improvement is evident, motivation to continue is sustained and our self-concept is strengthened.

Psychologists suggest that ability and effort are two major internal causative factors of success. While we are unable to expand our ability rapidly, we are able to increase our accomplishments markedly by applying more effort, and, in so doing, we exercise some control over our destiny.

Summary

The aerobic exercise instructor should not underestimate the application of sports psychology in maintaining a course of instruction that is consistent, improves continually, and serves as a source of pride for the individual. Some of the most important applications are made before the class begins. The informed instructor can cope with any state of anxiety or fatigue by relaxing and mentally preparing in a relatively quiet and private location prior to the class.

A wise instructor has carefully sequenced all events of the class and simply moves into the location and implements the plan. It is during this mental-sequencing process that the beginning, the middle, and the end of the class are thought out and put in order. The key sequence measure here is the music; it keeps the time and sets the rate of energy expenditure for the class. The instructor uses any adaptive behavior necessary to control his or her emotions as the sequence is implemented.

Each class is brought to a distinct ending, and following this closure, the instructor should evaluate the effectiveness of the session in meeting the established goals. Objective assessment of performance and instructive criticism of one's efforts are the mark of the professional instructor. The intrinsic motivation to do this is the basis for personal growth and pride.

References

Benson, H. *The Relaxation Response*. New York: Morrow, 1975.
Gallway, W. *Inner Tennis*. New York: Random House, 1976.
Kaus, D. *Peak Performance*. Englewood Cliffs, NJ: Prentice-Hall, 1980.
Neal, N. "Mental Imagery and Relaxation in Skill Rehearsal." *Scholastic Coach*, December 1981:50.
Nideffer, R. *The Ethics and Practices of Applied Sport Psychology*. Ithica, NY: Movement Publications, 1981.
Nideffer, R. and Sharpe, R. *How to Put Anxiety Behind You*. New York: Stein and Day, 1978.
Singer, R. *Motor Learning and Human Performance*, 3rd Ed. New York: Macmillan, 1980.
Stuart, R. Ed. *Behavioral Self-Management*. New York: Brunner/Mazel, 1977.
Suinn, R., Ed. *Psychology in Sports*. Minneapolis: Burgess, 1980.

Chapter 13

Sports Injury Prevention

Rose Snyder, MS

The majority of injuries affecting aerobics instructors and participants occur in the musculoskeletal system. Of the three general categories—sprains, strains, and overuse syndromes—overuse syndromes are by far the most common and the most preventable.

Gradual progression and overload, proper body mechanics, proper equipment, and adequate warm-up and cool-down are vital to injury-free participation in aerobics activity. They are also critical aspects of effective injury management and in the safe return to activity following injury. The major concepts related to this area are:

- Gradual progression and overload, proper body mechanics, proper equipment, and adequate warm-up and cool-down are factors in injury prevention.
- Beginning participants in an aerobics program should limit their participation to two or three 20–30 minute sessions per week.
- Aerobics instructors should limit their classes to three per day and 12 per week.   **[I.A: Frequency of Workout]**
- Standing with hyperextended knees may cause knee and/or low-back pain.   **[I.C: Body Alignment]**
- Forceful squatting should be avoided.
- Stretching should be pain free.

Gradual Progression and Overload

No matter how well-trained or conditioned a body is, it can be pushed to a point of fatigue and breakdown. Obviously, untrained muscles fatigue more rapidly and may be injured more quickly, but instructors and advanced participants are not immune from the repetitive overstresses encountered in aerobics.

For beginning participants, a 20-30 minute class every other day will provide an improvement in cardiovascular condition, as well as allow the body to gradually adapt to the stresses placed on it. According to AFAA guidelines, aerobic instructors should limit their number of classes to three per day and a total of 12 per week. Participation in aerobics seven days per week is not recommended. At least one day is needed to allow the body to recover and repair itself.

Be aware of the signs of fatigue and overuse:

- pain in the joints, tendons or muscles, especially if accompanied by a slight loss of motion
- swelling
- numbness, tingling, or burning in an extremity
- difficulty sleeping
- a general feeling of tiredness
- an increase in the number of colds or minor illnesses

These are signals for impending injury. Decrease your activity to a pain-free level. Rest or substitute an activity (such as swimming or cycling) that has fewer impact forces.

Proper Body Mechanics

Proper posture and body mechanics are important. The body should be held naturally erect but relaxed. The shoulders should be level and back, and the abdominals held in firmly. The arms and legs should be straight, but not in a hyperextended (locked) position. Hyperextension of the elbows and knees places an additional stress on the ligaments about these joints. Standing with the knees locked will also promote an excessive curve in the lower back (lumbar spine), which may cause back pain.

Exercises requiring a deep knee bend or a squat are potentially harmful to the knees. When performing an exercise requiring a squatting posture, follow these principles:

- Avoid a full squat, particularly a forceful, bouncing squat.
- Do not squat if you have pain or swelling in the knees, or if you have a knee injury or arthritic condition.
- When doing a squatting exercise, keep a good base of support (feet should be a comfortable width apart). The feet should be flat, with the toes pointed forward or slightly out to the side at approximately a 15° angle. The body weight should be centered so that a straight line could be drawn through the center of the thighs to the knees and from the knees to the great toes. Keep the back relatively straight.

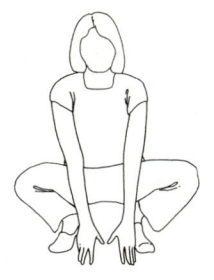

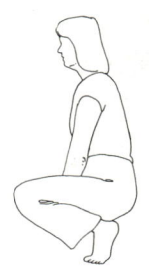

Equipment (Shoes)

It is important that aerobics participants wear proper footwear. Shoes should fit comfortably but snugly. The cushioning must be adequate to protect the leg and foot from the stress of high-impact loads, but also rigid enough to support the foot with a correctly placed arch support built in or provided as a removable insole.

Additional shock-absorbing insoles may be purchased and worn to further dissipate the shock. People who have flat (or pronated) feet may require the additional support and control of an orthotic device. These may be purchased ready-made or, if indicated, custom-made.

Proper Warm-Up and Cool-Down

Proper warm-up and cool-down consist of gentle, static stretching, each stretch held for approximately 15 seconds. It should be comfortable and pain-free. Static stretches are especially important for those individuals returning after an injury, because as muscles and tendons heal, they will shorten slightly. Instructors should recommend and encourage additional gentle, static stretching after the class particularly for those individuals who are sore or are very naturally tight. Ballistic stretching or bouncing should be avoided, because forced stretching creates a stretch reflex response that causes the muscle to contract, therefore inhibiting increased flexibility.

Static stretching should be used, because:

- There is less danger of tissue damage.
- The energy requirement is less.
- There is prevention and/or relief from muscular distress and soreness.

Summary

The injuries which occur in aerobics are overuse or overstress in nature. Gradual progression is the key to prevention and to a safe return following injury. Other factors such as proper body mechanics, proper shoes, and an adequate warm-up and cool-down consisting of gentle, static stretching are also important.

Commonly Asked Questions

Q. Which factors influence injury prevention?
A. Gradual progression and overload, proper body mechanics, proper shoes, and adequate warm-up and cool-down.

Q. List four or more signs of fatigue and overstress.
A. 1. Pain in the joints, tendons or muscles, especially if accompanied by a slight loss of motion.
2. Swelling.
3. Numbness, tingling, or burning in an extremity.
4. Difficulty sleeping.
5. A general feeling of tiredness.
6. An increase in the number of colds or minor illnesses.

Q. Describe the proper squatting posture.
A. A good base of support with the feet shoulder-width apart. The feet should be flat, with the toes pointed forward or slightly out to the side. The body weight should be centered so that a straight line can be drawn through the center of the thighs to the knees and from the knees to the great toes.

Q. What are the AAFA guidelines regarding the recommended number of classes per day and per week that an instructor should teach?
A. A maximum of three per day and 12 per week.

Chapter 14

Common Injuries In Aerobics And Their Treatment

Rose Snyder, MS

The number of people involved in aerobics for regular exercise is increasing. Unfortunately, this increase is also generating numerous patients seeking physicians' advice and treatment for aerobic-related injuries.

The repetitive nature and the impact-loading to the extremities in aerobics can and do cause many chronic injuries to the musculoskeletal system, commonly called overuse injuries. An overuse injury results when the body does not have sufficient time to adapt to the repetitive microtrauma. This inability to adapt leads to breakdown in the soft tissues and, occasionally, the bones (of the lower extremities). The major concepts related to this area are:

- The majority of injuries suffered in aerobics are overuse injuries.
- An overuse injury results when the repetitive microtrauma is such that the body does not have sufficient time to adapt to it.
- The majority of injuries that occur affect the lower extremities.
- Early treatment of an injury involves the use of local ice, gentle stretching and strengthening exercises, a decrease in activity to a pain-free level, the substitution of other activities, temporary cessation of activity, or use of aspirin.
- Forcible squatting, twisting, or sudden hyperextension of the knee may result in a ligament sprain or a cartilage tear of the knee.
- Proper body mechanics is essential to minimizing the incidence of low back pain.
- An acute injury should be seen within one to three days after injury.

148 ESSENTIALS OF AEROBIC EXERCISE

- Persistent pain, unresponsive to ice, aspirin and decreased activity, should be evaluated by a physician after 10–14 days.
- Allow approximately two weeks for every week of disability when returning from an injury.
- Specific rehabilitative exercises for the affected parts is necessary prior to return to activity.

Specific Injuries

Foot and ankle

Metatarsalgia   Weight-bearing is shared by the metatarsal bones in the foot (figure A.21). Frequently, in response to excess loading forces, this area may become very painful, particularly if the individual has a high-arched (or cavus) foot.

Treatment includes using a well-padded shoe and additional padding under the heads (front part) of the metatarsals. A soft, molded insert with a slight arch may also be used. Activity should be reduced to a pain-free level or discontinued until the symptoms subside.

Stress fractures   These are caused by excessive impact-loading on the bones of the foot. They are unable to remodel to the stress quickly enough, and an actual fracture line may be visible within two to three weeks. A stress fracture may occur in any of the bones of the foot, but are most

Figure A.21   The foot

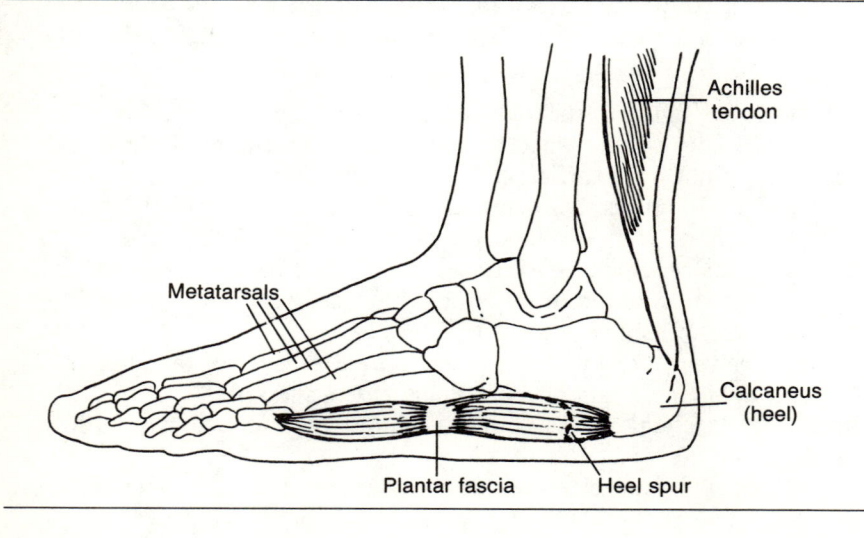

commonly found in the metatarsals (figure A.21). There will be pain and tenderness localized to the fracture site. Frequently, the pain subsides with rest from activity. In the later stages, the pain may be persistent and swelling may be present.

Treatment aims to decrease activity to a pain-free level or to cease exercise temporarily. Use ice locally to control pain and swelling. Check shoes to be certain that they are not worn and are well cushioned. An additional shock-absorbing insole may be added. Pain that does not respond to a decrease in activity should be investigated by a physician. If the diagnosis of stress fracture is made, substitute swimming and/or cycling to allow the bone(s) to heal. Return to activity should be very gradual with a shock-absorbing insole placed in the shoes to dissipate the impact forces.

Plantar fasciitis Mistakenly called heel spurs, this is a condition characterized by aching and occasionally a burning pain in the front part of the heel (figure A.21). Tight achilles tendons, a high-arched (supinated) foot, or a flat (pronated) foot are predisposing biomechanical factors.

Treatment consists of the application of ice, use of adhesive strapping or orthotic arch supports. Achilles tendon stretching exercises should be instituted. The use of heat before and ice after activity can be tried. A doughnut-shaped pad or shock absorbent heel cups may also be worn over the tender area to relieve the pressure.

Persistent heel pain should be examined by a physician. Oral anti-inflammatory agents or injections, custom-made orthotics, or surgical release of the plantar fascia (a last resort) may be used in selected cases.

Tendinitis This is an overuse injury common in individuals with poor muscle tone and flexibility and/or poor foot mechanics. It is an inflammation of the tendon of a muscle which may progress in stages from pain only after activity to chronic pain and dysfunction before, during, and after activity.

The most common sites of tendinitis are the achilles tendon behind the heel and the peroneal tendons on the outside of the ankle. Prevention is much easier than treatment. Gradual progression, gentle stretching before and after activity, and proper fitting, well-padded shoes are important. A reliable shock absorbent insert is also helpful.

At the early signs of pain, decrease the activity, ice the area for 15 minutes immediately following activity and two or three more times per day (see Icing section that follows). For achilles tendinitis, a 1/4- to 3/8-inch heel lift may also help. Oral anti-inflammatory drugs such as aspirin may be beneficial. The inflammation of tendinitis will result in decreased motion and strength, so appropriate stretching and strengthening exercises must be done.

If the tendinitis is due to a malalignment of the lower extremities, an orthotic appliance may be useful and may be obtained from an orthopedist or podiatrist.

Ankle sprains   These are acute injuries that may occur in aerobics, involving a stretching or tearing of one or more of the ligaments at the ankle. The majority of sprains occur to the "outside" or lateral ligaments.

Symptoms range from a mild aching the next day to immediate pain, swelling, discoloration, and dysfunction. Treatment depends on the degree of the injury, but acute (early) symptom management follows the RICE principle:

- rest (crutches if necessary)
- ice
- compression with an elastic wrap
- elevation of the extremity to a position higher than the heart

Following the acute stage or after immobilization has been discontinued, the rehabilitation program consists of cold soaks or a contrast bath (alternating hot and cold soaks for 20 minutes), range-of-motion, isometric, progressive-resistive, and balance exercises. Return to aerobics is allowed when a full, pain-free range of motion and strength equal to the noninjured side is achieved. Taping the ankle or the use of a nonelastic ankle brace is advisable for four to six weeks following a moderate to severe ankle sprain. Activities such as swimming or cycling should be substituted to maintain cardiovascular condition during the rehabilitative phase.

Leg and knee

Shin splints   More accurately known as posterior tibial tendinitis, these are characterized by pain located on the posteromedial (inside) border of the tibia (figure A.22). The condition can be precipitated by tight calf muscles, overuse, improper or well-worn shoes, and hard, unyielding surfaces. Shin splints are also related to the amount of pronation occurring at the ankle joint.

Treatments include ice massage to the affected area for 10–15 minutes, stretching of the calf muscles, and strengthening of the anterior tibial (front shin) muscles. If the shin splints are caused by excessive pronation, orthotic arch and heel supports may be indicated.

Stress fractures   These may occur in either bone of the lower leg (the tibia or fibula). At first, they may be difficult to differentiate from shin splints, but exquisite point tenderness at a specific site on the bone should make one very suspicious of a stress fracture. The exact diagnosis can only be made through radiographs or a special radioisotope scan. Regular x-rays may not show evidence of a stress fracture for three to four weeks.

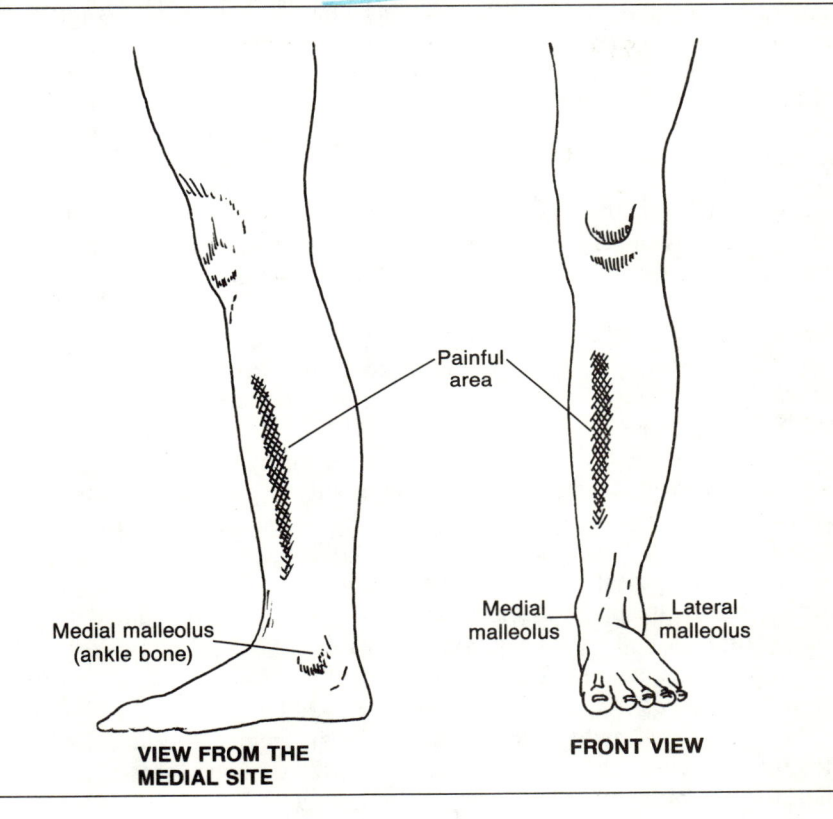

COMMON INJURIES IN AEROBICS AND THEIR TREATMENT 151

Figure A.22 Shin splints or posterior tibial tendinitis.

Painful area

Medial malleolus (ankle bone)

Medial malleolus

Lateral malleolus

VIEW FROM THE MEDIAL SITE

FRONT VIEW

Treatment of a stress fracture to the fibula or tibia is similar to that of a metatarsal stress fracture—rest from activity. Generally casts are avoided. The individual should continue swimming or bicycling during the healing phase.

A return to aerobics may be permitted in three to four weeks after x-rays show evidence of healing, and there is no tenderness to palpation.

Compartment syndromes The muscles, nerves and blood vessels of the lower leg are encased in four separate compartments. With vigorous exercise, the space in one of the compartments (usually the anterior compartment) may be compromised causing increased compartment pressure. The signs of an anterior compartment syndrome are pain, swelling, warmth, redness, and tenderness over the front of the shin. There is also associated numbness and tingling over the dorsum (top) of the foot as well as weakness of the anterior tibial muscles with a resulting foot drop.

An acute compartment syndrome, not quickly relieved by icing and discontinuing the activity, requires immediate medical attention. A chronic, or exertional, compartment syndrome will have the same symptoms but then can be relieved by rest. If the symptoms are persistent or worsen, medical evaluation is required.

Treatment consists of surgical release of the fascia surrounding the compartment.

Knee pain   Infrequently, an acute, internal derangement may occur, and a cartilage or ligament in the knee may be torn. The mechanism of injury may be a twist with the feet fixed, a rapid, forcible squat, or a sharp hyperextension.

Symptoms will include immediate pain and dysfunction accompanied by rapid swelling of the joint, usually within 24 hours. Proper treatment includes the use of ice, compression, elevation, and examination as soon as possible by a physician.

Usually knee pain is a direct result of overuse or overstress coupled with some common anatomical irregularities that result in pain around the kneecap (patella). Some of the common malalignments include pronated feet, bow legs, knock knees, and very loose kneecaps. Tight thigh and lower leg muscles may also contribute to the problem.

Pain may occur during or after activity. There may be associated swelling in the knee joint as well as a sensation of giveway. Squatting may result in increased symptoms and should be avoided if there is any pain or history of knee injury. Aerobics may not be the recommended activity for individuals with certain diagnosed arthritic conditions. The instructor should make inquiries prior to class and refer anyone with arthritic conditions to their physician for examination prior to beginning any activity.

Treatment includes the use of local ice following activity, additional gentle stretching to the quadriceps and hamstring muscles of the thigh, quadriceps strengthening in the form of straight leg raises to improve tone and patellar tracking (figure A.23). A patellar stabilizing brace may be useful until the quadriceps are strengthened. Orthotics may be used in the shoe if there is an accompanying malalignment at the foot.

When resuming aerobic activity, attention must be paid to proper body mechanics and weight distribution.

Hip and thigh

Hamstring strains, though infrequent, may occur. Treatment includes the use of ice and an elastic wrap for support. After the acute phase has passed, gentle strengthening and stretching are instituted. Heat may be used prior to activity, but ice should be used following activity if any soreness or swelling exist. Return to activity is permitted when full, pain-free range of motion is achieved.

Figure A.23 Quadriceps strengthening exercises.

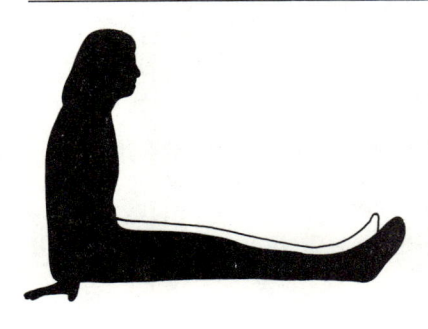

1. Isometric Quad Setting. Sitting or reclining on a flat surface with legs out straight, flatten knee to table by contracting the anterior thigh muscles. Attempt to slightly lift the heel as you pull the patella (kneecap) toward your hip.

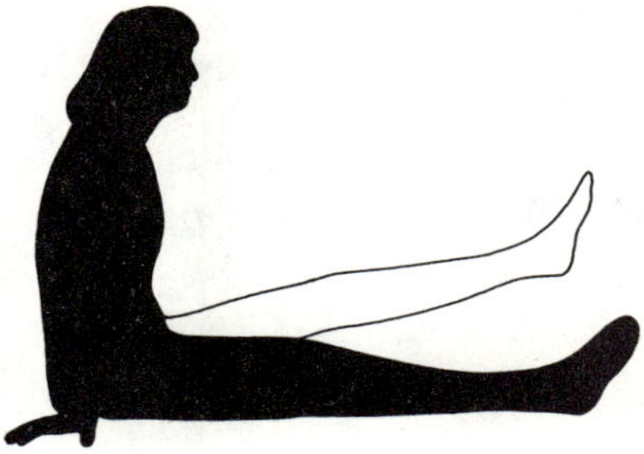

2. Straight Leg Raising. Be sure leg is completely straight before lifting it off of the table. Use a 12 second count; begin with a quad set for 4 seconds, lift the leg up to a 45° angle (approx. 12") and hold for 4 seconds, lower the leg and relax for 4 seconds. Repeat the exercise 20–50 times every hour. Resistance in the form of sandbags or weighted boot may be added up to a 10° maximum.

Stress fractures are rare, but they may occur in the hip or the femur bone in the thigh. They represent a potentially serious injury. Persistent pain in the hip or thigh, not relieved by rest and stretching, requires a medical evaluation including x-ray and radioisotope studies to rule out a stress fracture.

Back pain

Back pain may be precipitated by many factors. Among the more common ones are:

- tight hamstrings
- weak abdominal muscles
- weak back extensor muscles
- excessive or diminished lumbar (low back) curve
- poor posture
- use of improper body mechanics

In aerobics, the impact of each step is transmitted along the spine. These forces, coupled with any of the above factors, will cause pain. Following a physician's examination, exercises to strengthen the spinal muscles and/or abdominals may be prescribed. Care must be taken to avoid vigorously twisting the back with feet planted, excessive arching of the back, or standing with the knees hyperextended.

Icing

Using ice for 24–48 hours after an injury is very helpful in decreasing swelling and pain. However, icing may also be prescribed following the acute stage of your injury. It may also be used for conditions where inflammation or irritation of a ligament or tendon is found, i.e., tennis elbow, tendinitis.

There are two reasons why icing is a useful treatment:

- Applying cold for 10–15 minutes will cause the blood vessels to constrict and decrease the blood flow. *Result:* swelling will decrease and pain will be lessened (due to the numbing effect).
- At about 15–20 minutes, the skin temperature gets to about 59°F and a reflex (automatic) increase of blood flow occurs. *Result:* the increased blood flow has an increased healing effect.

> Icing = less swelling and pain and greater healing

How to ice

You may either freeze water in small paper cups, then peel back the paper as you gently massage the area for 20 minutes, *or* make an ice bag out of two plastic garbage bags (use the type you would have in your kitchen container). Place one bag inside the other and fill about half full of ice. Use crushed ice or ice cubes you have smashed a little as they will fit better and not be so heavy.

Next, add about 1½–2 cups cold water to bag. Tie the bag tightly. It helps if you twist the top of the bag several times and then wrap tape around the top snugly to prevent leakage.

When To See A Physician

Don't underestimate an injury. The saying, "no pain, no gain," is not entirely true. Respect pain as an indicator that something is not right. Reduce your activity to a pain-free level or intensity. Pain from an acute injury which is accompanied by considerable swelling and/or loss of function should be evaluated within one to three days. Pain which comes on gradually should be evaluated if it persists longer than 10–14 days despite a reduction of the activity and the use of local ice and aspirin.

Return To Aerobics

Return gradually to aerobics following an injury. A rule of thumb is to allow two weeks of gradual increase in activity for every week of disability. Try to find a substitute activity that you can do pain-free to maintain your cardiovascular condition while temporarily disabled. Remember to include specific stretching and strengthening exercises for the injured area in the rehabilitation process.

Summary

The repetitive nature and the impact loading to the extremities which occur during aerobics exercise can cause chronic, overuse injuries to the musculoskeletal system. Some of the common injuries include: tendinitis, plantar fasciitis, stress fractures, and patellar pain. If caught early enough, many of these injuries can be self-treated by decreasing activity to a comfortable level, the use of local ice, the use of aspirin, and appropriate rehabilitative exercises. Orthotics or shock-absorbing insoles may be useful. Pain, swelling, discoloration, loss of function, and bony point tenderness should be investigated by a physician.

Commonly Asked Questions

Q. What is the primary cause of overuse injuries?
A. Repetitive overuse or repetitive microtrauma.

Q. What is involved in the early treatment of an overuse injury?
A. The use of ice, decreasing the activity to a pain-free level, the use of aspirin, gentle stretching and strengthening exercises.

Q. Name four common injuries of the foot.
A. Metatarsalgia, plantar fasciitis, tendinitis, and stress fractures.

Q. What may be done to the shoe to alleviate the pain of the achilles tendinitis?
A. The addition of a ¼ or ⅜ inch heel lift to each shoe.

Q. What constitutes early treatment for an acute injury?
A. RICE—rest, ice, compression, and elevation.

Q. What are shin splints? What are some of the causes of shin splints?
A. An overuse injury affecting the lower leg, specifically, the posterior tibial muscle (a type of tendinitis). Shin splints may be caused by tight calf muscles, overuse, improper or well-worn shoes, hard, unyielding surfaces, excessive pronation at the ankle joint.

156 ESSENTIALS OF AEROBIC EXERCISE

Q. What are the signs of an anterior compartment syndrome?
A. Pain, swelling, warmth, redness, tenderness over the front of the shin, numbness on the top of the foot, weakness of the anterior tibial muscles (foot drop).

Q. What are the mechanisms for a knee ligament sprain or cartilage injury?
A. A sudden hyperextension, twisting of the knee with the foot fixed on the ground, a rapid, forcible squat.

Q. When would orthotics be used to treat knee pain?
A. If the knee pain results from a malalignment at the foot, e.g., excess pronation or supination (high arch).

Q. When and under what circumstances should a physician be consulted for an overuse injury?
A. If pain which comes on gradually persists for more than 10–14 days despite a reduction of activity and the use of ice and aspirin.

Part B

Developing an Aerobic Program

Chapter 1

Fitness Testing and Exercise Prescription

William C. Day, Ph.D.

The ideal way to get someone started on an exercise program is to evaluate his or her capacity for exercise, then design a program suited to that individual's fitness level, medical condition, and activity interests. This is the norm for specialized programs dealing with "high-risk" individuals such as coronary heart disease patients. It is not as prevalent among programs geared to the general population.

Exercise instructors should be familiar with the basic principles of fitness testing and exercise prescription. This information will not only enhance the level of professionalism but also may be helpful in interpreting test results and prescriptions and in advising program participants about testing and prescription services available in the community.

In this chapter, basic information on different areas of testing is presented—including exercise testing, cardiorespiratory fitness, muscular strength and endurance and flexibility testing. This chapter also covers the fundamentals of exercise prescription for each of these aspects of physical fitness. The purpose is to make the reader familiar enough with fitness testing and exercise prescription so as to be able to discuss it with potential program participants. It is not meant to be comprehensive. The References offer an opportunity to explore in greater depth.

Fitness Testing

Exercise testing

Exercise testing—also known as stress testing, graded exercise testing, or treadmill testing—doubles as a cardiorespiratory fitness test and a medical test for the diagnosis and prognosis of coronary heart disease. A person's physiologic responses to gradually increasing intensities of exercise are evaluated by using a treadmill or cycle ergometer as the instrument for controlling and quantifying the amount of effort expended. Typically, the person's heart rate and blood pressure are measured during each stage of the test. In addition, an electrocardiogram is constantly monitored, along with any physical signs or symptoms that might be elicited by the exercise. If there is no response that might cause the test to be stopped sooner, the person is usually encouraged to keep going until shortness of breath or muscle fatigue makes it difficult to continue.

The level of cardiorespiratory fitness is indicated by the level of work load, speed, and grade reached by the end of the test. A person who has a high capacity for moving blood and oxygen to exercising muscles, and who uses the oxygen once it's delivered, will reach a greater work load before becoming fatigued than an individual with a lower aerobic capacity. Some clinics or laboratories actually measure the amount of oxygen used by the person at each work level. Most simply estimate it based on the predictable and linear relationship between work load and oxygen consumption during either treadmill or cycle ergometer exercise.

The terms used to describe the highest level reached are *aerobic capacity, functional capacity*, or *functional aerobic capacity*. For practical purposes, these are synonymous and reflect a person's fitness for prolonged large muscle exercise such as running or cycling.

These exercise tests also determine the heart's ability to function normally while a demand for increased cardiac output is placed on it. This is evaluated by monitoring heart rate and blood pressure, as well as changes in the EKG pattern and any other signs or symptoms—such as chest pressure or pain—which might suggest an impaired oxygen supply to the heart muscle.

A frequently asked question is "Does a person need an exercise test before participating in an exercise program?" First of all, it must be understood that the exercise test is far from perfect in its ability to determine who will and who will not develop cardiac problems while engaging in exercise. That's why organizations such as the American College of Sports Medicine have established guidelines for determining who should be exercise tested prior to starting an exercise program. Generally, an exercise test is not necessary for those under 40 years of age who are without symptoms and at low risk of having cardiovascular disease prior to beginning an exercise program. On the other hand, the test is recommended for those who have cardiovascular, pulmonary, or metabolic disease (such as diabetes), and for those over 35 years of age who have identified risk factors for cardiovascular disease.

Most hospitals and clinics offer exercise testing services, as do many private physicians. In addition, a number of YMCAs, Jewish Community Centers, private health clubs, and similar organizations have this service available to their members and, in many instances, the general public. Many college and universities offer exercise testing through their allied health science or health and physical education schools. In addition, the local chapter of the American Heart Association may provide a listing of facilities within its area.

Cardiorespiratory fitness

Several tests of cardiorespiratory fitness are available. Most of the non-clinical variety fall into one of three categories:

- heart rate response to submaximal exercise (cycle ergometer or treadmill)
- heart rate recovery from standardized work load (step test)
- performance tests (1½ mile run/walk)

Heart rate response to submaximal exercise

Either a treadmill or cycle ergometer is used for this type of test. Heart rate and often blood pressure and the participant's rating of the level of exertion experienced are recorded at one or more submaximal work loads lasting three to six minutes. The heart rate response is used to estimate the aerobic capacities of individuals, using the assumption that the maximal heart rate is predictable based upon the person's age. Generally, persons with high aerobic capacities will attain relatively high work loads before reaching a given submaximal heart rate, while those less fit will reach that heart rate at lower work loads.

Although these are effective tests and offer an objective means for measuring progress and motivating exercise program participants, they do have limitations and precautions attached to them. They are not medical tests and are not used for detection of the presence or absence of disease. Persons with cardiovascular, pulmonary, or metabolic diseases as well as those at high risk should be cleared by a physician prior to taking this type of test. There are many individuals who have a low exercise heart rate response due to medications they are taking or the presence of cardiac disease. Obviously, using the heart rate response to estimate aerobic capacity would be inappropriate in these people. Finally, even among healthy individuals, there is some variability in the maximal heart rates for a given age group—so that the estimated aerobic capacity for a given person could differ from the actual measured results of a maximal exercise test.

Given the limitations, these tests do give reproducible results and help categorize a person's fitness level. Also, they give objective evidence of the relative success of the conditioning program.

The testing should be done by trained and, preferably, certified test administrators. Many organizations which feature adult fitness programs—such as YMCAs, Jewish Community Centers, private health clubs and fitness centers and colleges and universities—will have these tests available.

Heart rate recovery tests

These tests measure the speed of recovery of heart rate toward its resting level after exercise. The most widely used form of exercise is stepping up and down on a bench. The size of the bench and the rate of stepping vary among the different protocols available. A popular test is the 3-Minute Step Test which uses a 12-inch step and a rate of 24 steps per minute—a work rate that is within the comfort range of most healthy young to middle-aged adults. Other tests which use a higher step and a faster rate may be too difficult for many unfit people.

This type of test may be useful to broadly categorize a person's level of fitness. It carries the same limitations with respect to heart rate response as those listed for the submaximal exercise heart rate tests. One disadvantage is not knowing what is happening while the person is exercising. Also, the recovery heart rate is not as good a predictor of aerobic capacity as the heart rate actually measured during exercise.

The same precautions should be followed to clear people for these tests as those suggested for the submaximal exercise heart rate tests. The level of training required to actually administer these tests is less than that required for the cycle ergometer or treadmill tests—but there should be qualified people available for proper interpretation. Many of the same organizations mentioned earlier may also be able to administer these tests. Often, a college or university in the area has students trained in test administration.

Performance tests

Tests such as the 1½ mile run/walk, in which a person attempts to cover the distance in as short a time as possible, are very good estimators of aerobic capacity—but carry the obvious risk of subjecting the participants to maximal exercise without benefit of monitoring any of the variables which can be closely watched during clinical exercise testing. Obviously, only young, healthy individuals who are without symptoms and at low risk should attempt this strenuous test.

Muscular strength and endurance

In simple terms, muscular strength is the maximum force that can be generated by a muscle or a group of muscles. Endurance is the ability of the muscle or muscle group to perform repeated contractions.

With the advent of isokinetic testing and training equipment (Cybex), strength testing moved into the "high tech" age. An isokinetic exercise or movement is one in which the speed of muscular contraction is held constant while the person applies maximum force through the entire range of motion while attempting to perform the movement more quickly. (The testing equipment won't allow the person to move faster than the preset rate, and if the rate of contraction becomes less than the preset rate, no resistance is encountered.)

Although this is an impressive and effective way to test strength and endurance, the equipment is expensive and its use, for the most part, has been confined to the evaluation and rehabilitation of sports injuries. It does have the advantage of being able to quickly and accurately assess most major muscle groups and thereby identify strength imbalances which may exist between opposing muscle groups. Sports medicine and physical therapy clinics are the most probable sources of information on the availability and advisability of isokinetic testing.

There are several practical approaches to testing strength and endurance. Strength can be evaluated by having a person successfully perform one repetition of a given movement with the highest possible load. This is called a 1RM or one repetition at maximal effort. Administration of this type of test requires careful selection of appropriate loads and adequate rest between efforts so that fatigue doesn't become a factor. Also, careful selection of people for whom this is a safe procedure is important. For example, it would not be advisable for persons with heart disease or high blood pressure to be performing maximal efforts.

Muscular endurance can be measured by having the person repeat a movement at a given resistance as many times as possible. The resistance could be either a percentage of maximum (50% of 1 RM) or a fixed load (40 lb for women and 70 lb for men). Also, it could be a load which has been adjusted to the person's body weight. A commonly used exercise for evaluating both upper body strength and endurance is the bench press—using either free weights or a bench press exercise machine.

Finally, there is a category of strength and endurance tests which requires little or no equipment. Examples include push ups, pull ups and sit ups. One problem with this form of test is the difficulty that exists in standardizing the execution of the movement. Another problem is that people with low muscular strength or excessive body fat may be unable to perform even a single repetition.

Obviously, careful screening is advisable before allowing a person to perform any of these tests. Along with the high-risk individuals discussed earlier, caution must be taken when testing persons with injuries or with bone and joint conditions which might be aggravated by the exercise.

Flexibility

Flexibility—the range of movement of a given joint of the body—can be assessed with instruments such as a goniometer or with simple tests requiring little or no equipment, such as the Sit and Reach Test.

A goniometer is a device with two arms that rotate about a fulcrum with a scale showing degrees of movement. The fulcrum is carefully positioned at the point of rotation of the joint, and each arm is accurately placed along the body parts above and below the joint. The range of movement of that joint is then measured.

This type of testing is not the norm, however. It, like isokinetic strength evaluations, is more likely to be used in sports medicine, orthopedic and physical therapy clinics and in college and university research laboratories.

The most popular of the practical, low cost tests is the Sit and Reach Test. It assesses the flexibility of the lower back and hamstring muscle groups. The person sits on the floor with legs extended and spread slightly apart. He or she then reaches forward as far as possible without bending the knees or bouncing. The reach is measured with a yardstick placed on the floor between the legs or on a box against which the feet are placed.

Tests such as Sit and Reach can easily be administered in most facilities. The main requirement, other than the minimal equipment necessary, is a trained test administrator.

Exercise Prescription

The concept of prescribing exercise as one would prescribe medicine evolved from the early cardiac rehabilitation days when it was recognized that exercise, in order to be safe and effective, had to be carefully regulated for each individual's capabilities and needs.

Aerobic exercise

The prescription for aerobic exercise is usually based on the results of an exercise test, though it is possible to give a reasonable prescription based upon submaximal testing. The major disadvantages of using only submaximal testing are that the person's actual maximal heart rate may be unknown and some clinical signs will go unmonitored. As long as the prescription is within the submaximal range tested, especially for low-risk healthy individuals, this should not present much of a problem.

Six considerations are important in prescribing an aerobic exercise program:

1. Type of activity
2. Intensity of effort
3. Duration of each session
4. Frequency of participation
5. Progressive increase in the amount of exercise performed
6. Precautions for avoiding injury.

Type   Whatever activity is chosen, it should involve the large muscle groups and be one which can be performed for a prolonged time period. Examples include running, walking, cycling, swimming and rhythmical aerobic exercise. Other considerations include the individual's interest in and skill at the activity and ability to fit it into his or her schedule.

Intensity   This is the most difficult part of the prescription to translate to the participant. As a general rule, the more unfit the individual, the lower the relative intensity of the exercise. Relative intensity refers to percentage of functional capacity. An unfit individual with a very low functional capacity may start a program as low as 40%–50% of functional capacity while a well-conditioned person may exercise at 80%–90% of capacity. To be effective, conditioning programs should eventually elicit intensities of 60%–90% of functional capacity.

The most widely used method for prescribing intensity is to give the person a heart rate range for exercising which will keep him or her within the desired percentages of functional capacity. The reason this method is effective is because heart rate increases linearly with increasing intensity of exercise. The technique recommended is described in another chapter.

The success of the heart rate method is dependent on the ability to quickly and accurately determine it. Also, there are many people who are taking medications which markedly lower both resting and exercising heart rates. The most widely used are the beta blockers which are prescribed in the treatment of hypertension and heart disease. Examples include Inderal, Lopressor, and Corgard. Therefore, it is important to teach participants to pay attention to other signals of overexertion in addition to heart rate. These include the levels of muscular fatigue and shortness of breath. Rating scales for the perception of exertion are frequently used for this purpose.

Duration   The length of the aerobic exercise period will vary depending on the intensity of effort and the functional capacity of the individual. The range will usually be from 15–30 minutes. When exercising at a low intensity, the duration should be relatively longer than in sessions in which the intensity is higher. Also, those with higher functional capacities are able to exercise longer at a given relative intensity than those with lower capacities.

Frequency   The number of days per week that exercise is prescribed will depend on the intensity and duration of each session as well as the person's functional capacity. For those with very low functional capacities, the recommendation might be one or more low intensity, short-to-moderate duration sessions daily. At the other extreme, those with high functional capacities who are training at relatively high intensities would be encouraged to limit these to three to five days per week to allow for recovery and to prevent injury. For those activities in which a high level of bone and joint stress occurs, such as running and aerobic dance, a day of recovery is recommended between sessions, especially for beginners.

Progression   The beginning stages of a program should last from a few to several weeks, depending on the fitness level of the person. During this phase, emphasis is on low intensity aerobic exercises, stretching and light calisthenics. The objective is to gradually accustom the body to the increased exercise with a minimum amount of muscle soreness and risk of injury.

Next, the intensity is increased to the appropriate level (i.e., 70% or greater). Duration is gradually increased over the next few weeks before the intensity is again increased.

Eventually, most people will reach a level of fitness with which they feel comfortable. Continuing to exercise at this level on a regular basis will maintain it.

Precautions   Exercise is not without risk, and certain basic precautions should be taken to avoid injury and discouragement. Some of these are:

- Wearing footwear and clothing appropriate for safe participation in the chosen activities.
- Warming up before and cooling down after each exercise period. Both the warm-up and cool-down include low intensity aerobic exercise (e.g., walking, and stretching exercises).
- Drinking adequate amounts of water before, during and after an exercise session. This is especially important in warm environments.
- Paying attention to environmental conditions and making appropriate adjustments in intensity and duration of activity.
- Not exercising within two hours of eating a meal.
- Curtailing activity and seeking medical attention if unusual symptoms such as chest pain or pressure or persistent musculoskeletal pain occur.

Muscular strength and endurance

There are a number of approaches used in prescribing strength and endurance exercises. The overload principle is the common denominator underlying all of them. Simply put, if strength or endurance is to be improved, the muscle or muscle group must perform more work than that to which it has become accustomed.

Several variables are considered in designing a person's program:

- *equipment*: free weights, variable resistance machines, no equipment (e.g., calisthenics)
- *exercise movement*: push up, bench press, curl, etc.
- *resistance*: amount of force exerted per movement
- *repetitions*: number of times the movement is to be repeated
- *sets*: number of units performed (resistance times repetitions)
- *frequency*: number of days per week

A commonly used system involves having the individual perform eight repetitions of an exercise with a resistance that produces a near maximal effort to complete the last repetition. The number of repetitions is gradually increased to 12 over several weeks. At that point, the resistance is increased, and the number of repetitions decreased to eight and the process is repeated. One to three sets are prescribed. Strength training is best accomplished by exercising on alternate days.

Flexibility

The general recommendation for flexibility exercises is to perform a slow range of motion movements for the various joints including the shoulder, trunk, hip, knee, and ankle, along with a series of static stretches for the muscle groups involved. These are particularly important as part of the warm-up and cool-down for aerobic exercise.

Summary

Fitness testing for individuals entering exercise programs ranges from medically supervised stress tests to timed performances of a run or walk. Tests differ depending on the fitness component being tested, the sophistication of equipment used, the skill necessary for their administration and the degree of medical supervision required. The selection of tests is based on the age, health and medical risk of the individual as well as the availability of qualified testing services within the community.

An exercise prescription is based on the medical condition, fitness level and interests of the individual. The art and science of exercise prescription involves designing a safe, effective program by selecting activities to be performed at the correct combination of intensity, duration and frequency, and by gradually increasing the total amount of exercise per workout.

References

American College of Sports Medicine. *Guidelines for Graded Exercise Testing and Exercise Prescription*. Philadelphia: Lea and Febiger, 1980.

Chow, R. and Wilmore, J. "The Regulation of Exercise Intensity by Ratings of Perceived Exertion." *Journal of Cardiac Rehabilitation.* 1984:4:382–387.

Cooper, K. *The Aerobics Program for Total Well Being.* New York: Bantam, 1983.

Ellestad, M. *Stress Test-Principles and Practice.* Philadelphia: Davis, 1980.

Froelicher, V. *Exercise Testing and Training.* New York: LeJacq Publishing, 1983.

Pollock, M. et al. *Health and Fitness through Physical Activity.* New York: Wiley, 1978.

Chapter 2

Class Design and Conduct

Marti Steele West, BA
Linda Shelton, BA

The preceding chapters have outlined the major developmental and physiological areas that dictate aerobic class conduct. It is important to note that the AFAA exercise guidelines are recommendations based on correct body alignment, mechanics, and form as governed by physiological parameters and are designed to produce the most effective and safe workout within a one-hour time period.

Too many instructors are uninformed, usually because of a lack of training, of proper alignment or correct techniques. Sometimes instructors rely on exercises that are more fun than effective or that have been handed around from instructor to instructor. The reason that many of these are ineffective is because the exercise is not specific enough to offer enough resistance to produce muscular work within the various ranges of motion possible. Remember, quantity does not equal quality. Twenty-five side-lying leg lifts properly executed can do more for body toning of the outer thigh than 400 of them in the wrong position.

In this chapter, we will closely examine the design and content of a one-hour aerobic exercise class, breaking it down into the following categories:

- pre-class procedure
- warm-up
- upper body
- aerobics/post-aerobic cool-down
- waist exercises
- lower body
- abdomen
- static stretch

170 DEVELOPING AN AEROBIC PROGRAM

The format for this chapter follows the outline of the Basic Exercise Standards and Guidelines. Please refer to these guidelines (at the beginning of this book) for the recommended order of activities to include in a class.

Within each of the above sections, the following topics will be discussed as appropriate:

- time allotment
- which muscles are being used
- purpose of the exercises
- examples of specific exercises
- variations and transitions
- injury prevention
- risk factors
- adaptive techniques

Class Format

In order to provide a both safe and effective workout, care must be taken to design a class that follows a physiologically sound progression. Not only will the student benefit by avoiding possible injury, but the class will flow from one exercise to the next in a smooth, coordinated fashion.

AFAA recommends the following progression:

1. Pre-class instruction
2. Warm-up: A balanced combination of rhythmic limbering exercises and static stretching
3. The following exercises performed in a standing position, preferably in this in order:
   a. Standing leg work (not recommended immediately following aerobics)
   b. Arms, chest and shoulders
   c. Aerobics and cool-down
   d. Standing waist work
4. Floor work, in order of preference:
   a. Legs
   b. Buttocks
   c. Hips
   d. Abdominals
5. Static stretching and cool down

The above sequence is desirable not only because it is physiologically correct but, as mentioned earlier, it will keep the flow of the class smooth. By completing all of the standing exercises before the floor work, you will avoid creating "exercise gaps" caused by getting up and down off the floor.

If, however, the above sequence does not fit the policy of the exercise studio, or your personal preference, the progression may be changed so long as these following basic guidelines are observed:
- Always begin class with a warm-up period.
- Always end class with static stretching.
- Always follow aerobics with a sufficient cool-down period.
- Upon completion of strengthening exercises within a specific muscle group, briefly stretch those muscles before proceeding to the next group.

Pre-Class Procedure

Health screening
Your most important responsibility as an instructor is to provide your students with a safe and effective exercise program. This responsibility begins the moment they walk in the door. How do you know that it will be safe for an individual to participate in your class, no matter how safe your instruction? Obviously, we can't demand a complete physical examination with a stress test of every student, but we can provide some basic guidelines and screening methods to help protect their safety. [III.A: Medical Clearance] These should be discussed with all new students under 35 who have been physically active and who will generally need little or no medical supervision. For those who have been inactive, however, regardless of age, a physical exam is desirable before beginning an exercise program.

Finding the target zone
To many new students terms such as "aerobics" and "heart rate" will have little meaning. Briefly define aerobics [VI.A: Aerobics] and its purpose and explain how to find one's individual target zone. Demonstrate how to quickly find the pulse and explain at what point in the class you will ask them to find it. If a target heart rate chart is used, point out purpose and the procedure.

Shoes
If some class members are without shoes, AFAA strongly recommends they obtain and use proper shoes as a means of reducing the risk of injury to feet, knees and shins. This should be explained to the class, and the criteria for appropriate shoes discussed.

Introduction
Introduce yourself and announce the level of the class. Unless class level is specific, i.e., beginner or advanced, it is best to teach at an intermediate level and explain to the class how to adjust the individual exercises to their particular level of fitness and experience. In other words, try to give both a beginning and advanced version of your exercises, while performing at an

intermediate level. Motor skill, flexibility, intensity and duration capabilities of individuals are all factors to be considered.

As the class begins Explain that the class is non-competitive and that all participants should work at their own levels. Make sure the class is aware of the danger signs. [I.H: Danger Signs] In case of any other sharp pain experienced while exercising, the activity should be discontinued immediately and discussed with instructor following class. Remind students that breathing should follow a consistent rhythmic pattern throughout the class. The activity will reflexively dictate rate and depth of respiration. Do not restrict inhalation to the nose. Inspire and expire through the nose and mouth in a relaxed fashion.

The Warm-up

Purpose

The warm-up period is crucial to a successful workout for several reasons. Basically, it will help prepare the body for more vigorous exercise by increasing the flexibility of muscles, tendons and ligaments, thus allowing for a full range of motion while minimizing the possibility of injury. Without a sufficient and properly executed warm-up period, smooth, full range movement is not possible and the incidence of injury is much higher due to possible sudden movements which may cause straining or even tearing of a muscle or tendon.

Progression of movement

The warm-up period should last a minimum of 7-10 minutes and should consist of a balanced combination of static stretching and smoothly performed, rhythmic limbering exercises. In order to maintain a smooth flow, one should follow a specific order. Warm up from either the head to the toes, or vice versa (i.e., don't skip from the neck to the ankles, to arms and back to the calves). Currently, the most controversial issue in the exercise field seems to be whether static stretches should precede rhythmic warm-ups, or vice versa.

Muscle groups

In a correctly performed warm-up period it is important that all of the major muscle groups be used. However, it is especially important that those muscle groups which will be placed under the greatest stress in the more vigorous exercise to follow, be carefully and fully warmed up. An example of this would be the attention paid by a pitcher to the gradual and complete warm-up of his pitching arm, in addition to a general body warm-up. The warm-up period should be a gradual rehearsal of the same movements that will be performed more forcefully and through a wider range of motion in the activity to follow.

We recommend that all of the following muscle groups be warmed up at the beginning of class with, as mentioned above, special attention directed to those areas performing the hardest:
- head and neck (suboccipital group)
- shoulders, upper back, arms and chest (trapezius, deltoid, biceps, triceps and pectoralis major)
- rib cage, waist and lower back (external oblique, latissimus dorsi)
- front and back of thigh (quadriceps and hamstrings)
- inner thigh (hip adductors, gracilis)
- calf (gastrocnemius, soleus)
- feet and ankles

Type of movements

As mentioned earlier, the warm-up period should consist of a balanced combination of static stretch and rhythmic limbering exercise. A complete discussion of stretching technique will be found in the chapter on flexibility. The type of movement that we would term rhythmic limbering would include exercises smoothly performed at a moderate pace that directly involve different types of movements of the bones in the joints. Some examples would be small arm circles, leg circles, knee lifts, high reaches and small kicks. Movements should be gentle and controlled. All ballistic and jerky movements should be avoided, as injury could occur.

Do's and Dont's

1. Do warm-up and stretch the lower back before attempting any lateral movement of the upper torso, e.g., side bends.
2. Don't do traditional straight leg toe touches to stretch the hamstrings. Hyperextension of the knee joint places undesirable stress on the lower back and on the knee itself. Always roll down and come up with knees relaxed.
3. Don't do the plow as this position has the potential for injury to the vertebrae and discs of the cervical spine. Only under controlled circumstances should "the plow" be used for therapeutic purposes, and even under the direction of a qualified therapist its use is still very controversial.

The Upper Body

Purpose

In many exercise regimens, particularly those performed by women, we find that the upper body is often neglected. Strong, firm muscles in the arms, chest and shoulders are important to help maintain correct body alignment and posture. Another benefit to women is that strengthening of the pectoral muscles will help provide natural support for the breasts. Major muscles which should be the focus of upper body work include: biceps, triceps, pectoralis major, deltoid and trapezius.

Progression and time

A minimum of five to seven minutes of specific upper body exercise is recommended. These exercises should be performed with the lower body stationary or with limited movement. Upper body exercises may be performed before, during or immediately after aerobics. If performed during aerobics, the footwork should be kept very simple (e.g., an easy jog), in order that the arms, and/or chest and shoulders may be the area of concentrated work. Also, it is important to remember that arm exercises, particularly large arm movements, may significantly elevate the heart rate.

Correct performance

As mentioned in the chapters on conditioning, muscle strengthening requires repetitive movement against a resistance. In the case of upper body work, it is important to understand that consciously creating tension in the working muscle will help provide the necessary resistance. Movement that does not involve a consciously created tension or resistance within the working muscles will not provide the desired training effect. For instance, performing an arm curl by simply raising and lowering the lower arm (moving the lower from one point to another), would require many more repetitions to achieve the desired training effect than working the biceps and triceps and the lower arm up and down against resistance.

The position for performing upper body work should be with the body correctly aligned, abdomen held firmly and the shoulders not pulled up, backwards or forwards. Arm exercises performed while bending forward may be included for variety, however care should be taken to keep knees bent and to not remain in this position for an extended period as many participants will not have sufficient quadriceps strength to support the upper body and they could risk straining the lower back.

The speed at which exercises are performed is important. [I.D: **Speed, Isolation, and Resistance**] Performing a movement for every beat of the music is not necessary and, depending on the particular exercise, perhaps not very safe or effective. Try executing movements on every other beat (half-speed) as a means of providing a more controlled exercise.

Aerobics

As we have seen, an aerobic exercise class does not consist entirely of exercises providing an aerobic training benefit to the participant. The term *aerobic exercise class* has become the popular name to designate an exercise class containing an aerobic workout.

Why aerobics?

Your students will want to know why all this sweating and hard breathing is necessary. As we discovered in previous chapters, there are many reasons for participating in aerobic exercise. The following is a simplified explanation of aerobic exercise that is useful in discussions with your class.

Aerobic exercises are those which create an increased demand for oxygen over an extended period of time, such as jogging. Anaerobic literally means "without oxygen." Aerobic exercises train the heart, lungs and cardiovascular system to process and deliver oxygen quickly and efficiently to every part of the body. As the heart muscle becomes stronger and more efficient, it is able to pump more blood with each stroke and in fewer strokes, thus facilitating the rapid transport of oxygen to all parts of the body. An aerobically fit cardiovascular system will allow the individual to work longer, more vigorously and recover more quickly.

How long?

Although there is some controversy regarding the length of time that we must perform an aerobic activity, 20 minutes of continuous aerobic activity working with the target heart rate zone is considered the minimum time necessary to achieve a training benefit. Time allowed for rhythmic activities preceding and following the aerobic workout should be considered in addition to this 20 minutes.

How often?

In order to improve one's fitness level, four times a week is considered the optimum number of aerobic workouts. Three times per week will maintain and possibly improve the fitness level, and with only two times per week one will generally witness no major improvement and possibly a decline in overall fitness, depending on the activity level of the individual. An individual who was sedentary before beginning an exercise program will see an improvement in cardiovascular capability with very little training.

If students are only taking your class twice a week, or if they desire to train four or five days a week, they may use a different aerobic training method such as jogging or swimming. Exercising six to seven days a week, unless following a strictly monitored training program allowing for easy and hard days and varied exercise activities, can lead to certain overuse syndromes including fatigue and possible stress-induced orthopedic injuries.

Correct alignment

Correct body alignment is important in order to prevent unnecessary stress and possible injury to the feet, ankles, shins, knees and back. As with most exercises performed in an upright position, the abdominals should be held firmly and the shoulders carried in a relaxed position, back and down—not tense, not hunched forward. Do not lean forward, as this can contribute to shin splints, but do keep body weight balanced forward over the entire foot and not backwards on heels.

Foot placement and surface considerations

Heels should always come all the way down to the floor. Don't jog on your toes, as this shortens the calf muscles and Achilles tendon. Aerobics should ideally be performed on a wooden floor with a cushion of air beneath (not wood laid directly on concrete). This type of floor has a certain amount of "give" to it and is much less stressful on the bones and ligaments of the feet, ankles and legs. If jogging on concrete is unavoidable, mats should be used. In any case, well-fitting shoes designed for aerobics that provide sufficient support and cushion should always be worn.

Breathing

Steady rhythmic breathing (using both nose and mouth) which fits the exercise and does not impede mechanics should be used. Remind your students that aerobic means "with oxygen." Watch out for breath holders and periodically include definite times for students to inhale and exhale. Providing instruction will help the student develop his or her own breathing patterns in response to the intensity level of the activities performed.

Aerobic warm-up

The warm-up period should be approximately three to five minutes long. During this time the student will experience a gradual increase in heart rate and warm up the knees and ankles. Movements performed during this period should involve the large muscle groups in continuous, moderate, rhythmic activities. Examples would be: step-touches, with low arm swings, walking, gentle lunges and arm work with a very low level jog. Try to avoid lateral (side to side) moves during the first three minutes, allowing ankles and feet to become sufficiently warmed up. The goal is to start slowly and gradually increase both the intensity and the range of motion of your movements. This period can be a good opportunity to exercise the arms, chest and shoulders, while providing the necessary transition of a warm-up for your aerobic workout.

The aerobic workout

The next 20 minutes are the core of your entire class. Instruct carefully during this period in order to maximize potential benefits while minimizing possible hazards. A primary consideration, beyond providing a sufficient aerobic warm-up period, is knowing how to personalize the aerobic workout to fit the needs of the individual student. Obviously, most classes will contain students of varying fitness levels. Not everyone will be able to safely perform the same movements and derive the same benefits. Your job as an instructor is to provide the proper instruction and motivation that will encourage each student to work at an appropriate training level.

The two major variables which you must teach your students to adjust on an individual basis, are *intensity and range of motion*. Duration, as mentioned earlier, is basically set at 20 minutes. Intensity and range of motion are both inextricably tied to and basically measurable by monitoring the heart rate. For instance, a student who upon monitoring heart rate discovers that she is not working hard enough to be within her target zone, can rapidly increase her heart rate and intensity by making larger arm movements and/or lifting the knees higher as she continues the footwork pattern. The opposite would also hold true for an individual who is working too hard.

Two simple equations will help you remember:

- Smaller steps, smaller arms movements, less force applied for each movement = lower heart rate.
- Larger steps, larger arm movements, greater force applied to each movement = higher heart rate.

For the instructor teaching students of various fitness levels, we recommend that you teach your entire class, and particularly your aerobic workout, at an intermediate level, but always provide the necessary instruction to allow both the beginner and the advanced student to individualize the exercise to fit their particular demands. Strive to create a non-competitive atmosphere in which the goal is not to "keep going, keep kicking, higher and higher," but rather to encourage the students to work for themselves, seeking the ideal training level and learning more about themselves by listening to their own bodies, not just the words of you, the instructor.

Monitoring heart rate   In previous chapters, we discussed target heart rate zone and its application in an aerobic workout. As indicated below, monitoring an individual's target heart rate will provide a method of personalizing the workout to fit individual fitness requirements. In practical application, the pulses should be located immediately following vigorous exercise. Have students keep walking while taking heart rate. Count to 10 and multiply by 6. This number should be in your individual target zone. If it is higher or lower than the acceptable limits of your range, you will need to adjust the intensity of your exercise as described in the preceding section. Ideally, heart rates should be taken five minutes after the beginning of active aerobic work, and at least once more before beginning to cool down. Recovery heart rate should also be taken five minutes after the cessation of vigorous aerobic work. As an instructor it is important for you to respond to how a participant looks or says he or she feels during an aerobic workout. Signs to look for that indicate one is working too hard include: extremely labored breathing, nausea, lightheadedness, or the appearance that they are forcing themselves with every movement. These individuals should be urged to slow down. Generally, participants should be working at a level where they could carry on a conversation. In other words, not panting or gasping. Experienced students who are used to taking their heart rates will generally be able to perceive the exertion level they are working at without stopping to take heart rate, as they have learned to correlate how they are feeling and how hard they are breathing with their heart rate. Monitoring your class by perceived exertion alone is not recommended, however, as many students, particularly beginners without experience of monitoring their heart rate, have a distorted or inaccurate perception of how hard they are working relative to their heart rate.

Type of movements   As mentioned earlier, one should gradually increase the intensity and range of motion of movement during the aerobic workout. This also includes complexity. Whether using a choreographed routine or a series of combination moves interspersed with jogging, those movements requiring coordination of both arms and legs should be entered into slowly, starting with either the arms or the legs and then adding the other. Build upon your moves instead of trying to teach a complicated combination movement all at once. Let your students feel pleased and comfortable with their own accomplishments, not simply overwhelmed with your agility and coordination. Care should also be taken to observe the orthopedic considerations discussed earlier. Straight leg jumping or continuous hops on one foot should definitely be avoided as they are extremely stressful to the knees.

Peak movements are generally defined as any large movement using both arms and legs that require a greater amount of oxygen be delivered to the working muscles (such as swinging the arms to touch the toes during high leg kicks). These movements should not be attempted in the first three to four minutes of aerobic work and should not be maintained for more than 30 seconds to one minute. Following peak movements, one should work at a lower intensity activity such as jogging. In essence, this is a type of interval training which is characterized by periods of high intensity work interspersed with activities requiring a moderate energy expenditure.

If one were to perform peak movements continuously, a major portion of energy would be supplied through the anaerobic production of lactic acid. Once lactic acid production is initiated, levels will rise and cause exhaustion within only a few minutes. However, during *intermittent* exercise, the maximum benefit to the muscles and cardiovascular system is derived before lactic acid has a chance to accumulate. A brief rest period is all that's needed to lower these levels, thus preventing exhaustion.

Post-Aerobic Cool-Down
Purpose
The third and final phase of the aerobic workout is the cool-down period which immediately follows vigorous aerobic work. The importance of this phase cannot be overstressed as many potentially hazardous cardiac irregularities occur following, not during an aerobic workout.

During the aerobic workout, the heart rate and breathing rate were elevated in order to meet the body's oxygen demands. However, during approximately the first three minutes of the aerobic workout, the immediate energy requirements are met through the anaerobic breakdown of ATP, and oxygen consuming reactions do not supply the energy needs until the body reaches steady-state. An oxygen debt is created during the first few minutes of exercise which must be repaid during the recovery period. After moderate steady-state exercise this debt is completely paid and oxygen consumption has returned to the resting level within one or two minutes. During this recovery time the exerciser should continue performing rhythmic movements with the limbs in order to help return the flow of blood to heart.

Without a gradual cool-down period, the blood which is pooled in the extremities immediately after an aerobic workout, can't get back to the heart and the brain where it is needed. By stopping abruptly, the large muscles which were pushing the blood back to the heart during exercise are no longer doing this job and as much as 60% of the blood can remain pooled below the waist. This venous pooling will cause a drop in blood pressure and decreased blood flow to the brain, possibly causing dizziness, lightheadedness, nausea, or cardiac irregularities.

Exercise method
Keep your class moving for three to five minutes following the aerobic workout. Appropriate movements would include walking and step-touch sequences, both including moderate arm movements. The same continuous rhythmic movements that are used in the aerobic warm-up could also be used to gradually decrease the exercise level.

Breathing during the recovery period should be relaxed with the rate and depth dictated by physiological reflexes. Students should learn to be aware of their own oxygen requirements and learn to regulate their breathing accordingly. After approximately three to four minutes, the calves, quadriceps and hamstrings should all be stretched before proceeding.

Heart rate
After five minutes of cool-down activities, the heart rate should equal less than 60% of your maximum (220 minus your age, multiplied by .6). If the

heart rate is still elevated, the individual should continue walking slowly until it has dropped sufficiently.

Taking a recovery heart rate can show if the cool-down period has been sufficient and if you were exercising at a level that was too intense. The length of time that it takes for the heart rate to return to resting value is generally indicative of one's aerobic training.

In an aerobically fit individual, the heart rate will recover to its resting level more quickly than in an untrained individual. For your students this can be a good method of monitoring their progress if they elect to chart their recovery heart rate and the improvement in recovery time. This will be the first place evidence of cardiovascular training improvements can be seen.

Waist

Many individuals seem to have some confusion about waist exercises, and proceed as though the waist was comprised of one large encircling muscle that could be magically drawn in. In reality, the muscles that when toned and strong define the waist area are the internal and external oblique muscles. Thus the most effective waist exercises are abdominal curls with a lateral twist, as described in the preceding sections.

Standing waist exercises are very popular though not very effective. The rhythmic quality of the movements involved makes these exercises ideal for aerobic warm-up or cool-down.

The problem with many waist exercises lies in the injuries that could occur to the lower back because of improper alignment and mechanics.

To avoid injury to the lower back while performing standing waist exercises, the following guidelines should be observed:

1. Always align the body correctly. Stand tall and yet keep posture relaxed, not tense. Imagine a "midline" running from the top of your head down through the middle of your body. Try to keep your body balanced in relation to this imaginary midline. Abdominal muscles should be held firmly in an up, shoulders back and down.
2. As the upper body is moved to the side, make sure that the shoulder doesn't drop forward or pull backward. The shoulder should drop directly to the side.
3. Don't hyperextend the knees. Hyperextension of the knees causes the lumbar spine to arch inward, placing the lower back in a position to support the stress of upper body's lateral movement. Hyperextension also places excessive stress on the ligaments of the knee joint. Keep knees slightly relaxed or soft and aligned over toes.
4. Don't reach to the side with both arms extended up over the head. All of the weight of the upper body in this position is held by the lower back.

CLASS DESIGN AND CONDUCT   181

   5. Do not jerk, move too quickly, or throw the upper body. This is especially true if performing a twisting exercise. Remember: hips forward and square, knees relaxed and aligned over toes.

Purpose

Approximately 10–15 minutes of your class time should be devoted to exercises that strengthen the muscles of the hips, thighs and buttocks. Not only are these exercises important cosmetically, but strengthening the hamstrings and the shin muscle (tibialis anterior) can prevent a muscular imbalance caused by the strengthening benefits to opposing muscles during the aerobic workout.

Outer thighs

Exercises to strengthen the outer thighs (tensor fascial latae) and hips (gluteus medius) and upper buttocks (superior gluteus maximus), are generally performed while standing, lying, or kneeling. In any of the three positions, the leg is lifted to the side and out away from the body (abduction), and returned in a smoothly controlled motion. As in all exercises, the movement should not be jerky or rely on momentum to accomplish it.

In a standing position   Outer thigh exercises performed in a standing position generally require the use of a chairback or ballet barre to help the student balance without leaning in the opposite direction. The body should be held upright with the posture correct and the feet facing forward. Without turning the knee outward, lift the leg to a maximum of 40° off the floor, and smoothly return it. The opposite hand should be used for support on a barre if needed.

Lying on the side of the body   The body should be in a straight line with the top arm squarely on the floor in front of the body. The lower leg should be relaxed. Care should be taken that the hip bones are in a vertical position and not leaning to the front or back. Just as when performing the movement in a standing position, the left should not exceed 40°, and the leg should not turn out.

As a student becomes more advanced, the leg can be worked gradually around to extend out in front of the body. This should not be attempted before developing sufficient muscular strength and control to maintain the correct alignment while performing the movement.

On the knees, hydrant position   In this position it is most important that the lower back does not arch inward to the floor. Hold the abdominals firmly and the back flat. The head should be held as a natural extension of the spine, not dropped forward or arched backwards. Place the hands facing forward and keep the body balanced. Do not lean to the opposite side to compensate for the work of the muscles. Test for correct position by lifting working leg and opposite arm at the same time.

The upward movement of the straight leg or the bent knee should be small, again only 40° at the maximum. A larger motion requires the movement of the hip and decreases the effectiveness of the exercise.

Inner thigh

The most effective exercises to strengthen the inner thigh (hip adductors), begin from the basic position. Start by lying on the side with the hips in a vertical position (as described above for outer thigh, lying on side). The upper body is either lying down or supported. The upper leg comes over the bottom leg and the foot is positioned on the floor, facing forward. Wrapping the hand around the ankle will help hold it in the correct position. In an easier variation of this position the upper leg is brought over the lower and the knee rests on the floor. Care should be taken to keep the hips correctly aligned. From either position the lower leg is then lifted toward the ceiling (adduction), with the inside of the thigh facing upwards. Again, as the leg is lowered, the movement is controlled.

Many people erroneously perform a seated leg lift to the front for inner thigh work. This type of leg lift principally involves the quadriceps and is not an appropriate exercise for the inner thigh area.

Buttocks

Exercises for the buttocks generally work the gluteus maximus and often the hamstrings. These exercises fall into two major categories: those performed on the hands and knees involving the lifting of the extended leg, and those performed on the back, knees bent and feet flat with the buttocks slightly raised and then lowered. Both positions can be very effective, yet potentially hazardous to the lower back if performed incorrectly.

Leg lifts These exercises strengthen not only the gluteus maximus, but the hamstrings as well, an important consideration in light of the tremendous work the quadriceps perform during aerobics. The injury potential, however, cannot be overstated. It is imperative that these leg lifts be performed correctly so as to avoid injury to the lumbar spine.

On the hands and knees with the weight evenly distributed, extend one leg directly behind the body. The back should be flat and not arched in. Lower the foot to the floor. Raise and lower the extended leg in a controlled, non-throwing manner. *Do not raise the leg above the hips.* Lifting the leg up as high as you can go causes a tremendous amount of compression of the vertebral discs in the lower back. Any time the leg extends higher than the hips, one should drop down to the elbows and strive to keep the back in a straight line.

Pelvic lifts   When performed properly, pelvic lifts can be a wonderful exercise for the gluteus maximus. It is important to remember that height, in this and in many exercises, is not the goal.

Lying on the back, knees should be bent and feet flat on the floor. The middle and upper back should be held firmly against the floor as though a thread running through your body was pulling the bellybutton to the floor. Smoothly tilt the pelvis forward while contracting the buttocks. Release and repeat. Do not arch the back up off the floor.

Abdomen

Purpose

Exercises designed to strengthen the muscles of the abdomen are an important element in any exercise program. Strong abdominal muscles will not only provide the cosmetically pleasing effect of a flat stomach and slender waist, but more importantly, strong abdominals will adequately support the trunk and help prevent low back pain. The muscles involved include the rectus abdominis, which is primarily responsible for bending the upper body forward, and the internal and external obliques, charged with rotating, lateral and forward bending of the trunk. Strengthening the rectus abdominis will help flatten the stomach while strengthening the obliques and serve to slim the waist.

Hip and thigh flexors vs abdominals

When choosing abdominal exercises it is necessary to understand that many so-called abdominal exercises do not actually require the greater effort of the rectus abdominis, but instead rely on the psoas major and iliacus muscles. These powerful hip and thigh flexors, when contracted, will bend the body forward with little effort of the rectus abdominis. Any exercise that requires the lifting of one or both legs while lying on the floor is relying on the hip and thigh flexors. The contractions of these muscles also causes the pelvis to rotate forward, which in turn causes the lower back to sway off the floor. Any exercise done in this position would place an enormous strain on the lower back and provide very little benefit to the abdominal muscles.

Correct method

Exercises should be selected that will provide maximum strengthening potential to the rectus abdominis and obliques without involving the hip flexors. The most effective exercises for strengthening the abdominal muscles are abdominal curls. Variations on the abdominal curl should be performed for four to eight minutes. To correctly perform an abdominal curl use the following guidelines:

1. Lie on back with knees bent and feet planted firmly on floor.
2. Press the lower back firmly into the floor. Do not arch the back.
3. Do not strain forward with the chin or neck or jerk the head up and down.
4. Curl up slowly. Swinging movements that seek to rely on momentum are not only ineffective but can potentially cause strain to the neck. If your music is too fast to allow for correct performance of abdominal curls, execute movement at half speed, on every other beat.
5. Perform the curl only to a 20° or 40° angle. To sit all the way up to 90° requires the iliopsas muscles to complete the last half of the sit-up.
6. Breathing is important while performing abdominal exercises. Exhale while contracting the abdominals at the point of finishing your greatest exertion. Example: Exhale at the top of the curl, inhale when you lie back down.
7. *Never* perform double leg lifts! Not only are they ineffective in working the abdominals, but they place an enormous strain on the lower back.
8. Strengthen the internal and external obliques by performing abdominal curls while reaching to the opposite sides of the body.

End of Class Stretches

Progression

The final 7–10 minutes of your class should be spent performing static stretches. Static stretching is most effective at the end of your class, when all of the muscles are warm. If performed gradually and in a nonballistic manner, static stretching can be performed at this time with very little risk of injury.

The basic rule to follow when structuring your end-of-class stretches is that it is important to stretch the muscles that have been involved in strengthening exercises. As an example, don't neglect to stretch the quadriceps (which worked vigorously during aerobics), in favor of the hamstrings. The back is another area that is important to stretch, but often forgotten.

Just as at the beginning of your class, your final stretch routine should flow from head to toe or vice versa. Try to utilize one basic body position for several different stretches and then make smooth transitions into the next stretch, gradually stretching the whole body.

All of the same rules regarding nonballistic stretch would apply here. The wonderful part about stretching at the end of class is the relaxed feeling it can create and the extent of the stretch that can be achieved. This is the time to carefully work for increased flexibility by holding your stretches for at least 30 seconds, and taking the stretch perhaps a bit farther than would be safe at the beginning of the class. This period can also be used to teach relaxation techniques and create a calm, refreshed feeling within your students.

Heart rate

As your stretches are finished and the students prepare to leave, it is often advisable to take a final heart count. This would be advisable for those individuals who had a slower than average heart recovery time following aerobics, or for any individuals with related risk factors. Again, the recovery heart rate equals 60 percent of maximum (220 minus age, multiplied by .6). If not below this level, the individual was probably exercising too intensely and should work at a less vigorous level during the next class. Cool-down stretches should be continued until heart rate has lowered.

Saunas and hot tubs

Although the warmth might feel wonderful, saunas and hot tubs, even hot showers, should be avoided immediately following exercise. The heat causes the blood vessels to dilate and this, along with the fact that blood tends to pool in the extremities following vigorous exercise, causes the heart and brain to receive less blood.

Chapter 3

Body Shaping

Lauve Metcalfe, M.S.

Today, millions of Americans are learning to enjoy the benefits of optimal health through regular physical activity. Male and female, young and old are challenging themselves to become the best they can be. The life-style of the future is clearly one for lean, fit, trim individuals who desire to look their best, feel their best, and be their best.

While men have been the major benefactors of physical fitness in the past, women's involvement in fitness activities has grown astronomically in the last decade. This growth is due largely to participation in aerobic classes, sporting events (from road races to marathons and triathlons), and even body-building. Our society has become serious about exercise, and this quest for perfection is bringing both men and women to higher levels of physical and mental health.

This increased awareness of health and fitness has led to an improved quality of life for many individuals and, in addition, rewarded them with lean, trim bodies to show for their hard work. However, while this fitness phenomenon is taking place, there is a large percentage of our population that has only experienced frustration and failure in its efforts to obtain a shapelier form.

To illustrate this point, let's examine an all-too-common scenario.

Susan happens to catch a glimpse of herself in the mirror as she dresses for work one morning. Anxiety quickly spreads through her as she realizes that the shapely figure she was once so proud of in college has somehow converted itself into a pear shape. The excuses for her appearance have always been so easy to pass off on external events—getting married, having a baby, and now the job that has commanded so much of her attention these last few years have made the guilt easier to bear.

In desperation, Susan begins a new fad diet and vigorous exercise routine. After a week she feels sore, weak, and irritable. Depressed, Susan drops her exercise class and continues the drastic diet. After a few more weeks, she notices some weight loss, but her figure looks flabby and soft, not at all what she had imagined. And so, with her stamina shot and an overall sense of defeat, she breaks her diet and quickly regains her lost weight—and then some.

What Susan and countless other men and women need is a sensible program to reshape their physiques or figures. This approach must be a combination of healthy eating patterns and an exercise program that includes aerobic activity, strength training, and flexibility. Body shaping is not a simple task, but with a sound knowledge of the elements needed to make one shapelier, the desired results can be achieved. The changes that occur will not be temporary changes, but changes that will last for a lifetime.

Myths and Misconceptions

Before developing our body-shaping program, let's look at some common myths and misconceptions concerning physique and figure.

Myth: Aerobics is the only exercise I need

Aerobic (with oxygen) exercise is an excellent method of improving your cardiovascular system, respiratory system, and overall fitness level. Your body burns fat as fuel when engaged in low-to-moderate intensity aerobic exercise for a sustained period of time—walking, running, cycling, and swimming are aerobic exercises. Aerobic exercise is important in developing a high level of fitness, but should not be done to the exclusion of the other components of fitness: muscle strength and flexibility.

Strength training is a necessary ingredient to an exercise program because it increases muscle tissue to give shape and contour to your physique or figure and assists in accelerating your caloric expenditure.

Flexibility is responsible for increasing joint range of motion and elasticity of the muscles, in addition to decreasing the risk of injury and pulled muscles.

A balanced program of aerobics, strength training and flexibility exercises is essential for one to achieve his or her optimal potential.

Myth: Weight training by females will develop "massive" unattractive muscles

Females do not possess the male hormones that cause massive muscle development. While a strength-training program will increase muscle tissue on one's body, the result will be added shape and definition to the figure. How extensive a female's muscle tissue can be developed is determined by heredity, body build, and the intensity of the strength-training program.

Myth: Weight training will make me heavier

Emphasizing overall body weight is very misleading when beginning a strength-training program. Exercise—particularly a strength program—increases lean body mass (muscle tissue) while decreasing body fat. Muscle tissue has a higher density than body fat, so the scales may not change drastically, but the physique or figure may improve dramatically.

Myth: I'm too old to strength train

The benefits of strength training are particularly valuable in suppressing and reducing age-related bone loss and the effects of osteoporosis (loss of bone mass to the point where fractures occur with relatively minor trauma) as we age. Research has shown that muscle weight is an important determinant of the size and suppleness of our bone mass. Increases in the levels of calcium in the bones has been reported along with increases in muscle tissue associated with strength training. This is of particular interest to women because of their accelerated loss of bone mass following menopause.

Myth: You can sweat pounds off

Sweating is good for you, but it does very little to help you lose weight. One should never use artificial methods such as saunas, rubberized suits, or other such devices. The weight that you will lose is primarily water and body fluids that could be damaging. The purpose of sweating is to keep your body cool. The human body has a marvelous thermostat mechanism, yet it malfunctions if the humidity gets too high or the sweat can't evaporate. It is important when exercising to take in a sufficient amount of water to replenish fluids that are lost and to wear loose, "breathable" clothing. Never try to sweat pounds off; it could lead to dehydration, heat stroke, or hyperthermia.

Myth: Exercise will help spot reducing

Different regions of adipose tissue (fat) are subject to the influence of sex-specific hormones. Females tend to protect fat stores on their hips, thighs, and buttocks, while men protect fat around their stomachs. Spot reducing does not work. By exercising muscle that is located underneath fat deposits, you will tone up the particular muscle exercised, but the fat will not disappear unless food intake is decreased or activity is increased. When fat is burned, the loss is in equal proportions throughout the body. The benefit of aerobic exercise is that it burns fat, and strength training adds shape and contour once the layer of fat has been removed.

Myth: My appetite will increase as a result of exercise

Appetite is a psychologic desire for food that is influenced by a variety of factors both physiologic and psychologic. The control center for food intake (appestat) is located in the brain and functions like a thermostat. Exercise can stimulate eating behavior but the increase serves to maintain body weight. Regular exercise assists the appestat to adjust caloric intake to energy needs.

Myth: Fat changes to muscle, and muscle changes to fat

Fat and muscle are two entirely different substances. Fat cannot change to muscle, and muscle cannot change to fat. If a person with nicely developed muscle tissue stops exercising, the muscle itself will become smaller (atrophy) from lack of use. This person is likely to gain body fat if he or she remains inactive and continues to maintain the same eating habits. Conversely, a person with a high level of body fat who begins an exercise program and proper eating habits will lose body fat and gain muscle tissue.

Everyone wants to have a well-proportioned, shapely body. The problem that arises between this desire and the reality that stares back from the mirror is not a lack of will power. Commonly, it is a lack of information such as evidenced in the scenario and the myths described, and lack of education regarding how to develop a body-shaping system that is successful for individual needs.

Prior to pursuing a plan to shape up one's body, an understanding of some basic factors influencing physique or figure is needed. The most significant would include:

Heredity The genetic make-up of our system is predetermined. Little can be done to change the length of our bones, or the size of our skeletons. We inherit one of three general body types:

- *mesomorph*: predominance of muscle on the body
- *endomorph*: primarily round, chubby build
- *ectomorph*: appearance of a lean and thin body

There are many variations of these three body types. Most individuals tend to be a combination of two classifications, such as a mesomorphic-ectomorph (a strong muscular but very lean build), or a mesomorphic-endomorph (a strong muscular "hefty" build). Regardless of the general characteristics, *all* body types can improve their shape through the combined effects of good nutrition and an exercise program.

Percent of body fat Fat is simply stored energy. Food energy is expressed in calories, which are units of heat energy. Heat energy is used by the body in order to function properly. If not all the calories that are taken into the body are used, the remaining calories are stored as fat. As fat stores increase, the percentage of body fat increases proportionately. Authorities differ as to what the "ideal" percentage of body fat should be.

It is generally considered desirable for an adult female to have 18%-22% fat, and an adult male 12%-16% fat.

Lean body mass   Muscle tissue is the lean active tissue which burns calories during exercise, after exercise and during its normal resting state. It is a major contributor to basal metabolism, and it makes an essential contribution to physique and figure because it provides shape and definition to the body. For example, strong, well-defined quadriceps and gluteal muscles contribute significantly to a shapely upper thigh and firm, round buttocks.

Basal metabolic rate (BMR)   BMR is the body's system of generating heat from calories consumed in order to function properly and meet the demands of a 24-hour period. The primary use of the calories (energy) consumed is in heat production. At rest, without doing any physical work, all energy consumed must be converted into body heat or stored as fat.

Increasing the BMR is often the missing link in understanding obesity and the body's ability to convert energy to heat or store it as fat. Significant strides have been made in research recently to provide methods of increasing BMR. The amount of muscle tissue in one's body is a major factor in elevating BMR.

Posture   Posture is one of the most underestimated components of an improved physique and figure. How you carry yourself, and the position of your head, shoulders, and hips for proper alignment can often be the single most dramatic flaw in personal appearance. Proper alignment enhances the bustline, can expand the chest, make one appear taller, flatten the stomach, and reshape the buttocks. Posture is directly associated with flexibility and a balance between various muscle groups. Proper alignment of the body reduces strain on those muscle groups that withstand the effects of gravity. Low-back problems are often associated with poor posture habits.   [I.C: **Body Alignment**]

Now that you have an understanding of the contributing factors influencing one's physique, let's review the role of nutrition and exercise.

Nutrition

Most people operate under the premise that they can reduce body fat simply by dieting. While this assumption seems harmless enough, many individuals purposely subject themselves to strict diets that can cause a tired, haggard appearance or even malnutrition and serious eating disorders. The fact is that unless one reduces body fat with a balanced nutritional eating plan and an appropriate exercise program, the desired goal of having a firm, well-toned, healthy physique or figure may be beyond one's reach.

Dieting alone—that is, placing yourself on a restricted diet, a self-imposed starvation diet, or deliberately underfeeding yourself in order to lose unwanted fat—can be extremely hazardous to your health, both physically and psychologically.

The body perceives this self-imposed decrease in calories as a warning that something is wrong. Not certain when it will be fed again, it hoards calories and automatically reduces the need to burn calories. BMR slows down to conserve fuel. That is just what you don't want to happen. This caloric deprivation leads to a decrease in muscle tissue as well as body fat. During a fast or a very restrictive diet, you can actually lose more muscle than fat. The result can be very poor muscle tone and an unattractive soft appearance.

Underweight persons who are attempting to put weight on their bodies by dieting alone have a tendency to be overfat due to lack of physical activity. These individuals try to gain weight by increasing the amount of food they consume. While they will gain weight, because they are overeating and engaging in minimal activity, the added weight is primarily fat.

The American Medical Association recommends that the public give primary emphasis to the achievement and maintenance of the most desirable body composition. Body composition refers to the ratio of fat and lean body mass making up the body. A balanced body composition should be accomplished through regular exercise and proper eating patterns.

The body performs best when it is regularly stressed by appropriate physical activity and, at the same time, properly nourished. Exercise combined with a healthy diet is more effective than diet alone. Strict, long-term diets make it difficult to maintain the concentration or energy needed to perform a quality workout.

A Review of the Components of Fitness

Importance of aerobic exercise   [VI: Aerobics]

Aerobic exercise improves the cardiovascular and respiratory systems, and the individual's physical work capacity. It burns fat as fuel and thus assists in maintaining a desirable level of body fat.

Importance of flexibility   [I.G: Full Range of Motion]

Flexibility is needed to move the body and its parts through a wide range of motion without undue stress to the muscle attachments or anatomical structure. Flexibility is essential in maintaining correct posture, preventing low-back problems, and reducing the chance of injury.

Importance of strength training

Strength training is needed to develop muscle that is lean and functional, while at the same time aesthetically attractive. Regular strength training is beneficial for this purpose. As muscle tissue increases, your caloric expenditure is accelerated.

Energy expenditure is elevated not only during exercise but also for a period of time afterwards. The length of this time depends on the intensity and duration of the exercise and the individual's level of fitness. Research has reported 10% elevations in BMR for as long as 48 hours following exercise. This adds to the energy cost and contributes to the body fat loss more than the energy expended during the exercise alone.

Body shaping through strength training

Most women find that the amount of physical activity they participate in slowly declines after high school or college. Traditionally, women have never been encouraged to develop their figures, particularly upper body musculature. As a result of this inactivity and muscle disuse, they tend to become "bottom heavy," posture sags, and low-back problems appear. Later in life, the combination of these symptoms and lack of muscle tissue contributes to loss of bone mass and the early onset of osteoporosis.

Strength training not only maintains muscle tissue, it strengthens the musculature and bone mass to prevent these problems. Strength training stretches the chest muscles and strengthens the back to maintain good posture, and strengthens the abdominal muscles to minimize low-back problems. This adds a valuable dimension to a workout and makes a large contribution to reshaping one's physique or figure.

Equipment

There is currently a wide variety of equipment available designed to develop the musculature and give added definition to body parts. To achieve the greatest benefit from strength training, it is best to utilize free weights and exercise machines to tone and shape your body. Increasing muscle tissue requires that you overload muscle groups at a level of intensity sufficient to generate growth. As you grow stronger through training, the resistance (weight) must be increased in order to progressively overload the muscle group.

An increase in muscle tissue and definition will result from the greater resistance and the general intensity of the workout.

Free weights vs machines   There is some controversy over the selection of free weights vs machines for strength training: which is better? Both methods can produce positive benefits in strength, muscle size, body fat reduction, and muscular endurance. The advantages of machines over free weights are primarily a matter of experience and personal preference.

The following are some practical advantages free weights have over machines:

- *Dumbbells and barbells* are effective in developing the smaller synergistic (helping) muscles and stabilizer muscles of the body.
- *Free-weight exercises* more closely match the neurological patterns of associated sport skills because of joint kinesthesis (range of motion), leverage similarities, and bodily involvement.

Barbells and dumbbells are versatile, less expensive, and take up less space (a plus for home usage).

Balance does become a factor when using free weights. One must control the movement of a free weight more carefully than a machine, creating better neuromuscular command for an exercise. This recruits more muscle fibers, making the muscle network stronger.

Cost and accessibility can be key issues. In order to work out with machines, it is usually necessary to attend a fitness center or school facility which often involves paying a membership fee. Free weights can be purchased for minimal cost and used and stored at home. Ideally, one would receive the greatest benefits with a combination of free weights and machines.

Ankle and wrist weights   These usually range from one to three pounds and can be a good introduction to weight training. Ankle and wrists weights provide the body with an "overload" to assist in recruiting more muscle fibers than body weight alone. Combined with an aerobic exercise routine, ankle and wrist weights can increase heart rate and begin to shape body muscle. These weights are particularly useful when doing high repetition strength work.

The value of understanding the advantages of different types of equipment is the realization that it is possible to develop a sound and effective body-shaping routine with a combination of ankle and wrist weights, dumbbells and barbells. A routine that is versatile and adaptable to your specific needs and personal goals can be achieved.

The program

Frequency   You should schedule your workouts two to three times per week or on an every-other-day basis. The days you are not strength training should be your aerobic days.   [I.A: Frequency of Workouts]   However, if you are concentrating on high repetition, low-resistance work (such as activity with ankle and wrist weights), daily workouts would not cause undue overload. Make sure you have sufficiently warmed up and that the exercises are within your ability and fitness level.

Intensity   Intensity simply means how hard you work and is measured by your exercise heart rate. It is very much a function of your level of conditioning at any given time. Begin slowly, to avoid muscle soreness and ensure that your muscles are properly warmed up. As you progress and achieve improved levels of muscular fitness, you may increase the efforts you are putting into your exercise. Generally, muscles should be challenged so that they are fatigued in order to gain the desired results. However, you should never demand so much from yourself in a workout that you feel excessive soreness the next day. Progress only as quickly as your exercise heart rate permits. Remember, the key is to begin slowly and progressively increase the level of intensity over time.

Time You can accomplish a great deal in 20–30 minutes per workout, if it is at a sufficient level of intensity and periods of rest and recovery between exercises are minimal.

Repetitions and sets—how many? A repetition is an individual full cycle of an exercise, taking the body part through the full range of motion. (*Example*: For a sit-up beginning on the floor, curling up to a 45° angle and returning to the floor is one repetition.) 10–15 repetitions is usual.

A set is a group of repetitions performed in sequence with no noticeable break. This is followed by a rest or recovery period and then another set of repetitions. Sets in the range of two to three are suggested.

There are three basic methods to increase the training intensity and therefore, the effects of an exercise:

- performing a greater number of repetitions with a specific weight
- increasing the weight and performing a specific number of repetitions
- doing an established number of sets and repetitions with a specific weight using a shorter rest interval

Rachel McLish and Dr. Lynne Pirie, female body-builders, suggest that a beginning program involve one set of 10–12 repetitions per exercise for the first week's workout. The second week, two sets are done, and the third week and the weeks thereafter, a total of three sets is recommended.

In the beginning, you may feel awkward with the execution of the movement, but after a few repetitions you will be more comfortable. It is important to choose a beginning weight that will allow you proper form. Once you feel your form is maintained, you can advance to higher weights.

Breathing

It is important to maintain a constant breathing pattern. **Never hold your breath.** There is no set rule for developing a breathing pattern. Most individuals find it more natural to exhale during the exertion and inhale during the recovery part of the lift. Experiment so that you can discover what is comfortable for you. [II.E: Breathing]

Rest interval This is the time when you allow your cardiovascular system and muscles to recover before you begin another set of repetitions or a different exercise. In the beginning, the rest interval until you feel sufficiently recovered to continue will be longer. As you increase your general level of fitness, you will want to reduce the rest interval to as short a period as possible. If you have difficulty keeping the rest interval short, the amount of weight used may be too heavy. Decrease the weight and add more repetitions. This will not only enhance the intensity of your workout, but will add a cardiovascular benefit to your muscle toning and strengthening program.

Training Tips

Proper form

Form is extremely important in strength training. If you find yourself lifting a weight too quickly, jerking it, or swinging the weight in order to perform the action, you may be increasing the chance of injury and decreasing the effectiveness of the exercise. It is important to isolate the muscle group that is being exercised. If you are unable to control the weight throughout the movement, you are probably lifting too much weight. Drop down a few pounds and see how your form improves. Concentrate on moving the dumbbell or barbell slowly along the full range of motion. Stopping before the completion of this range will give only partial benefits. Focus on lowering the weight a bit more slowly than you raised it. This will help ensure a full contraction throughout the movement.

Work out with a partner

For safety reasons as well as motivation, it is best to have another person present during a workout. This can be accomplished easily in an exercise studio or fitness center, but for home workouts it may be necessary to plan ahead.

A partner can be a real asset as a motivator, a spotter and someone to critique your form. Also, knowing that you have a responsibility to another individual makes skipping a workout more difficult.

How much, how often?

Strength-training programs vary in format depending on what an individual is trying to achieve through his/her strength work. A program designed to build muscle mass, definition, and bulk could be an extremely intense workout on an every-other-day basis.

Another format may be a split routine that works different muscle groups on consecutive days. There is as much variety in strength-training routines as in the types of exercises that can be performed.

Training with heavy weights increases muscle mass. For those areas of your body for which increased mass is desired, heavy weights with low repetitions will produce the best results.

Lighter-weight, higher-repetition workouts don't build as much mass, although the shape, contour, firmness, and detail of the muscle are accentuated.

For the individual concerned with basic body shaping, concentration should be focused on developing a sequence of exercises to enhance each muscle group. The initial focus should be on adapting a routine that fits into your schedule, can be done regularly, and is enjoyable.

Developing your program

In developing a training routine, emphasis should be placed on overall body conditioning and should be concerned with the development of all major muscle groups of the body in order to maximize the potential of one's physique or figure.

If an area is ignored or one particular area is overemphasized, the overall appearance may turn out unbalanced. Once you feel comfortable with various exercises, you will be able to add to or delete from your program, and concentrate on developing or reducing specific body parts.

There is no one "successful" method of training. You should be aware of potential problems that can be avoided. To decrease the possibility of overtraining, begin with one basic exercise per body part (shoulders, back, chest, abdominals, biceps, triceps, buttocks, thighs, calves). Once you have mastered a set routine, blend in your own variations to keep up your interest. Some strength-training professionals suggest that it is best to train the torso muscle groups before the arms and legs. Others prefer to alternate between an upper body and a lower body exercise to increase the cardiovascular benefit. These techniques and a wide variety of others are more of a personal preference than principle. The bottom line is to develop a program that works all muscle groups, provides the intensity to generate muscle tissue growth, and is fun, so that you look forward to working out.

The warm-up   Prior to beginning your program, a warm-up and a stretch period are necessary to minimize injury and muscle pulls. A warm-up should consist of three to five minutes of brisk walking, jumping rope, stationary cycling, or mild calisthenics to increase respiration, elevate body temperature, and stretch ligaments and connective tissues.   **[IV: Warm-Up]**

The stretch   The stretch period will enable your joints and muscles to limber up and become more flexible. To stretch, slowly ease into the desired position until a "stretch sensation" is experienced. Back off slightly from this stretch position and hold for 10-30 seconds. Never bounce into a stretch position, but stretch slowly and rhythmically.   **[IV.C: Stretching]**

The exercises   The exercises selected are intended to exercise the various body parts and are only a sample of a wide range of exercises available. For a more in-depth exercise routine, you may refer to the books at the end of the chapter for reference. The exercises will utilize ankle and hand weights, dumbbells, and barbells so that you may visualize a progression that is best suited to your situation.

CHEST EXERCISES

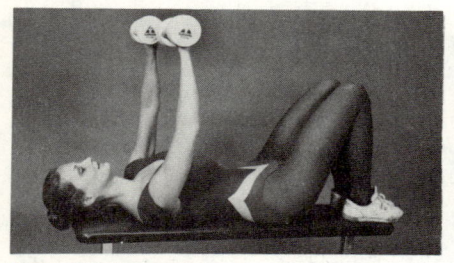

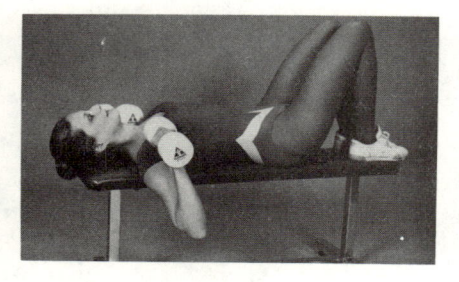

Dumbbell Bench Press
Emphasis: Develops chest (pectoral), shoulder (deltoid), and back of upper arm (triceps) muscles.
Execution: Grasp two dumbbells and lie with back flat on bench. Bend your knees, placing feet on bench. Push weight to straight arm's length directly above shoulders, palms facing forward and dumbbells touching. Slowly bend arms, keeping elbows wide and lower weight until it touches slightly below your shoulders. Press weight back to starting position. Repeat.

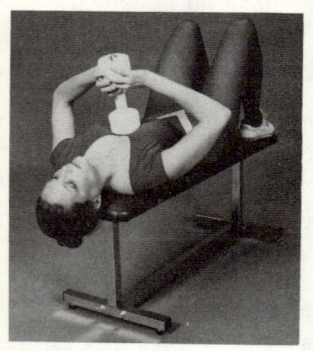

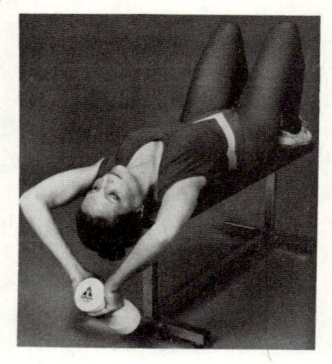

Bench Pullover
Emphasis: Stretches back muscles (latissimus dorsi).
Execution: Lie lengthwise on bench, bending knees and placing feet on bench, with head just over edge of bench. Rest your palms under the upper part of the dumbbell, and hook thumbs around the handle. Position the dumbbell against your chest. Slowly, with bent elbows, pass the dumbbell over your face and extend back towards the floor. Go as far as comfortable. Slowly return to starting position, keep elbows close together. Repeat.

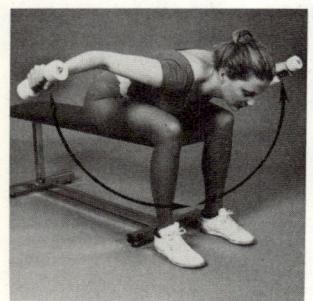

BACK EXERCISES

Seated Bent Laterals
Emphasis: Strengthens upper back muscles (trapezius) and back portion of shoulder muscle (deltoid).
Execution: Sit on edge of bench with feet shoulder-width apart on floor. Grasp two light dumbbells and bend forward at waist until your torso is resting on your thighs. Arms are in front of your calves, elbows slightly bent and palms facing in. Slowly raise the dumbbells in a semi-circular arc out to the side until they reach shoulder level. Slowly lower back to starting position. Repeat.

BODY SHAPING **199**

SHOULDER EXERCISES

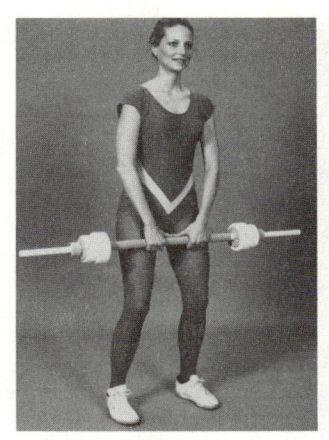

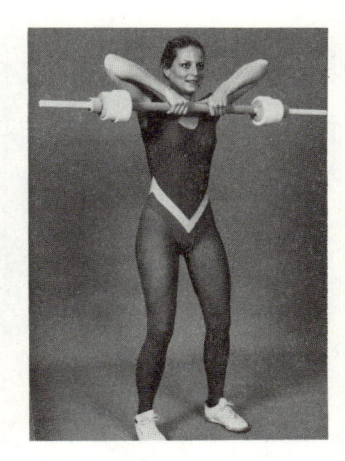

Upright Rows
Emphasis: Develops shoulder (deltoid), upper back (trapezius) and biceps muscles of the arm. Great for "rounded shoulders" posture.
Execution: Grasp bar in hands with index fingers 4–6 inches apart, palms facing body. Stand erect with feet shoulder-width apart, knees slightly bent. Your arms should be down at your sides, with bar resting on upper thigh. Keeping elbows above hands throughout movement, slowly pull bar up till hands touch your neck/chin area. Shoulders are rotated back slightly. Chin up. Slowly lower weight to starting position. Repeat.

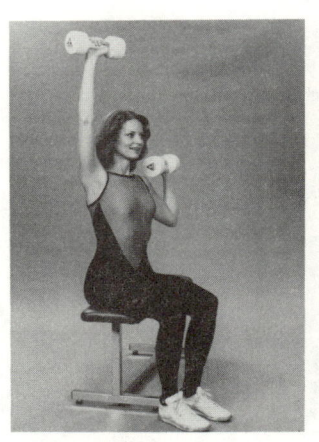

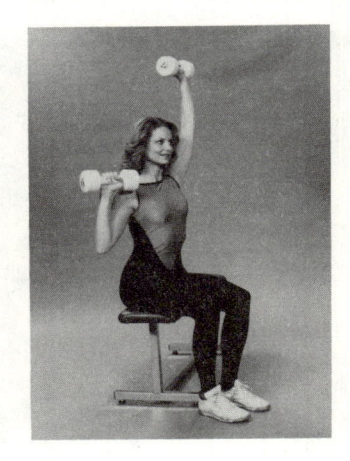

Seated Dumbbell Press
Emphasis: Strengthens shoulder (deltoid) and back of upper arm (triceps) muscles.
Execution: Sit comfortably on a bench and pull dumbbells up to your shoulders. Rotate hands so palms are facing forward. Push one dumbbell directly upward until it is at arm's length above your shoulder joint. As you begin to lower the weight, start to press the other one to arm's length. Continue to alternately press and lower weights.

ARM EXERCISES

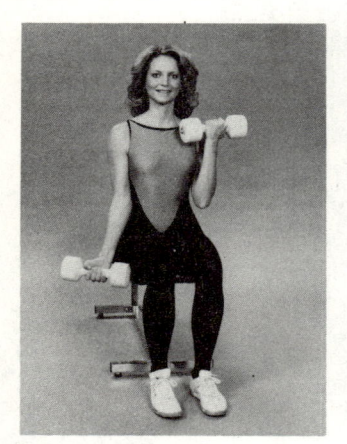

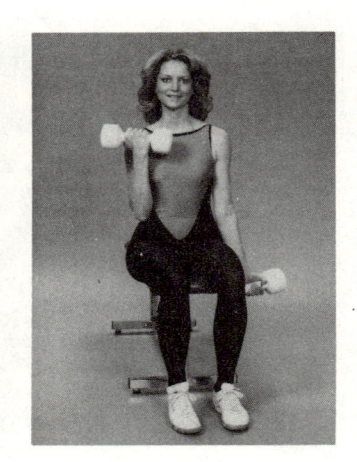

Seated Dumbbell Curls
Emphasis: Develops the muscles of the upper arm (biceps) with a secondary emphasis on the forearms.
Execution: Sit comfortably on a bench with arms at side, elbows slightly bent. Grasp dumbbells, palms facing upward, and slowly raise one dumbbell up to your shoulder. As the weight is being lowered, raise the other dumbbell to the opposite shoulder. Alternate sides. Repeat.

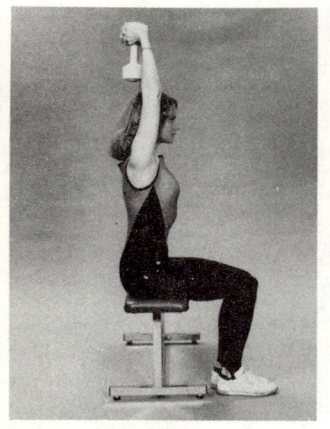

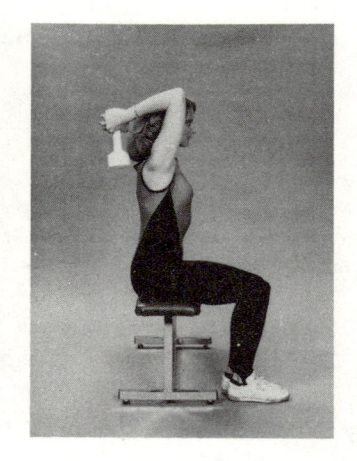

Seated Tricep Extensions
Emphasis: Strengthens back of upper arm (triceps) and upper back (trapezius) muscles.
Execution: Sit comfortably on a bench. Place your thumbs and index fingers around the upper part of a dumbbell and extend overhead with elbows slightly bent. Slowly lower the weight behind the head, bending at the elbow as far as possible. Keep elbows close to the ears. Press weight up to starting position. Repeat.

ARM EXERCISES (continued)

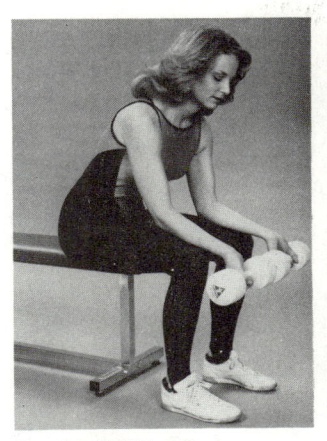

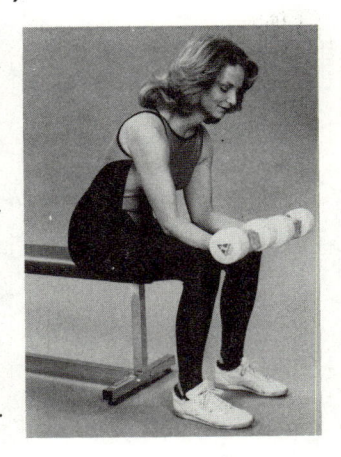

Dumbbell Wrist Curls
Emphasis: With palms facing up, wrist curls strengthen the flexor muscles of the forearm. With palms down, the exercise stresses the smaller muscles of the forearm.
Execution: Grasp a dumbbell in each hand. Sitting on the end of a bench, rest your forearms on your thighs so that the wrists are off the edge of the bench by your knees. Relax and drop your wrists down as far as possible, then curl the weight up as high as possible. Repeat.

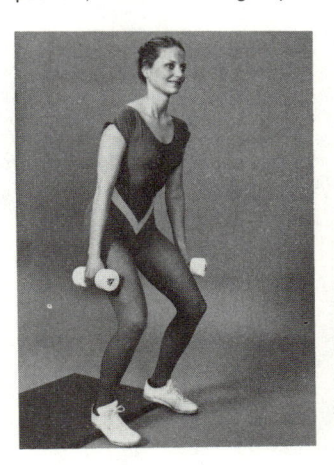

Partial Squats
Emphasis: Develops the muscles of the thighs (quadriceps), buttocks and hips.
Execution: Hold a dumbbell in each hand. Spread feet shoulder-width apart with toes pointed slightly outward, knees bent. If possible, elevate heels one to two inches by standing on a board. Slowly lower buttocks, leaning forward slightly until you reach a 45° angle. (Do not go into a full squat position or let thighs go beyond a parallel position to the floor.) Slowly resume the standing position, keeping knees slightly bent. Exhale on the way up, inhale on the way down. Keep head erect, focus eyes straight ahead. Repeat.

THIGH AND HIP EXERCISES

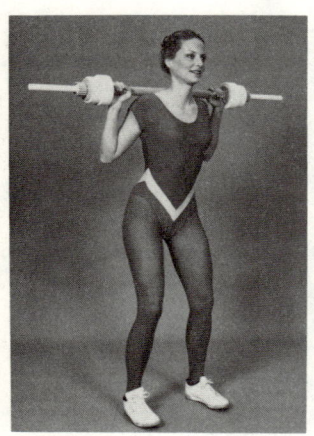

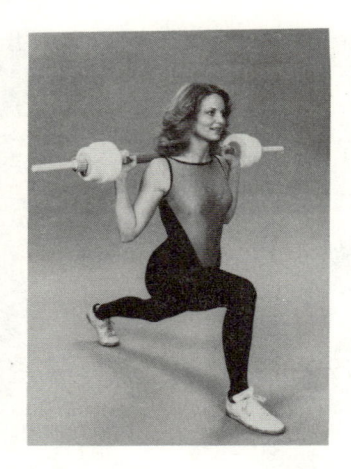

Lunges
Emphasis: Develops quadriceps, buttocks, hamstrings, and overall shape of thighs.
Execution: Place barbell behind neck and grasp bar comfortably at shoulders, palms facing forward. Stand with feet shoulder-width apart and toes pointed directly forward, knees bent. Keep head up, focusing eyes straight ahead. Keeping torso erect, step forward approximately three feet with your right foot. Left leg is slightly bent. Slowly bend right leg until it reaches a 45° angle. Your right knee should be slightly ahead of, and directly above your right ankle. Back is straight with head up. Push off with right leg and return to starting position. Repeat with opposite leg.

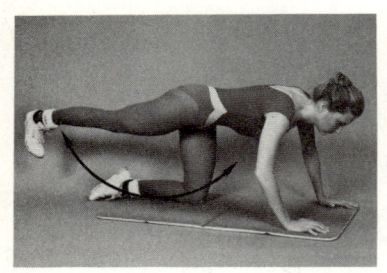

Rear Leg Lift
Emphasis: Strengthens and tones buttocks, hips and lower back.
Execution: Strap on ankle weights and kneel on padded surface. Arms are shoulder-width apart, elbows slightly bent. Back is straight, and remains straight throughout exercise. Bend right leg and bring knee into chest area, do not round back. Slowly extend right leg backward while keeping hips square, tightening buttock muscles to give a straight linear appearance with back. Foot is flexed. Return to starting position and repeat, alternating sides.

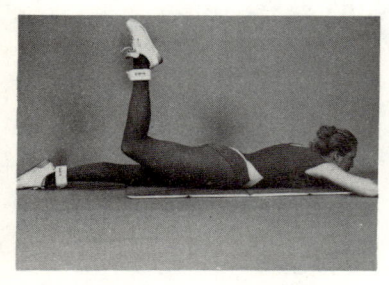

Buttock Lift
Emphasis: Firms and tones buttocks muscles.
Execution: Lie face down on padded surface, with ankle weights on. Arms are bent at the elbows and supporting the head. Hips are on floor and remain on floor during the exercise. Left leg is in relaxed position in alignment with body. Right leg is bent at the knee with toe pointed. Raise right leg toward ceiling tightening buttocks, and keeping right hip on floor. Hold. Slowly lower. Repeat, alternating sides.

BODY SHAPING

THIGH AND HIP EXERCISES (continued)

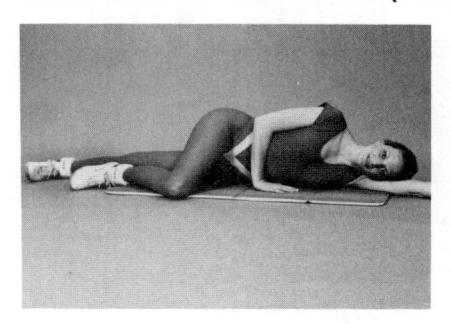

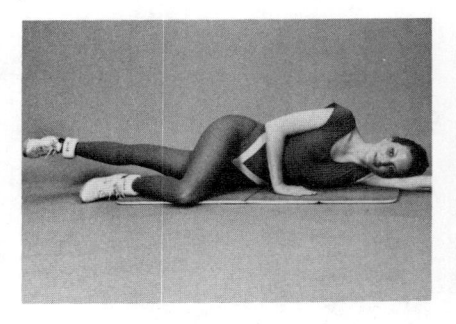

Inner Thigh Lift
Emphasis: Strengthens and tones inner thigh muscles.
Execution: Strap on ankle weights and lie on left side with left arm extended. Head relaxed, bend upper leg (right) bringing knee toward abdomen and to rest on floor. Flexing lower leg (left), raise it as far as possible toward ceiling. Hold. Slowly lower. Repeat, alternating sides.

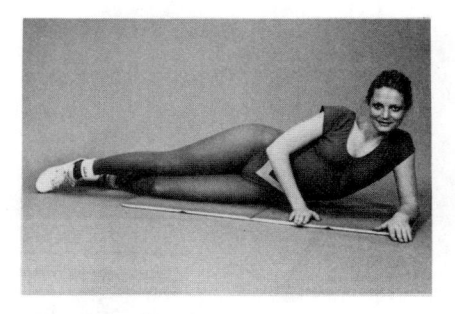

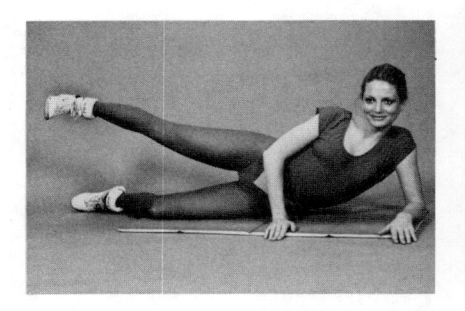

Outer Thigh Lift
Emphasis: Firms and tones outer thigh muscles.
Execution: Strap on ankle weights and lie on your left side on a padded surface. Body weight is supported by left forearm, right arm, and left hip. Keeping your hips in alignment, bend bottom leg slightly and use as support. Upper leg (right) is extended with knee facing forward. Raise upper leg up toward ceiling with foot flexed. Hold. Slowly return to starting positon. Repeat, alternating sides.

LOWER LEG EXERCISES

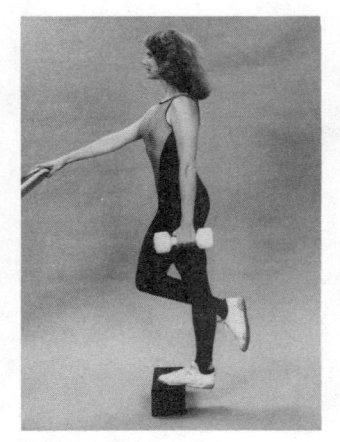

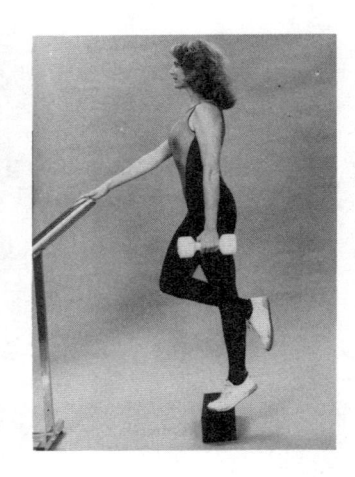

One-legged Calf Raise
Emphasis: Develops calf (gastrocnemius) muscles.
Execution: Place toes and ball of your left foot on a block of wood or stair riser. Place dumbbell in left hand, and bend right leg to keep it from assisting the movement. Grasp a sturdy upright for balance. Drop left heel as far down as possible, while standing erect, chin up. Slowly rise up on the toes of your left foot as high as possible. Lower body back to starting position. Repeat, alternating sides.

ABDOMINAL EXERCISES

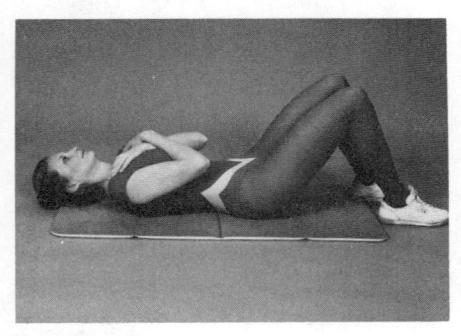

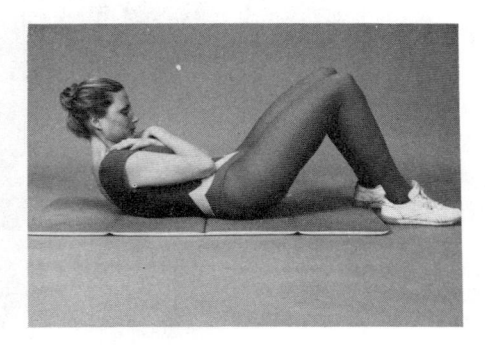

Bent Knee Curl
Emphasis: Strengthens abdominal muscles.
Execution: Lie on your back with knees bent on a padded surface, feet firmly on floor and hands across chest. Slowly curl head and upper back off the floor keeping chin tucked into the chest area. Lower back should remain on floor. Slowly return to the starting positon. Repeat.

BODY SHAPING

ABDOMINAL EXERCISES (continued)

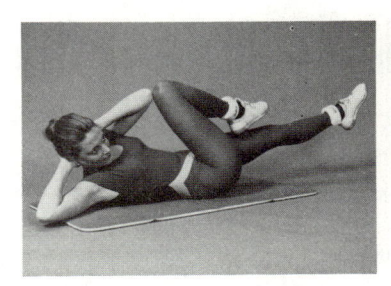

Elbow to Knee Twist
Emphasis: Strengthens abdominal muscles, tones side muscles.
Execution: Lie on padded surface. Strap on ankle weights. Clasp hands behind the head. Curl forward and twist, bringing right knee in toward left elbow. Left leg is extended. Mid-back should remain on mat during exercise. Twist body and bring left knee to right elbow with right leg extended. Continue to alternate sides and repeat.

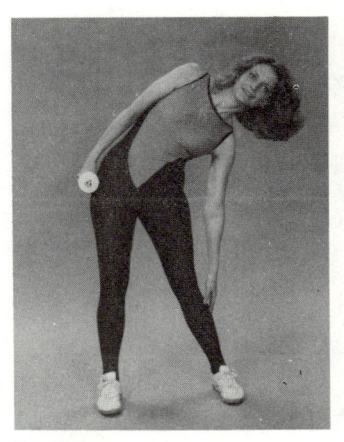

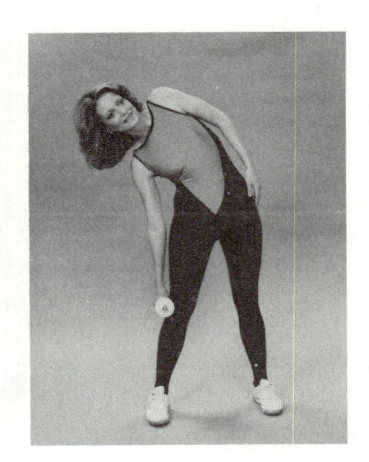

Tic-Tocs
Emphasis: Tones up side muscles (internal and external obliques).
Execution: Stand upright with feet shoulder-width apart, knees slightly bent. Extend both arms comfortably at the side with one dumbbell in the right hand. Slowly move upper body to the left as far as is comfortable, preferably so the left hand moves below the left knee. Move torso back to the right as far as comfortable, preferably with the dumbbell reaching below the knee. Repeat. Alternate sides.

Maintaining motivation

Everyone who exercises regularly knows that there are times when you just don't feel up to putting your body through another workout. Even the most dedicated athletes have periods of inactivity.

There may not be any universal cure for these "exercise blahs," but there are some strategies to help keep on the right track:

Establish a plan Regularity of training and a clear plan for achieving your goals are the fundamental components to your success in body shaping. It is important that the plan put together is *your* plan, designed to fit your personal needs and interests. While it is desirable to follow basic strength-training principles, be creative!

Remember what body parts you are working, the sequence, and what exercises you will perform. With a plan, you won't be wasting valuable time and your training will be more consistent.

"The will to succeed is worth nothing unless you have the will to prepare."

Record keeping Devise a training diary that charts your workouts: aerobic, strength and flexibility, length of the workout, time of day, your mood, even your food intake. This helps track progress and monitor your improvement.

After several weeks, you'll discover patterns emerging that may surprise you. For example, there may be a certain time of day that you have more energy or a particular time when your sweet tooth is aroused. By becoming aware of your body signals, you might schedule a healthful snack to avoid a binge, or plan your workout during a part of the day that is less stressful.

Goals Goals are best put on paper as specific items (e.g., "I want to improve my posture") and then written out as a plan of action ("To do this, I will work on stretching my chest muscles by doing strength training, practice walking taller and straighter, and never slouch in a chair"). By having a more specific plan, your goals will be easier to accomplish. You should make all goals realistic, and even break them down into three-month plans to help you maintain your momentum. Initially, you may have to set up weekly or even daily goals that clearly define your workout progression to keep you motivated.

It is interesting how goal setting brings you closer to your inner self. You may realize that the goals you originally put on paper have changed after several months. This can be a positive step. You need to carefully analyze your plan of action if you find yourself constantly changing them or falling short. They are meant to be an incentive to give guidance and stability to your program.

Quality workouts, not quantity   At times you may find yourself less than thrilled to step into the workout arena. It is important to listen to your body and assess whether the problem is physical or psychologic. If you are physically drained, you may be better off not exercising and taking a rest day. Your body may be signaling that it's on overdrive and needs a rest. If your "get up and go got up and went," you may be psychologically burned out.

Before cancelling your exercise, try some deep breathing and relaxation techniques prior to working out. Escape to a quiet area, lie down, relax and take a few deep breaths. Close your eyes. Imagine yourself at your very best (110%), going through a fantastic workout. Focus in on the image—the every detail of what you're wearing, the room, the music played. Feel the electricity of the workout—how wonderful and smooth your body feels. Imagine that it is the best you've ever done. Keep the image in your mind's eye. Repeat your deep breathing, stretch, and open your eyes. If you're still not psyched to give your workout a go, reread your goals and plan of action. Think how important those goals are. Bill Squires, a college track coach, offers the following thought to his runners: "Success is that place on the road where preparation and opportunity meet. But too few people recognize it because it comes disguised as sweat and work."

Reward yourself   After a good workout, or once you have successfully met your goals, celebrate. Treat yourself to a movie or a new outfit or even buy yourself some flowers. But be careful not to undermine all your hard effort by rewarding yourself with sweets or forbidden foods. If you *must* treat yourself to a treat, remember: moderation is the key.

Accepting the Challenge

The fundamental key to developing a physically fit and well-toned physique or figure is essentially understanding balance—the balance between proper nutrition and regular exercise and the balance that exists within an exercise program between aerobic activity, strength training, and flexibility.

Exercise brings out the best in all of us. It strengthens our bodies, invigorates our minds, and adds life to our spirits. Once this philosophy is understood, accepted, and practiced, there is little difficulty in sustaining this pattern throughout life.

The challenge is yours—to achieve a high quality of living that comes from a balanced, healthy life-style. It is a challenge to become the best you can be, to take charge of your life and accept responsibility for your health—a challenge worth the effort that will bring all of the rewards of total well-being.

Summary

Body shaping requires an understanding of balance in a program—balance between good nutritional habits and a regular fitness program, and a balance within the fitness program of aerobic exercise, flexibility, and strength training.

Many myths and misconceptions on this subject have developed, including lack of knowledge of the benefits of strength training and muscle development, the effects of age, weight loss, and the difference between muscle tissue and body fat.

Among the factors influencing physique and figure are heredity, percent of body fat, lean body mass, basal metabolic rate, and posture.

Eating habits play an important role in reducing body fat. However, dieting alone can do more damage than good by causing a loss of lean body tissue. Therefore, an awareness of the careful balance between caloric consumption and caloric expenditure, and increased levels of activity and enhanced muscle tissue is necessary to develop ideal body composition.

The primary components of exercise include aerobic activity, flexibility, and strength training. All three are necessary for optimal fitness and health.

Strength training contributes significantly to one's overall fitness level by increasing the strength of the bones, ligaments and muscles; increasing lean body tissue, muscle mass and bone density, and increasing the individual's overhead caloric burn.

In developing a strength-training program, one must consider frequency, intensity, and time. The program should be well-planned, with specific exercises for all body parts. Attention should be directed to proper form, breathing, rest intervals, and how much and how often one trains.

Maintaining a consistent program is often a challenge. Keys to motivation include establishing a plan, keeping a record of your workout, setting challenging, yet reasonable goals, emphasizing quality, not quantity, and rewarding yourself for your accomplishments.

Both free weights and exercise machines are effective tools to tone and shape the body. Each has benefits, and the decision to use one or the other or a combination of both is often a matter of personal preference and convenience.

References

Body shaping
McLish, R. *Flex Appeal*. New York: Warner Books, 1984.
Pirie, L. *Getting Built*. New York: Warner Books, 1984.
Schwarzenegger, A. *Arnold's Bodyshaping for Women*. New York: Simon & Schuster, 1979.

Weider, J. *Bodybuilding and Conditioning for Women*. Chicago: Contemporary Books, 1983.

Zane, F. and C. *The Zane Way to a Beautiful Body*. New York: Simon & Schuster, 1979.

Flexibility

Anderson, B. *Stretching*. Fullerton, CA: Anderson-World, 1975.

Nutrition and exercise

Astrand, P. *Textbook of Work Physiology*. New York: McGraw-Hill, 1977.

Bailey, C. *Fit or Fat?* Boston: Houghton Mifflin, 1978.

Lamb, L. *The Health Letter*. San Antonio, TX: Communications, Inc., 1984.

Nash, J. *Taking Charge of Your Weight and Well-Being*. Palo Alto, CA: Bull Publishing, 1978.

National Strength and Conditioning Journal, P.O. Box 81410, Lincoln, NE 68501.

Sharkey, B. *Physiology of Fitness*. Champaign, IL: Human Kinetics Publishers, 1979.

White, P., Ed. *Diet and Exercise: Synergism in Health Maintenance*. Chicago: American Medical Assoc., 1982.

Chapter 4

Motivation and Habit Training

Barry M. Devine, Ph.D.

Mankind's ability to deliver and recover satellites in space and to walk on the moon suggests that the task of selecting and implementing a physically healthy life-style should be simple. That logic seems to end at the psyche of the human animal. While more than 90% of all individuals believe in exercise as part of a healthy life-style, less than 15% exercise regularly. Clearly, there is a need for motivation, guidance, emotional support, stimulation, and careful planning on the part of the aerobic instructor.

The scientific history of our species can be traced back two million years. During this history, mankind has practiced some sort of organized agriculture for 10,000 years and has lived in urban settings for only about 800 years. Looking back, then, we realize that our heritage includes 99.5% of a history as primitive hunters and gatherers—hardly the best preparation for life in the 20th century. Furthermore, futurists tell us that the accelerating rate of change suggests we will be even less prepared to meet the demands of the 21st century.

Scientific evidence has made it eminently clear that regular exercise is a vital component of a healthy life-style—one which enables us to enjoy the best possible quality of existence in this advanced society. Some recent trends in healthful life-styles are quite encouraging, for example:

- More people than ever are participating in exercise programs.
- More than 30 million people have stopped smoking.
- Nutritional habits are changing with more awareness of content and effect.
- The incidence of heart disease and other cardiovascular disorders has decreased.

On the other hand, we have much to accomplish in the immediate future, as indicated by the following facts:
- Developed western countries have the highest incidence of cardiovascular disease in the world.
- More than 60% of adults in the population of the United States are overweight.
- One-third of the population over 17 years of age still smokes regularly.
- The US population will spend more than $200 million this year to lose weight the "no-work way," and will spend nearly as much to improve physical fitness without effort.

The aerobic exercise instructor has the challenging responsibility of generating enthusiasm for a regular exercise program among class participants. The remainder of this chapter is directed toward an understanding of this problem, and the development of a strategy the instructor can utilize to assure that class participants get the guidance and supervision they need.

Health professionals report that 30%–50% of individuals who start an exercise program will drop out within the first ten weeks. In a moment, we will examine the reported reasons that so many people are not able to reach their exercise program objectives, but first we need to be aware of the cultural climate in which we grow up.

This society tends to glorify the athlete, while both implicitly and explicitly telling the nonathlete that he or she is not of great worth. The emphasis on winning rather than losing for the 10-year-old teaches that to "exercise" (without competition) is to lose. Largely missing is the attitude that while everybody cannot be an athlete, all normal individuals can and should have adequate health and physical fitness, i.e., it is not necessary to be an athlete to experience the benefits of exercise.

While today young girls are much more likely to be encouraged to be physically active, we must remember that many adult women did not receive that support and encouragement when they were younger. Many of them seek a quality exercise experience in their adult years after perhaps decades of sedentary life. These women obviously require special guidance and encouragement; their appearance is being judged by today's standards, but for most of their lives, their appearances were suited to a different and less demanding standard.

At the same time, we have many males seeking a quality exercise experience in middle-age after finally accepting the fact (often delivered by a physician and extensive laboratory tests) that they will not survive much longer unless they modify their "successful" but indulgent and sedentary life-styles.

Questions to be answered in the text:

MOTIVATION AND HABIT TRAINING   213

- What are the commonly reported reasons for the attrition of people from exercise programs?
- What are factors which *do not* appear to influence attrition from exercise programs?
- How can the instructor maximize motivation so as to prevent attrition?
- What subjects are appropriate for the instructor to discuss in class to educate participants about exercise?
- What can the instructor do to assure that his/her classes are conducted safely?

Reasons Reported for Attrition From Exercise Programs

Perhaps we all expect a degree of uncertainty and hesitation among those joining a new class, especially if it is the beginning of an exercise program. This can soon be followed by feelings of dejection and frustration when no signs of "instant fitness" are apparent. Modest discomfort experienced in the early stages of a program, such as dry mouth and labored breathing, finally disappears in time. Likewise, normal muscle soreness and stiffness is to be expected after workouts and should be anticipated at the beginning. However, it should be noted that any excessive discomfort (such as nausea or pain) while exercising is a reason to stop exercising. A situation of this sort should be reviewed before commencing the next class workout. The most common reasons for a cessation of the exercise program are as follows:

- *Insufficient time*. This is usually associated with numerous commitments and is the most common reason reported. When questioned further, individuals reporting this reason are usually found to make time for watching television and engaging in other passive activities. Nearness of the exercise facility appears to play a part here.
- *Lack of self-discipline*. The importance of peer and "significant other person" support is very important in this area.
- *Lack of interest. Boredom*. The unique growth of aerobic exercise classes is closely related to the fact that music is a wonderful tool to keep up interest. Interest will fade if the intensity of the activity is inappropriate for the participant. Freedom from illness or injury is another factor that will help maintain interest.

Surprisingly, it appears that the following factors do not have a significant effect on adherence to exercise programs:

- general health awareness
- attitude toward physical activity
- level of physical fitness

- previous athletic experience
- socioeconomic status

Strategy To Maximize Motivation In Your Class

Clearly, the quality of supervision and guidance offered to the exercise program participant is critical to his/her compliance with the program and completion of objectives. What follows are specific strategies to ensure that the instructor provides the guidance and supervision that will keep each participant motivated.

Educate class members on the essential facts about exercising

Information on flexibility, weight loss/body composition, strength, cardiovascular condition and relaxation should be explained. Appeal can be made to the participants' desire for excellent health and an attractive appearance. Subjects such as injury prevention, the importance of warm-up and cool-down, proper equipment, modifications for environmental changes in temperature and humidity, should be included. Make a point of answering questions of individuals in a class whenever possible, and providing directions to obtain answers you are unable to provide. Make it clear that the benefits of exercise cannot be stored. They are lost as quickly as they are gained.

Supply directions regarding fitting exercise into busy schedules

Make it convenient. Indicate all the class times available, even suggesting additional times to management if necessary. Suggest exercising at a regular time to make it a fixed part of routine. Research indicates that attrition is less common among those who exercise in the morning. This is undoubtedly due to the fact that mornings are less likely to be interrupted by the unforeseen. This is not to say that all persons should be advised to exercise early in the day, because some individuals are simply not comfortable doing so. Exercise programs later in the day enjoy the unique feature of being able to effectively ease the tension of the day. Morning schedules have the advantage of being cooler during the hot months.

Offer personal support to your class participants

Try to influence peers and/or "significant others" in the lives of participants to be supportive. Tell participants to invite guests to observe or join an appropriate level workout. Exercising with a partner or several friends may be a very influential in keeping all members of the group exercising.

Make certain that your class is a safe workout

Be sure that all participants are properly warmed up, observe proper sequencing and special do's and don'ts.   **[IV: Warm-Up]**   Convince older people that age is not a barrier to exercise, as long as proper directions are followed. The environment in which classes exercise must be properly equipped and lighted—an atmosphere in which the instructor can make a nonthreatening workout environment. Participants must be able to relax as they commence their warm-up sequences. To be safe, it is best to curtail exercise if suffering from a minor illness, even if the individual is feeling strong. This assures that the stress of exercise will not inhibit recovery. If a participant misses a week of exercise, it is appropriate to pick up at the same level when rejoining the class. For each two weeks of exercise missed, advise the participant to drop back one level of intensity by class.

Do not forget to make your class enjoyable

Establish an atmosphere of friendliness and personal warmth. Keep classes moving. Maintain high energy and interest. **[III: Pre-Class Procedure]** Take a personal interest in class members, try to learn names, especially of newcomers. Make a point to communicate with each participant in every class, even if it is only by eye contact. Introduce yourself at each class session and state the level of the class you are about to instruct. Ascertain that class members are wearing appropriate footwear, and be sure to underscore the non-competitive nature of your class. Often the sole reason a person is motivated to continue exercising is the satisfaction derived from your personal association with him or her.

With these important demands upon the instructor, it is not surprising that the AFAA Standards recommend that an instructor teach no more than three classes per day and no more than twelve in one week. **[I.A: Frequency of Workouts]**

Be careful to support the commitment of each class member

Each participant in an exercise program needs to be encouraged to make a six-week commitment at the outset. This is an adequate time to experience the "training effect," providing appropriate frequency, duration, and intensity are observed. Once the benefits of the program become apparent, it is easier to set new goals and to maintain motivation. Progress will come gradually and only as a result of patience and persistence.

Each program participant should be urged to think about his or her level of physical fitness changing with each session. Charting progress can be a very motivating technique in this regard. Girth measurements of waist and hips, resting heart rates and body weights are variables that can be measured and charted. Owing to changes in body composition brought about through exercise, body weight measures can be misleading. Sensitizing exercise participants to the fit of their clothing is another motivating awareness. Finally, regular aerobic exercise program participation should lead to a reduction in resting heart rate of one beat per minute for each two weeks during the first 16–20 weeks of the program—awareness of this factor should serve to increase the motivation.

Reward the patience and persistence of your class members

Habits are established by the repetition of behavior, so it is important for the participant in an exercise program to have a positive experience at each exercise class. Encourage participants to reward themselves after each workout. Rewards can vary from a leisurely shower to a self-administered massage, from a manicure to a leisurely hour of reading, from the purchase of a new article of exercise clothing to a movie with a friend. The essential factor in this association is to reinforce a behavior positively, thereby making it more attractive to repeat until the habit is more completely bonded.

Summary

Mankind does not have a long history of living in an environment even remotely similar to that of today. Accordingly, the bodies we possess are not well suited to the demands placed upon them. A regular exercise program is essential if we are to meet those demands and enjoy all the benefits of this unique time in history.

Our society is giving more attention to healthful life-styles, but too few people have adopted regular exercise programs. It is the responsibility of the aerobic exercise instructor to ensure that participants in classes do not lose motivation and withdraw from the program prematurely. Individuals select a class exercise program because they want the benefits of exercising with a group under the direction of a leader; we must provide the guidance and direction they expect.

Cultural values and expectations have made it difficult for many individuals to maintain an active life-style. As values and expectations are changing, many of these people are seeking membership in aerobic exercise programs. The instructor needs a strategy to maximize the motivation of all members of each class. The strategy hinges on providing education regarding exercise, guiding class members to fit exercise into their varying schedules, offering personal support, ensuring safety, making the session enjoyable and suggesting rewards to ensure the commitment. We should realize that many individuals will remain in a program solely because of the rapport that has been established with the instructor. Each class then needs to be exciting, stimulating, challenging, satisfying, enjoyable, and productive.

References

Alter, J. *Surviving Exercise*. Boston: Houghton Mifflin, 1983.
Bailey, C. *Fit or Fat*. Boston: Houghton Mifflin, 1977.

Garrison, L. and Read, A. *Fitness for Every Body*. Palo Alto, CA: Mayfield Publishing, 1980.
Hockey, R. *Physical Fitness*. St. Louis: Mosby, 1981.
Pollock, M. and Wilmore, J. *Health and Fitness Through Physical Activity*. New York: Wiley, 1978.
Shepro, D. and Knuttgen, H. *Complete Conditioning*. Menlo Park, CA: Addison-Wesley, 1976.
Ulene, A. *Feeling Fine*. London: Magnum Books, 1977.
Vodak, P. *Exercise—The Why and the How*. Palo Alto: Bull Publishing, 1980.

Part C

Professionalism and Aerobics

Chapter 1

Professional Conduct

Marti Steele West, BA

The fitness industry is in the midst of a scientific revolution. Recent advances in the field of sports medicine are impacting upon the daily workout of thousands of consumers in everything from technically sophisticated weight training systems, to greater shock absorption in shoes. For the first time in sports history, the public has access to many of the same training aids as the professional athlete. The exercising public is gradually becoming educated in what it means to be fit and how to achieve fitness safely. In other words, we are seeing the birth of the informed fitness consumer.

Increased consumer knowledge provides an additional benefit in that it creates a demand for quality, both in training apparatus and in instruction. Thus, for the professional fitness instructor, the responsibilities have grown as the public has increased its demands upon our knowledge, athletic performance, instructional techniques, and ability to provide emotional support. At times it seems as though one must be everything from nutritional counselor to physical therapist in order to satisfy the needs of the students. How then, in the face of these demands, do we define the role and conduct of professional fitness instructors?

Professional Responsibility

Perhaps the focus of our attention should be the word "responsibility." Above all else, we, as fitness instructors, have agreed to accept the responsibility for providing an appropriate training session, designed to improve and maintain the overall fitness of healthy adults. To a certain degree, our students place their physical well-being in our hands. Instruction of an exercise class, however fun it might be for the student, is serious business.

The first step in meeting this responsibility to our students is to qualify ourselves. It is our individual responsibility to seek education and training to the extent necessary for the type of class and population we desire to instruct. The degree of training and the type of credentials necessary will vary according to the fitness level and physical and medical considerations of our students (see associated chapters on this content). Once having achieved the necessary level of education, it is our continued responsibility to expand our knowledge base and remain abreast of current research.

However, qualifications set limits, and it should be our responsibility as professional instructors not to exceed the limits of our education and training. Unless specifically trained as a therapist, it is not the place of the instructor to prescribe exercise treatment. With adequate training, immediate first aid for a medical condition such as a sprained ankle can be our responsibility. Treatment for chronic back strain should not. The role of instructor carries with it a certain degree of authority in the eye of the public, and we must be cautious not to abuse our position by attempting to overstep our limits. Providing general information on everything from injury prevention to nutrition should be our responsibility. Treating specific injuries or prescribing specific diets is not within the jurisdiction of the general fitness instructor, who doesn't have the requisite education, training, and license to practice. As professional instructors, it is our role to instruct, motivate, and monitor our students. In addition, it is, as in any other profession, our responsibility to refer our students to another professional when his or her demands exceed our capabilities.

The respect that we gain as professionals will come not only from defining our roles and educating ourselves to fulfill those roles, but also from our ability to present ourselves in a professional manner. This presentation can be separated into the following two categories:

- how we are visually perceived as instructors
- our instructional technique

Visual Impact

The visual impact of the fitness instructor cannot be overstated. To the students, the instructor should exemplify the process of self-improvement. That is not to say that anyone 10 pounds overweight should not be instructing. Rather, through the instructor's own visible commitment to improving his or her own level of fitness, he or she demonstrates the effectiveness of the exercise program and provides motivation for the students.

Professionalism is also exhibited through an instructor's choice of attire. Clothing and shoes should be clean and appropriate to the activity. Wearing tights and leotards that are full of runs or too skimpy will create an image that at best can be described as distracting. Comfortable, well-fitting exercise clothes that allow the students to easily observe the body in the correct exercise positions is the professional choice for fitness instructors.

Instructional Technique

The conduct of the class itself and the manner in which one instructs is another aspect of professionalism. The instructor should take charge immediately. It should be made clear that the instructor is there for the specific purpose of instructing and aiding the students to reach their individual fitness goals, and that their cooperation is essential to the success of the class. Whatever rules are necessary to maintain control should be established. Normally these rules, such as not speaking in a disruptive manner during class, are unspoken, but at times one must openly confront an individual for the benefit of the class as a whole. Students should not be allowed to wander in and out, or ignore your instruction and "do their own thing" as this can be very distracting to the other students. (This would not include individuals who must adapt a particular exercise to fit their individual medical or physical needs.) The professional instructor should demonstrate that he or she is capable of taking responsibility for the authority of his or her position.

Perhaps the most difficult aspect of teaching fitness, particularly for the novice instructor, is realizing that the time spent instructing belongs to the students. It is the instructor's job to help, and not compete with the students. It is the instructor's responsibility to be well-prepared, and to lead the students through a safe and effective workout. The exercise class experience should be uplifting and motivational, instilling within the students the desire to take responsibility for achieving their fitness goals. Students should feel that every attempt is made to monitor their safety and progress and that their accomplishments are recognized.

Professional conduct for fitness instructors will continue to become more clearly defined as the roles gradually evolve. One aspect which will not change, however, is the responsibility one must assume for placing the fitness and safety of the student before all other concerns. Providing quality instruction shall continue to be the mark of a professional instructor.

Chapter 2

Certification

Marti Steele West, BA

By definition, a profession is a vocation or occupation which requires advanced or specialized training in the liberal arts or sciences. A professional is thus an individual practicing one of the professions. Accordingly, a doctor, lawyer, or a teacher would fit this description, but what of the fitness instructor? Where or how does he or she fit into this cadre of professionalism?

The key to understanding what makes a professional can be found rooted in the word "requires." In most all accepted professions, and certainly in all professions which place one individual in a position of giving instruction, information, or care to another, the practitioners have met certain established requirements. A registered nurse standing at our bedside administering to our care has, through both theoretical and practical training and testing, met certain requirements that provide evidence of an acceptable level of competency. School teachers, psychologists and dentists alike, are all called upon to demonstrate their knowledge and practical ability to perform their various jobs effectively and safely. In other words, they have all fulfilled the requirements of an accepted standard recognizable to the public.

The fitness industry, outside the arena of organized sports, has in the past not received much serious attention from either the medical or legislative community. Since the mid 1970s it has experienced a phenomenal period of growth, and yet it has only been in the past few years that either the consumer or the industry itself has begun to see the need for standardization within the field. As the science of exercise develops, and the public's workout becomes more and more technically and medically oriented, we are all discovering that firm thighs and a flat abdomen are not the only qualifications necessary to instruct a safe and effective exercise program. Too often the exercise experience for the consumer has been plagued by contradiction and misinformation, not to mention physical injury. In lieu of the governmental requirements and regulations which police most other professions, the consumer must rely on the fitness industry to regulate itself. Fitness instructors should join the ranks of other health care professionals and be required to meet certain standards. Certifying the achievement of these requirements through instructor certification programs can provide an accepted standard by which one can measure the professional competency of a fitness instructor. The public is thus served by being able to recognize the level of competency of its instructors, and the qualified instructors themselves will benefit from an increased respect for their skills and training. Certification can be the means by which the fitness industry designates the qualified instructor as a professional.

Certification, however, is not a magical solution to the unprofessional ills of the industry. The very fact that instructor certification is at this time not within the realm of government, but of industry, creates one very basic problem: what does certification mean when virtually anybody can "certify" an instructor? There are scores of certification programs available, and unfortunately, not all are created equal. The consumer and the professional instructor are thus both faced with deciding which, among the myriad of offerings, will be the one which sets an acceptable standard. How does one choose? By what criteria does one judge the validity of a given program?

First, and of foremost importance in examining the actual features of a given program, are the *standards* themselves and the *certifying body* behind those standards. Certification means that someone is validating the fulfillment of the requirements according to a certain standard. *Who has developed the standards? What are the credentials of the certifying body?* On what grounds should their standards of competency be accepted? In order to provide a valid certification, an organization must first establish its own integrity.

Secondly, one should examine the validity of the certifying process. How are the requirements met? Are both theoretical knowledge and practical skills tested? Does everyone who applies automatically become certified? Certification that makes no distinction between qualified and unqualified is of little value. Certification should provide proof of knowledge and ability, not of sufficient money to buy it.

Another important feature of a certification program should be requirements for continued education. In most professions all licenses and certifications have a certain term, and renewal depends on the professional's ability and willingness to continue his or her education. Encouraging continued education and training serves not only to enlarge the instructor's knowledge base, but to keep a rapidly growing industry up to date with the latest research.

Program curriculum can also be a discriminating factor among programs. While varying to accommodate specialized interests, instructor certification should require a basic theoretical understanding and/or practical competency in the following areas

- exercise physiology
- body composition
- safe and effective exercise methods
- cardiovascular and medical considerations
- CPR and first aid
- basic anatomy
- injury prevention
- sports nutrition and weight control
- effective instructional technique
- health screening

Programs lacking in certain areas of basic curriculum will not provide a general standard for measuring an instructor's overall competency.

Finally, one should examine a program in terms of one's own needs. From either the point of view of an instructor, or a consumer, different certifications will provide evidence of varying degrees of competency and areas of specialization. For example, to an instructor facing the possibility of working in several different clubs, perhaps in different cities or even in different states, a certification by a strictly local club or organization would be of little value. Likewise, an instructor working part-time at one club, in a small town, would have little use for a highly technical, national program, more suited to a practitioner in a clinical setting. As a consumer, one should seek to ascertain that the requirements of a particular certification are at least equal to the level of technical skill necessary to implement the individual's exercise regimen.

In response to the need for certification of a safe aerobics program that reflects standards and guidelines developed by experts in the fields of exercise theory and practice, AFAA has implemented a certification program. An overview of this program is described below.

Certification Program for Aerobic Exercise Instructors

The Aerobics and Fitness Association of America is an association of aerobic exercise professionals and enthusiasts, advised by a multidisciplinary Board of Advisors, dedicated to the promotion of safety and excellence in the instruction of aerobic exercise. It is our belief that the public deserves the following:

1. Safe and effective exercise instruction
2. A standard by which to recognize the competency of the personnel directly administering an exercise class.

To meet this goal, AFAA, under the direction of its Board of Advisors, has developed a nationwide Certification Program for Aerobic Exercise Instructors. The AFAA Certified Aerobic Instructor has demonstrated a basic degree of competency, adequate to instruct a safe and effective aerobics exercise class to healthy adults. The criteria for Certification by the Aerobics and Fitness Association of America are as follows:

1. Individuals must demonstrate knowledge of
   a. Anatomy and exercise physiology
   b. Cardiovascular/medical considerations of aerobic exercise
   c. Injury prevention
   d. Correct exercise execution and instruction
   e. Appropriate class format and instruction technique
   f. Sports nutrition
2. Hold current CPR Certification

Certification is by both written and practical examination. Certification workshops which offer instructors both a review of the required curriculum and the opportunity to participate in the examinations, are held approximately twice a month at sites throughout the United States.

AFAA Certification as an Aerobic Exercise Instructor is valid for a period of two years. Certification is renewed through AFAA's continuing education and recertification process.

Summary

One can state that certification of fitness instructors can help promote professionalism and protect the consumer. However, it remains the responsibility of the industry and the consumer to determine the validity or appropriateness of individual programs.

*Copyright © 1985 Aerobics and Fitness Association of America.
All rights reserved in all countries.*

Chapter 3

Continuing Education

Phyllis G. Cooper, RN, MN

Continuing education (CE) is the process of lifelong learning. It may encompass the learning of new information, behaviors, or skills, or it may be the expansion of knowledge, behaviors, or skills in a given area. Central to this process is the realization that CE is ongoing and involves adult learners. Understanding the elements of CE is essential to recognition and acceptance of this process. This chapter focuses on the process of CE in general and the rationale for CE for aerobic instructors in specific.

Lifelong Learning

Adult learners are influenced by an entirely different set of factors than those that influence the child learner. Most of these factors are a result of the growth and maturation process itself. Others are a reflection of previous exposure to an educational process. The classic work on adult learning is done by Malcolm S. Knowles, an adult educator and professor of education, who has laid the foundation for the theory of adult learning with his Andragogical Theory. This theory outlines the factors that influence adult learning. These factors are:

- A self-concept that is self-directed.
- A reservoir of life experiences.
- A readiness to learn because of a need to know.
- A problem-centered orientation to learning.

What this means is that learning will occur in response to a need, and that the person will seek the learning necessary to continued success in a job. But learning will occur only if the learner feels that instruction takes into account what the need is; identifies how the new knowledge or skill can be helpful for day-to-day practice; and takes into account the knowledge base and previous experiences of the learner. The learning must be relevant, useful, applicable and current.

A Plan for Continuing Education

Continuing education is the cornerstone of a successful aerobics practice. Whether you work in a small or a large facility or are a private trainer, CE has relevance for you. Because the fields of aerobics, sports physiology, and medicine are evolving, one's knowledge and subsequent practice must change to reflect the new discoveries. The continuing education process involves planning for the acquisition and application of new and expanding knowledge and skills. This plan should be concrete, not just a haphazard "I read this or that journal" or "Maybe I'll take this or that class." A plan for continuing education should include:

- at least one journal, read on a regular basis
- classes taken in a college or a university setting
- organized classes taken from a professional association
- informal classes or learning experiences occurring in the work place
- sessions where correct workouts can be practiced and reviewed for accuracy.

Role of the Professional Association

A professional association functions to maintain a certain quality of practice and to represent the professional who provides services to the consumer. In order to ensure that quality practice is maintained, most professional associations recommend or require that their members participate in continuing education. If the professional association also provides a certification for members, then the certification implies a level of practice that is safe and of a certain quality.

The Aerobics and Fitness Association of America believes that a professional must be a safe instructor who has a high-quality aerobics practice. To ensure the continuation of such standards, AFAA requires certain educational experiences before an instructor can be recertified. These requirements are listed below:

Aerobics and Fitness Association of America Criteria for Recertification

The Aerobics and Fitness Association of America, in response to the need of the AFAA Certified Aerobic Exercise Instructor for continuing education and professional growth, and in recognition of the right of the public to a valid, and thus current, standard by which to recognize instructional competency, has developed the following criteria for recertification as an Aerobics Exercise Instructor.

AFAA Instructor Certification is valid for two years. Within that period a Certified Instructor must submit proof of the following, in order to renew his or her certification:

1. A minimum of 15 hours of AFAA-approved continuing education classes from at least two different areas. Acceptable classes would include:
   a. Any AFAA courses offered for continuing education.
   b. Any courses offered by an accredited college or university in any of the following subjects or related subject areas
      - Exercise physiology
      - Anatomy and physiology
      - Kinesiology
      - Sports medicine
      - Nutrition
      - Physical therapy
      - Body composition
      - Sports injury prevention/treatment
      - Instructional methods
      - Facility management
   c. Other courses offered in the above or related subject areas offered by hospitals, clinics or other organizations may be valid. Acceptability of these courses will be determined by the AFAA Board of Certification upon petition to the board by the instructor.
   d. Courses offering only practical experience without class time devoted specifically to theory such as ballet, jazz dance or cheerleading class, shall not be acceptable.
2. Hold current CPR certification.

Copyright © 1985 Aerobics and Fitness Association of America. All rights reserved in all countries. (Reprinted with permission.)

As an area of practice evolves, so do the requirements for quality. It is likely that in the very near future the professional association, as well as employers, may require the aerobics instructor to show proficiency in a workout through a practical exam on a yearly or two-year basis. We expect doctors, nurses, and paramedics to perform practical aspects of their professions at a certain ongoing level of competence. Before long, the consumer will be asking for an assurance of the same quality of practice from the aerobics instructor.

Role of the Aerobics Instructor

As a professional, the aerobics instructor is responsible for participating in an organized approach to lifelong learning. The instructor needs to be aware of those areas of practice that are new or changing. He or she must take the steps necessary to enhance knowledge and skills in such areas. Participation in a professional association allows the instructor to have access to the latest developments in the field and to classes utilizing these new developments.

Summary

This chapter focused briefly on the process of continuing education. It dealt with the concept of professional responsibility as it relates to continuing education. The role of the professional association and aerobics instructor as it relates to CE were discussed.

Chapter 4

Instructor Training

Marti Steele West, BA

During the past few years, we have seen aerobic exercise become the chosen lifetime exercise for thousands of individuals. Hand in hand with this growth in popularity has been the rapid increase in the number of instructors. While many come from other fitness careers, the vast majority initially became instructors as a means of staying in shape themselves. Most instructors teach on a part-time basis and rely on another career for financial support. In surveys of instructors attending AFAA Certification Workshops during the program's first year, it was revealed that fewer than four out of every 10 instructors have had even one hour of formal education in exercise science. We are thus faced with the dilemma of creating educated professionals from individuals who are generally involved with the world of aerobics on an amateur basis. Many have neither the time, money, nor motivation to pursue long-term university level training in exercise science.

The question now becomes: how much education and training is enough? Is a college degree really necessary? If not, how can instructor competency be judged?

In 1983 the Aerobics and Fitness Association of America, with the publication of the *Basic Exercise Standards and Guidelines,* established a standard of acceptable performance for aerobic exercise classes with healthy adults. In the same year, AFAA Certification for aerobic exercise instructors was also created, thus providing the first worldwide standardized measure of instructor competency. Many other instructor certification programs now exist (see Part C, Chapter 2 for a complete discussion of certification), thus enabling the public and professionals alike to answer the question of how much training is enough.

During the past few years, we have seen the appearance of training programs designed specifically to prepare an individual to instruct an aerobic exercise class for healthy adults. Exercise classes for special populations (e.g., cardiac rehabilitation patients) usually require more extensive education and training and are not considered in this discussion of instructor training. These specialized programs are being taught through a variety of institutions, including universities, private organizations, and individual clubs. Examples of ongoing training programs include the AFAA Certified Instructor Training Program, the certificate program offered by the University of California at San Diego, the YMCA, and the programs offered by the International School of Aerobic Training, Fitcamp and Fitness Instructor Training, to name a few.

Most training programs provide the successful participant with some evidence of his or her competency, such as certification, that serves to identify the general skill level of the individual. At this point, however, with the required competencies varying from program to program, evaluation of a training program is still difficult and each program must be reviewed independently.

The evaluation of an instructor training program from either the point of view of a consumer, a professional, or a would-be instructor, should focus on several key points. Of primary importance is the actual course curriculum. The following is a general outline of subject areas that should be covered in an instructor training program:

- basic anatomy and physiology
- components of fitness
- principles of conditioning
- cardiovascular function
- CPR certification
- flexibility
- appropriate class format
- correct exercise execution
- basic nutrition
- body composition
- weight control and eating disorders
- fitness assessment
- risk factors
- danger signs
- medical considerations
- environmental considerations
- instructional technique
- motivation

- music
- legal responsibilities

The AFAA Certified Instructor Training Program is a 40-hour course that covers the subjects outlined in this chapter.

The amount of time which must be committed to a program and the manner in which that time is utilized are also important considerations. Teaching aerobic exercise requires not only correct theoretical and practical knowledge, but the ability to motivate and monitor one's students. Having sufficient time to practice teaching and receive constructive feedback from the trainer should be an important element in any training program. On the other hand, a program which deals too heavily with how to teach may be lacking in areas of theoretical knowledge. An appropriate allocation of time in a training program could be approximated as follows:

- For each class meeting, one-third of the time should be spent in lecture and discussion of theoretical material.
- The remaining two-thirds of the session should focus on trainer demonstration and participant teaching experience.
- For every hour of in-class theoretical study, there should be at least one hour of assigned and/or recommended reading and study to be completed on the participant's own time.
- The total course time should be no less than 25–30 hours, at an absolute minimum.

The deciding factor in the appraisal of any training program should be the quality of the finished product: the instructor. The reputation of a particular program for preparing instructors with an adequate level of core knowledge and safe, effective instructional techniques, will ultimately determine the professional acceptability of that particular program and any accompanying certificates. A training program will not exceed the quality of its training materials or the credentials and reputation of its trainers.

The ever-increasing demand for qualified instructors in the field of aerobic exercise can be met through specific training programs. Those courses which meet the criteria of appropriate curriculum, length and method of study and training, and have a reputation for providing a high quality of instruction, serve a valuable purpose in the fitness community by providing specific education at a reasonable cost in terms of both time and money. It remains, however, the obligation of the prospective instructor or class participant to evaluate the merits of each training program on an individual basis.

Part D

The Aerobics Business

Chapter 1

Starting Your Own Business

Sheila Cluff

Look past the glitter and glamour—there's a whole lot more to starting a business in the fitness industry than merely having a love of exercise and teaching classes.

You can learn the how-to's on your own from the suggested reading list at the end of this chapter. So, instead of listing references and quoting sources on managing employees, setting up profit and loss statements and discussing your financial needs with a banker, I want to share my experiences and the insight I've acquired regarding what it really takes to build a successful fitness business.

If you're in the market for never-fail advice or foolproof techniques, you'll be a very long time getting your enterprise off the ground. But the good news is that by understanding the following principles, which I'll explain in detail, you can reduce the risks, speed up the process and stack the deck in your favor.

The Basics

Concentrate on the *five basic essentials* you must have:

1. A reasonable amount of intelligence.
2. An adequate amount of capital.
3. An enormous amount of energy.
4. A hell of a lot of guts.
5. That "certain something," also known as luck *and* good timing.

Now, let's get started.

You must have a reasonable amount of intelligence

Answer "yes" or "no" to the following questions:

- Do you have the educational background required to meet the high standards in the fitness world?
- Do you have the confidence, flair and finesse to teach?
- Are you certified or taking classes to become certified?
- Do you have the genetic luck to move well to music and to be extremely energetic?
- Can you set an example and be an inspiration to students?

If you've just shouted "Yes," you've taken a major step toward a rewarding career in the fitness industry. Congratulations!

Take the time right now to establish your goals. Here are some questions to stir your thoughts: Where are you headed? Do you want to teach all the classes yourself? Or do you want to manage a score of teachers? Perhaps you really want to open your own center or start a spa.

For those who need to be in charge and adore it, in addition to having an entrepreneurial bend, this field is wide open. However, you must also realize that by being your own boss, you will not have the cushion of working for someone else. Leadership isn't for everyone. If you're going to succeed, there can be no doubt in your mind—you must definitely want to own your own business.

What will that business look like? Is it going to have a physical plant, a studio? Will you be able to start on a grand scale or is a smaller one indicated? Are you considering a tie in with a franchise organization? With a franchise, you are in essence your own boss, *but* you will be obligated to certain organizational rules/directives. Is that acceptable or will it crimp your creative style?

What will be your focus? Slanted toward the business community? Homemakers? Corporations and industry?

There are no right or wrong answers, and your ideas can go from one extreme to the other. This is where a reasonable amount of intelligence is essential.

I started with a very small consulting firm that catered to businesses, industry, recreation departments and school districts and used this as a footing to establish credibility in my locality. This is an excellent way to start if limited capital is a real consideration.

I'm a great believer in planning, and I urge you to set goals. Make small ones, medium-sized intermediate ones and don't be afraid to dream big— you need to know where you want to be five years from now. Get one thing straight this minute: prepare with intelligence and be positive. Say this sentence out loud: "This is going to be a growing business, and I will want to expand."

Do you know that you are a "product?" That's right, and you need to study the market in your town to calculate your chances for success. Are there other classes or gyms that constantly undercut each other? If you join them, will you have the capital to do battle? With a measure of innovative thinking, you could scoop the market leaving others behind. Could you offer

- a fit-to-ski program?
- a couples class?
- an exercise program for tots?
- a seniors or handicapped class?

Do your homework and gather information on the competition; then review *all* the details so your programs will be spectacular.

While setting up your goals, check out the labor market. Will you be able to hire competent teachers? Could a junior college provide some part-time staff members? Will an apprentice program enable you to reduce the financial burden of your budding business?

Use a reasonable amount of intelligence and get the answers. Successful people do not accept failure as an option. That doesn't mean there won't be setbacks, but when they occur, consider them as points for reflection, not signs that you have personally failed.

You must have a reasonable amount of capital

How much money do you have? How much can you afford to put into your business? Consider the options if capital is an issue. Do you want to be the sole owner or can you take in a partner? If you want to go it alone, could you borrow to allow yourself that luxury? Talk to the local banks and study alternative financing. Those who make it big refuse to take no for an answer. Personal loans or loans against your investments could be the best bet. Check out the options before you make a decision.

Have you thought about presenting a business plan and going after investors? What are the advantages and disadvantages of incorporation? Could you save capital through legitimate tax loss—by using that loss to your benefit? Research in every way you can how the Small Business Administration and various government agencies supply grants and low-interest loans to small business—it may pay off.

When considering a partnership, heed my words of warning: make certain that your idea of working hard is the same as your partner's. If your partner feels a stress-filled day is six hours long and your idea of a normal work day is sixteen, you're in trouble. The more you can iron out before forming any partnership, the more successful you'll be. Get everything down in writing, too, because money changes people. I also suggest making a list of "business expectations" adding even the smallest detail of how many hours you'll work, when you'll take money out of the business, and who'll do the bookkeeping.

One area that I have discovered a lot of new business owners neglect is the high cost of advertising. People must know you're out there and ads cost money. Graphic design is expensive. Have you priced stationery, insurance, utilities, taxes? Look at every facet of your proposed operation *before* you begin.

One way to do that is by following an existing fitness business. Scrutinize what the local gym is doing. Look at the quantity of their ads. Look at the editorial coverage they're getting. Listen for their radio advertising. Check what they're paying and realize that an ad budget is a must.

Now, let's talk about where you can SAVE money. Free publicity is a gold mine—and can be yours for the asking. Make a list of the local charities and offer your services. How about fund raisers? It makes sound business sense to give away services to get clients—don't underestimate this valuable tool. It works. Let's say you are sponsoring a fun-run for a civic group or helping to raise money for a specific city project—suddenly you have the opportunity to talk about your fitness business on local television and radio and to be included in press releases for the paper. Use your influence in the community to get editorial coverage without expense.

One resourceful business woman took on the challenge of making over a physically unfit local celebrity. The notable became ten pounds thinner and felt marvelous and our entrepreneur got a lot of publicity. In addition, she convinced the city to hold fitness classes for its employees and made the front page of the local newspaper (wearing her center's t-shirt of course).

Another creative exercise instructor formed a relationship with a charity in her town. For every new student the organization signed up to attend her classes, she donated a portion of the fee. She had the charity working for her and both came out on top.

Get the word out about how great your program is and your goals will slide into place. Yes, it may take some giving, but look at it as a powerful investment.

Another source for saving cash is bartering. Need business cards or flyers or stationery? Trade a month's free classes to the printing firm in exchange for the supplies. Bartering can get you advertising, services and products. You will have individuals in your center who won't be paying, but once they sample your program and see the outstanding results, they'll re-register and bring their friends along, too.

You must have an enormous amount of energy

Owning a business means there will be no one to tell you what to do and how to do it. There is freedom, but there are no established guidelines. You may have to work seven days a week in the beginning. In order to keep up that pace, you must practice what you preach. You must stay in peak condition and be alert at all times. It won't be an easy balance, either, because you'll have all the pressures of a new business to contend with. But once you neglect your own advice and start to get run down or out of shape, your credibility will dissolve—that means you'll lose the respect of your clients and your employees.

It really does take an enormous amount of energy to operate your own business and to reach your goals, and you must bring that energy into the business on the creative side, too. You'll have to constantly invent ways to improve, to make the techniques you teach "state-of-the-art," and to make sure you're a mile ahead of the competition. Mental energy is crucial.

To help in this area, sign up for seminars, go to motivational workshops, subscribe to professional journals, network with other business and civic leaders. Keep those creative juices flowing.

Keep your mind open. Just because something hasn't been done "that" way before, doesn't make it wrong. Think of the idea as unique or trendy, and it may help reap bigger profits. As a health and fitness business professional, you have the responsibility to keep abreast of the constant changes in our industry, or you must get someone on your team to do that for you. The only other option is to be left behind—this business moves fast.

Sure there will be days when you will feel out of step—learn to look at the alternative. If that doesn't keep you going, nothing will! Of course, you'll need a pep talk once in awhile, but that's when your enormous energy comes into the spotlight. You need to create enough energy for the highs and lows *and* for your personal life. It's a big mistake to put all your energy into the business because your relationships will crumble. Don't get so involved in your business that there isn't anything else in your life—the business won't run as well. Balance your personal energy output with your professional energy output.

Remember: you cannot be all things to all people. Make a smart move and get help. If you are starting a business and also running a home, hire some household assistance. Think of it as investment in the future and watch your business grow.

You must have a hell of a lot of guts

Any new business is risky and I won't depress you with the percentage of failures during the first five years of operation.

You've got to have guts to buck the odds. It can be really frightening to mortgage your home to get capital for your business and see those bills piling up. Are you the type who is able to stand the emotional tension associated with this enterprise? Please give some thought to that—it's a serious question.

When times were tough and I thought of giving up, *I worked harder.* You'll probably have to do that too. One of the most difficult decisions I had to make when I began (and had very little money) was to double my advertising budget. It hurt—but it worked.

You need confidence and the guts to move out of the crowd—not in a naive way—but with success-oriented self-assurance. No one said it would be easy, but knowing ahead of time that you will encounter hurdles could make your jump smoother.

It takes guts to sign a lease to rent a facility, especially when you will be legally obligated to make payments regardless of your student count. That can stress anyone, but guts will help you go on in spite of the ramifications. Otherwise, fold this book and quietly pick up the want ads.

Getting positive feedback from those close to you can be an asset—the world won't always think your smashing methods are as exciting as you may. An emotional support system will enable you to weather some of the storms. However, the hard work will be all yours.

That clearly brings us up to *criticism.* It can be nasty at times. Do you have the guts to listen even though you may not agree? It's a foolish business person who covers her ears to an opposing opinion. Listen and profit. You just may change your mind, or you may charge ahead as planned. But, have the guts to realize there is a positive and negative side to all businesses.

You must have that "certain something," also known as "good timing."

Everything else can be a snap, but unless your timing is perfect, you could end up being just one more statistic on a government business failure report. Sorry—you're still not home free. That "certain something"—call it luck or good timing—is a very real component of success.

When I started the Palms in Palm Springs, I had no control over a potentially disastrous situation. I opened weeks before the first snow storm Palm Springs had had in fifty years! It was the coldest winter on record *and* in the East, where I was depending on attracting a lot of guests, the weather was exceptionally balmy. That was bad luck. At the same time, the following year was the absolute reverse. It was gorgeous in Palm Springs and the East had a series of freezing winter storms.

Sometimes luck is a matter of researching the area when you plan to locate. Sometimes, it's who you know and not what you know. Sometimes, it's being in the right place at the right time.

Economic trends can have a major effect on luck or timing. One fact, you must never forget, is that people still consider health and wellness to be a luxury item. When times get tough, it's the exercise class that goes, not food or shelter or new shoes for the kids. But when times are good, people want new clothes and a fit and trim body to go with them.

It could be that you will have to suffer through low-economic periods—providing it makes good business sense—so that when the tide changes, you'll have a firmly established business. But there's no exact formula regarding how long to hold a business together—that's where your reasonable intelligence will help you.

Recognize the potential of good timing. If you see a trend—perhaps a new type of resistance equipment is catching on and your gym still has the old style—you need to review your budget to project what it will take to compete with the competition. You may also want to consider how long you can keep the old equipment and still keep your clients happy.

Good timing means staying one step ahead—thinking up classes that someone else can't totally duplicate. Create a uniqueness that will set you apart. Maybe you're the only person who is teaching classes for the blind, or who is using small hand weights, or who can offer child care. Being different could make you a winner.

Polish your skills. Do you need to learn how to effectively give a speech? Hire (or barter with) an acting coach to learn how to improve your public image. For example, let's say you are sponsoring a fund raiser and have been invited by the local talk show host to appear on her show. You'll have three minutes at the maximum to talk about the project and your center—learn to make that precious time count.

Timing and luck will skyrocket if you're identified as a "doer." People will remember you, remember your business and want to catch some of your vitality. Is being visible a matter of timing, luck, or old-fashioned common sense? That depends on who you ask!

Don't wait for luck to come to you—position yourself so you'll be ready when it happens.

Summary

Sure you'll get bounced around. Success does have a price tag, but being involved in the fitness business is truly addictive. Now you know what I consider the "essentials" to starting your own business, so what's holding you back? Get out and go for it!

Commonly Asked Questions

Q. What is expected of me as a teacher in a fitness business?
A. Everything you've got and more. You don't have the luxury of bringing personal problems into your class or business. *You* must be the

motivator. Your energy level must be high at all times. Students are intuitively receptive. They can instantly pick up on a lack of enthusiasm or a lagging desire to teach the class. You can never allow that to happen. You've got to be "on" every single moment—not as a performer, but as instructor and a guide.

Q. How do I know if I have the knack to run a business?
A. Have you been successful organizing a charity event? Do you enjoy leading and teaching? Are you creative beyond the call of duty in your present job, but prefer to do more on your own? If you can say yes, you probably have what it takes. Keep in mind that when you run the show, when you're the person in charge, *you can't call in sick.* Make sure you are convinced and can honestly say that a fit and healthy body will have a positive impact on your students' lives. If you can't, your dishonesty will be evident to everyone.

Q. What kind of sacrifices will I have to make?
A. In the beginning, there may be times when you'll have to forego personal enjoyment to take care of your business. You'll have to be prepared to give up time with those close to you. You may even have to work harder than you ever thought possible.

Q. How can I find good people to work for me?
A. Trust your instincts. Check references. Know that you will make a few mistakes—everybody does. Once you hire someone, create incentives to keep his or her motivation high, but you must realize that without your example, nothing will work. You have to perform as hard or harder than all of your employees.

Q. Why did you start your fitness business?
A. Fitness has a positive impact on life, and I wanted to help people discover that fact. Being a catalyst is very exciting. That's why I started and why I'm still so enthusiastic.

References

Financial Planning Manuals

Ellis, J. *A Financial Guide For The Self-Employed.* Chicago: Regnery, 1972. (An easy-to-read manual dealing in detail on issues such as partnership, incorporation, sole proprietorship, insurance, taxes, retirement planning and an array of pertinent topics.)

Smith, C. *Getting Grants.* New York: Harper & Row, 1980. (Gives the how-tos to open doors with the grant-making agencies.)

Stevens, M. *How To Borrow A Million Dollars.* New York: Macmillan, 1982. (A complete guide to the more traditional financing methods as well as the more "creative" alternatives plus how to sell yourself to obtain the necessary financing for your business.)

Tracy, J. *How To Read A Financial Report.* New York: Wiley, 1980. (If you need to know what those assets and liabilities mean because you are the business, this book supplies the answers.)

Vardaman, G. *Making Successful Presentations.* Amacom, 1981. (Beyond just making speeches, you'll need this information when you attract investors or take your business proposals to the bank.)

Krentzman, H. *Managing For Profits.* Washington: Government Printing Office, 1981. (Practical basic theory and day-to-day information the small business owner needs to make decisions and take action.)

Business Sense in Book Form

Brandt, S. *Entrepreneuring: The Ten Commandments for Building A Growth Company.* New York: Addison-Wesley, 1982. (Provides strategy for creating and managing a growing company, with business plans and how to implement the ten main operation procedures.)

Siegel, G. *How To Advertise And Promote Your Small Business.* New York: Wiley, 1977. (Concise, no-nonsense guide to advertising.)

Lane, M. *Legal Handbook for Small Business.* American Management Association, 1977. (Common sense info to set up and run your small business, including how to choose professional help.)

US Small Business Administration, Washington, DC 20416: Offers training, counseling and booklets on the topics below and many more:

- starting a small business
- developing records and bookkeeping systems
- locating sources of financing
- locating a business site
- developing customers

Most services are free.

Chapter 2

Legal Considerations

Randi S. Lewis, J.D.

Aerobic exercise injuries will occur in spite of the training or competence of the instructor and the caliber of the exercise program. Of course, the likelihood of injury is reduced when the instructor is highly trained and the program is medically sound. The reality is, however, that instructors and exercise clubs may find themselves open to questions on the safety, qualifications, and soundness of their programs. This chapter deals with two major concerns for any fitness business owner, instructor, or consultant: the liability aspects of business operations and the need for consumer protection.

Liability Aspects

Keep in mind that anyone can file a lawsuit against anyone else. All a person must do is prepare a complaint, pay a fee, and file it with a court.

In addition, even if a person proves he or she was injured while participating in an exercise class, he or she will not automatically win the lawsuit. To prevail, one must prove that the class instructor and/or the exercise club were negligent—that is, that their conduct fell below a certain standard of care—and that such neglect caused the injuries sustained.

The injured person will attempt to prove, for example, that the instructor taught the class improperly and perhaps was not qualified to teach, or that the exercise studio had a substandard training and exercise program, had no program at all, or hired unqualified instructors.

Although aerobic exercise injury lawsuits cannot be prevented, they can be successfully defended. And there are affirmative steps that can and should be taken to ensure that the liability of owners, operators, and employees is limited.

The intent of this chapter is to raise the consciousness of owners, operators, and instructors of exercise facilities. It lists a number of measures they should take to protect themselves from obvious legal liability.

This chapter does not, however, constitute a legal opinion or legal advice, nor does it pretend to define the standard of care by which an exercise program will be judged. Each athletic club and aerobic exercise class has its own unique style, to which the following suggestions must be tailored. If a specific inquiry or problem exists, it is advisable to seek legal advice.

Injuries may arise in any type of organized exercise class, including aerobics, Jazzercise, yoga, and aerobic dance classes. The term *exercise class* will be used as a generic term to encompass all organized exercise classes. For purposes of this article, the terms exercise studio, exercise facility, athletic club, and the like will be used interchangeably.

Exercise clubs/studios

Owners and operators of exercise studios should implement the following measures to lessen the likelihood of injuries and protect themselves from legal liability and financial loss:

1. Purchase liability insurance.
2. Develop a structured, medically sound exercise program.
3. Hire well-rounded, qualified instructors.
4. Require that every person who participates in an exercise class sign a disclaimer and release.

The best protection against lawsuits is liability insurance. If an injured student sues the studio or its instructor, the insurance company will pay for and provide defense of the insured, and it will also pay any settlement or judgment fees, up to the limits of the policy.

If the injury is serious enough and the judgment or settlement exceeds the limits of the policy, the exercise studio would be required to pay the difference. Since payment of a large differential could potentially drain the studio's assets, it is imperative that the limits of the policy be as high as the facility can afford.

In addition to purchasing liability insurance, the exercise facility should obtain an all-risk or comprehensive insurance policy to protect the facility and its equipment from such perils as theft, flood, and fire.

Program approval

Some exercise studios develop a structured program that all instructors are required to follow. Other clubs allow classes to vary from instructor to instructor. Whichever type of program your club follows, it is a good idea to have the basic program or exercises approved by one or more sports medicine professionals, such as orthopedic surgeons and physical therapists who specialize in sports medicine.

If the athletic club has the economic resources to go the extra mile, it may hire a sports medicine professional to assist the staff in developing different routines for the exercise and aerobics classes. In order to limit the club's liability, it is important to document in writing the sports medicine professional's contribution and approval. At a minimum, a letter of approval should be kept in the file.

The exercise program might be evaluated periodically. Each time such an evaluation in made, written approval of the updated program should be obtained from the professional consultant.

By obtaining and documenting the contribution made by the sports medicine professional, the exercise program is upgraded, and the members of the club will receive high-quality fitness training. This may also be a useful marketing tool, which will help justify an increase in membership dues. Additionally, a jury or court is furnished with documented reasons for it to find that the exercise club has taken the utmost care and responsibility in developing its exercise program.

Hiring qualified instructors

Hiring well-rounded, qualified instructors is another step toward limiting liability. Even if the instructors are already experienced and qualified, it is advisable to develop an instructor training program. The training program should preferably be approved in writing by a sports medicine professional.

The instructor training program should also be documented. One way is to compile a written training manual to be given to each instructor. One copy should be kept in the office at all times as a reference manual.

The manual should be approved by the same sports medicine professional who approves the exercise program. It should contain general guidelines regarding injury protection and require instructors to successfully complete a certification course.

Instructors should be required to join a local or nationally recognized professional association, and periodically update their knowledge and training regarding the latest developments in the exercise field.

This additional training requirement upgrades the exercise facility's program and demonstrates that the owners and operators are selective and responsible in hiring and training their instructors.

If, for whatever reason, the exercise club chooses not to obtain professional approval for the manual, it may be best not to compile a manual at all. It could prove to be a double-edged sword. The injured party's attorney could hire a expert in sports medicine to review the manual. If it contains information guidelines which are medically unsound, that would be brought out at the time of trial and could increase substantially the exercise studio's liability.

Trends toward state certification

In California, legislation has been introduced which, if enacted, will require every person or exercise facility providing instruction to disclose the minimum level of training and certification held by all instructors. Specifically, if would be a description of the instructors' training in sports medicine, exercise physiology, nutrition, recognition and prevention of sports injuries, first aid, and cardiovascular pulmonary resuscitation (CPR). The penalty for not disclosing this information is that the customer be entitled to a refund of initiation or membership fees.

This legislation is the beginning of a national trend toward requiring certification or licensing of aerobic exercise instructors. It will potentially upgrade the quality of exercise programs offered to the general public.

In addition, this type of legislation may ultimately establish a standard of care with which owners and operators of exercise facilities must comply and by which they may be judged. That is, it will be easier to demonstrate liability on the part of the exercise studio should the studio hire instructors who lack the basic training and/or certification.

It is also advisable to periodically give class participants printed or typed handouts containing information on how to protect themselves while performing certain exercises. However, the contents of the handout must be accurate and should avoid mentioning exercises that are the subject of controversy among experts in the sports medicine field.

Disclaimer and releases

In addition to providing informational handouts, the exercise club should seriously consider having each person who participates in an exercise class, whether a club member or a first-time guest, read and sign a written disclaimer and release form. This form should disclaim any liability for negligence on the part of the exercise club or any of its employees. The release might also describe the nature of the exercise program and request that each person consult a physician prior to participating in the exercise program.

At a minimum, the release should contain the following: language indicating that the participant acknowledges there is a risk of injury; a statement by the participant that he or she agrees to be solely responsible for any injuries sustained as a result of participation in the class; and a statement that the participant agrees to hold harmless the exercise club, the staff, and instructors for any injuries sustained while using the exercise facility.

Although a court could find that by signing the release, the participant assumed the risk of injury (especially where informational handouts are distributed as well), such a disclaimer and release signed by the class participant will not necessarily release the exercise studio from being held responsible for the injuries sustained.

For example, in some states or jurisdictions, such a release might be deemed to be invalid as against public policy. Other localities require that the disclaimer and release be conspicuously printed in certain sized type, or it will not be valid.

Still other laws require that the release set forth clearly to a person untrained in the law that the document has the effect of releasing his or her claim for personal injuries. Any release is more likely to be effective if written in plain, easily understandable language.

However, a release standing alone will not win the case for the exercise club. It may be used as one piece of ammunition in the defense of a lawsuit.

It is advisable to consult an attorney to prepare such a release so that the language and other particulars are prepared in accordance with the law of the state or locality in which the exercise facility exists.

Instructor liability prevention

There is nothing more disconcerting to an instructor than being sued by a student. Most often, it is alleged that the instructor failed to properly warm up the class. As a result, the student claims to have been injured while attempting to perform a stretching exercise.

What affirmative steps can the instructor take to lessen the likelihood of being sued, or more importantly, being held liable?

The instructor should take the responsibility of obtaining the proper training. Active membership in a highly regarded professional aerobic fitness association, such as AFAA, is advisable because it will help the instructor keep abreast of the latest developments and techniques in the field.

The instructor should update his or her training whenever the opportunity arises and implement that knowledge in the exercise routine. Certification should be prominently displayed. Receipts and certificates should be kept for documentation.

Since the allegation that the instructor failed to properly warm up the student is so common, great care should be taken in devising the warm-up and stretching routine. AFFA suggests, for example, that each exercise routine begin with static stretches and slow rhythmic movements which do not encompass a full range of motion or stretch a muscle to its maximum length.

The instructor should make certain that there are no exercises in the routine that would create a high risk of injury. While teaching the class, the instructor should demonstrate the exercises and explain why certain exercises are done in a particular manner. At the same time, the instructor should also explain why and demonstrate how improper positioning could cause injury. Common sense, of course, dictates that if a participant is having difficulty getting into a stretch, he or she should not be pushed further into that position.

Most importantly, supervision of the exercise class should be combined with the instructor's own personality and charisma so that the class is fun and enjoyable. The class should be conducted in a way that encourages participants to work at their own paces.

Before accepting a teaching position, the instructor should know whether the exercise club will idemnify and defend employees in lawsuits for personal injuries filed by class participants. Instructors who are presently working for an athletic club should also know whether their employer offers them this protection.

Typically, larger and well established facilities will have liability insurance that will cover instructors in the event of a lawsuit. Small or relatively new facilities may not have insurance or may have insurance which does *not* cover instructors. In such a case, the instructor should obtain a written indemnity agreement from the owner of the exercise studio.

The indemnity agreement is important because without it the instructor may be held personally liable for all or a portion of the judgment, and have to pay for an attorney to defend the case.

Instructors who are self-employed should follow the same guidelines as exercise studios in regard to requiring their students to sign a disclaimer and release agreement that releases the instructor from liability in case of injury. The instructor should be aware of the limitations and problems with the release.

Finally, both the self-employed instructor and the instructor who works for a club that will not provide indemnification should consider obtaining a personal liability insurance policy. The cost of some premiums is prohibitive fut AFAA provides an *affordable* liability insurance policy for both instructors and studios.

Consumer Protection

Aerobic exercise has become a way of life for millions of Americans. This national obsession has created a variety of health studio services.

Health clubs have become big business. Unfortunately, as many disgruntled consumers will attest, there are health clubs which sell memberships and then either never open their doors to the public or go out of business without notice.

This consumer fraud is becoming widespread. In the past several years, some states have enacted laws to make it more difficult to pull off these scams. It is expected that health club legislation will increase dramatically in the immediate future.

Before opening an exercise facility, one should become thoroughly familiar with local health club laws and any pending legislation. Failure to comply with the letter of the law may lead to severe penalties.

One bill recently enacted by the California state legislature provides not only a right to sue if injury occurs as a result of a violation of the health studio law but also an award of three times the amount of actual damages assessed, plus reasonable attorney's fees.

That severe penalty is indicative of the lengths to which lawmakers will go to protect consumers from fraud.

An upcoming trend in such legislation is the requirement that monies collected by an exercise studio before it opens be deposited in a trust account in a federally insured bank. If the facility does not open, the monies in the account would be returned to the consumers.

Some states already require new facilities that have actually opened to post a bond with the state which would be available to consumers in the event a facility goes out of business. Going one step further, proposed legislation in California would require that the contract between the athletic club and the consumer contain clauses providing for rescission of the contract and refunding of membership dues, as well as transferable memberships in appropriate circumstances.

Summary

A student who files a law suit against you will not necessarily prevail by merely proving that an injury occurred. The injured student must also prove that someone's conduct was negligent or fell below a certain standard of care and that such negligence was the cause of the injury.

The suggestions discussed in this chapter may help the owners, operators, and instructors of exercise clubs to refute a claim of negligence. If some or all of the suggestions are followed, it will be much easier to demonstrate that care was taken to develop a top quality aerobic exercise program and that the student's failure to follow instructions or taking of unnecessary risks was the actual cause of the injury.

Chapter 3

Equipment for the Aerobics Business

Terence Moffatt

Exercise equipment is becoming an integral part of the aerobics business. While machines that have been traditionally considered aerobic tools (e.g., rowing machines, exercise cycles and treadmills) are becoming even more important to aerobic training, so too are a number of anaerobic fitness products.

Free weights, such as hand-held weights and weighted wrist and ankle bands, have been incorporated into aerobic exercise routines in order to increase their cardiovascular benefits while promoting flexibility and toning muscles. Even circuit training on much larger single-station weight machines has been adjusted to provide very high intensity aerobic conditioning.

This chapter will provide information on the various types of weight training equipment utilized by some aerobic businesses and will also explore the latest developments and trends in home exercise equipment.

Aerobic Training Equipment for the Aerobics Center

An increasing number of aerobics center operators have begun to install several different pieces of exercise equipment. The growing appeal that some of this equipment has to a sophisticated clientele has been a factor in influencing these operators to install the gear, and the functional advantages of these machines can make them worthwhile investments. For example, clients usually don't have to be monitored while using the machines. Even initial operating instructions can be given quickly and easily. Because the machines are used individually, classes don't have to be organized.

Because the most popular machines at aerobic centers are relatively trauma-free, they can be used by people who are restricted from doing more rigorous exercises. These machines are widely used by people recovering from sports- or exercise-related injuries, and by those who are undergoing rehabilitation.

Exercise cycles, rowing machines, treadmills, and rebounders (minitrampolines) are the most popular pieces of aerobic exercise equipment installed at centers today. Most are relatively compact, making it easy to incorporate them into even the smallest facility. Versions of each are found in every price range.

The following section presents more specific information about this equipment and some of the other exercise machines making their way into aerobic fitness centers.

Exercise cycles Exercise cycles are today's most popular aerobic exercise equipment. Once used in fitness clubs primarily as a warm-up tool before strength-training exercises, they are now offered as an alternative form of aerobic exercise. Like many of the aerobic exercise machines, exercise cycles provide relatively trauma-free exercise. This makes them especially popular with exercisers who cannot perform more strenuous routines and people who may have suffered or are recuperating from an exercise- or sports-related injury.

Riding an exercise cycle, like riding a bicycle, not only enhances the cardiovascular system, but tones and strengthens most of the leg muscles, especially the quadriceps.

The exercise cycles available for club use vary greatly in price and sophistication. At the high end of the market are extremely sophisticated electronic models that measure calories burned, cycling speed, distance, heart rate, and time of heart rate recovery. But what exercisers really like about these high-tech cycles is that they provide a constant workout. By cycling at a preset level, the exerciser is assured that each workout is equally beneficial. The feedback that these machines offer is an important incentive to exercisers. These high-tech machines can be very expensive, costing as much as $2,000 each.

Of course, less expensive exercise cycles are available, and are for the most part just as functional. When selecting an exercise cycle for use in an aerobic business, it's imperative that it be sturdily built. Most equipment offered for home use will not stand up to the rigors of institutional use. Opt for commercially designed and built models.

Two things to look for on noncomputerized models include a weighted flywheel and a belt-braking resistance system. The weighted flywheel will provide a smooth, consistent cycling motion. The belt system provides even resistance and is easier to service than other braking systems. Expect to pay as much as $500 for a well-built, commercially designed machine.

Rowing machines   Rowing machines have been incorporated into aerobics businesses mainly because they have been so heavily promoted for home use. Consequently, more and more people know about them and ask to use them. Although the rowing machine is technically an anaerobic fitness item, providing a muscle-building and toning workout for the upper and lower body, it can be used for aerobic training if one works out on it long enough to provide cardiovascular benefits.

Like exercise cycles, rowing machines for institutional use are available in a wide range of price and technological sophistication. The most advanced rowing machines, like those built by Precor (Redmond, WA) and AMF American (Jefferson, IA), provide readouts of such things as elapsed time, stroke rate, total strokes, calories burned per minute, and total calories. AMF American's Benchmark 920 Rower features an electronic alternator that can be adjusted to 20 different resistance settings.

The feedback from these electronic rowing machines gives exercisers more of an incentive to continue their programs, especially if they need to determine even the slightest improvement to encourage them to continue.

Computerized rowing machines cost $600 or more. Noncomputerized rowing machines, however, will provide the same aerobic benefits at a much lower cost to the business operator. In addition, these simpler machines are less likely to need as much service as the more technically advanced models. Noncomputerized rowing machines for institutional use start at $250.

Whether the rowing machines you invest in are computerized or not, it is important that they be able to stand up to many hours of vigorous use. One important consideration on fixed-oar models is that they have heavy-duty and equally matched twin resistance-producing hydraulic cylinders.

Treadmills   Treadmills may be enjoying a revival in the marketplace, but currently their use in fitness centers and at homes isn't as great as that of rowing machines or exercise cycles. Nonetheless, treadmills, especially the motor-driven computerized models, are excellent alternatives to running in inclement weather or around small and crowded indoor tracks.

Basically, exercising on a treadmill provides the same cardiovascular and muscular benefits of running. One advantage to using a treadmill, however, is that the cushioned tread on many machines reduces the trauma that the body may experience while running on harder surfaces.

An advantage of motor-driven and computerized treadmills is that they can provide a constant and steady workout that can be easily measured and compared to previous exercises. On most of the electronic models, digital displays provide data on speed, distance, and time.

The heavy use these machines get—especially their motors—requires that they be very well built. Expect to pay as much as $3,000 for a reliable brand.

Nonmotorized models are useful machines. Even if not computerized, they usually have a speedometer and an odometer to provide the user some measurable data. Nonmotorized treadmills are substantially less expensive; they usually begin at around $600.

If you're thinking of installing treadmills at your facility, look for sturdily built machines that will be able to go the distance over and over again. A key consideration with motor-driven models is safety. Make sure they are equipped with easily operated emergency shutoff switches. Finally, all treadmills should be designed with handrails at the front or side.

Rebounders Rebounders, or mini-trampolines, were one of the first items that marked the turnaround of the exercise equipment market. These simple tools are not only fun, they provide a cushioned surface allowing trauma-free exercising.

Rebounders are still popular at aerobic centers and should be considered for use by all new or expanding operators. Although their design is relatively simple, it is important that they be examined carefully before purchase. A collapsing rebounder frame or failed landing mat could lead to serious injury. Reinforced landing mats are a must, and springs and frames should be made from heavy-duty steel.

The very competitive rebounder market has brought in a lot of inexpensive equipment that simply will not survive after extended use. Shop for a brand from a well-known manufacturer and expect to pay $100 and up.

Free weights Free weights, especially smaller, hand-held weights and weighted wrist and ankle bands, have become extremely important to aerobic training. Not only do they enhance the cardiovascular benefits, they increase the benefits to the body's musculature.

As a marketing tool, the use of free weights has been particularly helpful in attracting more men to aerobic training programs.

These weights are by far the simplest and most easily understood pieces of exercise equipment. If you are planning to invest in free weights for use at your facility—especially if they're going to be used in group situations—some care must be taken in selecting them.

Hand-held weights should have some type of texturized handle or other safety feature to prevent them from slipping out of the user's hands. Look for weights with either knurled handles or some sort of restrainer. A classic example of the latter is AMF American's Heavyhands, which have a padded loop that comes over the back of the hand to keep the weights comfortably secure. Triangle Health and Fitness Systems, a Campbell Soup affiliate, manufacture a soft vinyl dumbbell, which is washable and, if dropped, will not mar the floor.

The newest and most comfortable wrist and ankle weights are made by Triangle Health and Fitness Systems. These are made of soft vinyl and are easily attached with a Velcro strap. The advantage of these products is that that the arm muscles are less restricted (because the hands are free), enabling a greater flow of oxygen and nutrient-rich blood to the exercising muscles.

Hand-held weights are available in a wide range of prices. The simplest, cast-iron versions are the least expensive. Stainless steel and more sophisticated versions cost more.

Cross-country ski simulators Cross-country skiing is generally recognized as one of the best forms of aerobic exercise. A total body conditioner, cross-country skiing builds the entire body and greatly enhances the cardiovascular system.

Cross-country skiing simulators, while hardly able to recreate the experience of skiing through a snow-shrouded forest, do provide much of the same workout. Although these machines have, for the most part, been marketed directly to consumers for home use, they are turning up more and more in aerobic centers.

Versa Climber This is a relatively new piece of equipment best classified as a total body conditioner. It is, however, gaining popularity with the operators of aerobic centers. The machine simulates climbing a ladder, and it can be adjusted to provide different resistance settings. A computerized model of the Versa Climber displays exercise time, climbing time, and stroke rate.

Strength-Training Equipment for the Aerobics Center

Expanding your aerobics center with strength-training equipment, especially single- or multi-station weight machines, is a major move that requires careful consideration.

Cost is the primary factor to consider, because this equipment is very expensive. But space considerations are almost as important. Strength-training machines, for the most part, are large pieces of equipment. To set up an adequate strength-training center equipped with even a few pieces of gear requires a great deal of floor space.

Some pieces of strength-training equipment are more popular than others, and some aerobic centers have begun to install these machines at their facilities. Currently, the two most popular pieces of equipment are abdominal and lower-back machines. Most of the manufacturers of strength-training equipment have developed their own versions of these machines, and one, Nautilus, has even developed machines for home use.

Strength-training equipment varies greatly in how it provides resistance, but, generally speaking, the amount of resistance does not vary much from one brand of equipment to another.

Operators of strength-training centers say the key factors to consider when buying equipment are ease of operation and adjustment, simple maintenance and good warranties. Ease of operation is important so that neither your clients nor your instructors are intimidated by the equipment. Easy adjustment, whether it is seat height or work load, is important so that more people can use the machines in a shorter period of time. This will help to keep lines short during peak hours.

Easy maintenance means simple care. The less complicated the machine, the easier it is to take care of.

Warranties are obviously important. Strength-training equipment can sometimes break down, requiring what could be expensive repair. One fitness center operator recommends that strength-training equipment shoppers buy from long-time vendors with good track records. Such companies will be able to provide parts and service down the road.

As mentioned above, there are many different types of resistance systems on the market. Below is a quick look at two of the most popular.

Weight stacks   Most single- and multi-station weight machines provide resistance with adjustable weight stacks. These machines are generally easy to maintain and adjust. The companies that market machines of this type include Nautilus, Universal, Paramount, Polaris, and Eagle/Cybex.

Compressed air   Some types of equipment provide resistance with compressed air. What fitness centers like about these machines is that they can be set for extremely light work loads, making them easier to use for older clients or people undergoing rehabilitation. Changing resistance on these pieces of equipment is easier than with weight stack machines and also much quicker. One of the leading manufacturers of compressed air, strength-training machines is Keiser Sports Health Equipment.

Fitness Equipment for the Home

Personal trainers are increasingly called upon by their clients for information about equipment for the home. Here is some information on the latest trends in home exercise equipment and some overall suggestions on what should be considered before making a purchase. Many of the tips we offered on buying equipment for use in an aerobics center will apply here.

In fact, much of the commercial equipment is available to the consumer.

Exercise cycles intended for home use should have weighted flywheels, belt braking systems, and padded seats. A good exercise cycle can be purchased for $250 (for a nonmotorized model) to $4,000 (for a computerized cycle that is also equipped with a television to counteract boredom). Clients should be advised that anything selling for under $250 is probably not worth the investment.

Fixed-oar rowing machines should have sturdy hydraulic resistors, and the frame should be solidly built, to adequately support the weight of the exerciser. Excellent rowing machines are available for $250 and up. More sophisticated computerized models are retailing for $600 and up.

Clients shopping for treadmills should follow the same tips given earlier, especially regarding the safety features. Again, motorized models should have an emergency shut-off switch. All treadmills should have either front- or side-mounted handrails. Solidly built nonmotorized models begin at about $600. The better motorized models designed for home use retail for $1,500 and up.

Strength training equipment for the home

Strength training for home use has become very popular with the development of relatively compact strength-training machines. Currently, there are three basic types of these machines, which differ in the ways they provide resistance.

The most popular type of strength-training machine on the market uses a weight stack to provide the training load. These compact machines are designed to simulate many of the exercises done on a variety of single-station machines. Advise clients to shop for very sturdy steel-framed machines that will be able to support the weight load they carry. Also, if your clients are seriously interested in weight training, suggest that they invest in home units with weight stacks that can be increased. A serious trainer can progress beyond limited weight loads quickly. Look for some of the in-home versions of the brands used in fitness clubs. Universal, Marcy, and Paramount are some of the leading suppliers of this type of equipment for the home.

Another popular type of strength-training equipment uses heavy-duty elastized bands or springs to provide as much as 200 pounds of resistance. These machines are not as jarring to the body as some weight stack machines can be, but they cannot be adjusted as accurately to various weight settings. Another problem with them is that after repeated and extended use, the springs or elastized bands have to be replaced. The best known manufacturers of this equipment are Soloflex and Pro-Form.

The newest type of home strength-training equipment uses the exerciser's own body weight to provide the resistance. Sitting, kneeling, or reclining on a sliding bed, the exerciser pulls cables, which pull the bed up an inclined ramp. The steeper the ramp, the greater the resistance. Additional weights can be added to increase the workload. The leading manufacturer of this type of equipment is Total Gym by West Bend.

As the fitness field develops further, so will the center- and home-based equipment business. Size, quality and services offered by a single piece of equipment will improve, and the high-tech qualities now in expensive models will become standard. The most successful use of equipment is made by the wise shopper who analyzes personal and/or business needs, shops the choices, weighs the alternatives, and makes an informed decision.

Chapter 4

Common Sense Guide to Success

Michael Nicola

When Charles Dickens wrote, "It was the best of times; it was the worst of times," he might have been thinking of the fitness industry. For the worst of times, there are days when two of the teachers are sick, five others are tearing apart the sound system, and students are complaining about the lack of parking spaces. But these times are more than offset by receiving a letter from a student thanking you for turning her life around. Or watching a former "aerobiphobic" glide through the aerobics portion of the advanced class. The fitness industry, which is the cutting edge of self-expression, has both profound rewards and demanding challenges.

Like many other managers and owners in the fitness field, I left a successful but largely unsatisfying career that nearly disabled me with back problems. After having to see clients while I was unable to sit up in an office, becoming fit was not just a basic need for me, but approached a manic obsession.

In a very real way, that experience prepared me for the fitness business. Many promoters with only mercenary interests are moving into the field and trying to make a fast buck, but they are in for a difficult time. Success in this industry demands more than a smooth pitch and a pretty package. It must be based on deeper motivations than turning a profit. Instead, you have to want to deal with people's bodies, feelings and self-images in a gentle, restorative and caring way. To succeed, you have to be genuinely interested in upgrading the quality of their lives and your own and be truly sensitive to their needs. In this way, you will attract people to your establishment.

Editor's Note: Throughout this book, we have presented objective data on exercise instruction, fitness essentials, program development, and professional training. The chapter that follows is written from another perspective—the personal viewpoint of an experienced fitness business operator.

Strategies for Success

Genuine concern for others counts in this business because it is intensely service-oriented. You are dealing with self-images. Your clients want to feel that you are on their side, and the demarkations between owner, management, staff and client cannot be so structured that you lose touch with that process.

In order to create this feeling, you must have a clear and sincere purpose behind your operation. If you cannot state concisely why your business is different and important to the goals of the clients, chances are high that you will not succeed. The purpose of our studio, for example, is the creation of a nurturing environment where people can express themselves with their bodies. Like any successful purpose, this very clear statement continually keeps us on course. Whenever there is a question or problem, we match it to our purpose and make our decision accordingly.

We had a class in martial arts, for instance, that somehow just didn't seem to fit. As we discussed why, we realized that the class was about defending yourself, not expressing yourself through your body. Since it didn't fit the purpose of the entire studio, we dropped it. At the same time, we wanted to offer a movement class. Even though it was not an exercise class in the traditional sense, it was consistant with our purpose and belonged on the schedule.

Once you have a purpose, the next step is collecting the elements that can put it in action. These elements include:

- the right partners
- financial operations
- marketing and advertising
- member recruitment, motivation and retention
- legal aspects
- staffing and budgeting
- professional affiliation

The right partners

Going it alone results in a product that is too much a reflection of only one person's vision. To me, fitness is a business that demands input from different perspectives. The best way to get this is through partners who work well together.

When you look for a partner, you want someone who shares your sense of mission, and who will discuss openly, argue, resolve conflict—and go to the wall with you. You also want someone who has a different area of expertise. If your strength is marketing and motivation, you don't need someone else doing that. You certainly do need someone, however, who manages money well.

In this particular industry, a partnership must include at least three areas of expertise. One person must handle the context of the venture, and create the aesthetics or the space in which the business operates. Another must provide the actual content of the program, and a third should handle the money and practical affairs of the business. Ideally, there should also be a fourth person who observes and corrects the problems as they arise.

The partners must meet regularly to assess what is happening to the business and each other. These meetings are think tanks, and often the only time during the week that you can all get together and talk as a group. If the partnership is working well, you will be able to look at the problems and find results without pointing fingers. After all, your problems are common ones, so there is no reason to waste time with blame. Be reasonably sure about the partnership before you make your first move. In our experience, relationships that don't work in the beginning only get worse.

Financial operations

It takes a lot of money to run a fitness-oriented business. The more ambitious the operation, the more money it requires. But even a streamlined organization is not inexpensive to operate. Don't forget that you are dealing with people's physical health so that buying and hiring the best is not a question of choice. You simply cannot skimp on materials or staff in this industry.

Do not try to open if you are under or marginally capitalized with no reserves to rely on should an emergency arise. Concentrate on financing. If your vision is sound and your ability to communicate it precise, someone with money will say yes. Even then there are no guarantees, of course, but to give your life's blood without having the monetary staying power is damaging to you, the students, and ultimately, the profession as a whole.

Marketing and advertising

In advertising, my philosophy has always been, "If *you* wouldn't buy it, you can't sell it." It is much easier to market and advertise a product or service you are proud of and enjoy using yourself. After your first flush of success, it is a common mistake to rest on your laurels and lose sight of your original purpose. One way we avoid that is by having *all of the managers and owners regularly do at least one groundwork task that they find very tedious and sometimes unpleasant*. In doing so, we are forced to experience the studio just as a client would, and improve the product so that we can successfully market and advertise it.

I, for instance, hate working the juice bar, but I do it one day a week. This hands-on experience gives me an immediate awareness and sense of responsibility for each area of the club, including those that normally seem trivial or demeaning. It also keeps me in touch with the staff and the clients.

When they see me wait on them or see another of the owners scrubbing the floors, they find it hard to think of us as only owners—aloof and unapproachable.

How can you know what someone means when she says a particular teacher was boring, unless you experience the class yourself? Conversely, when marketing a new class, how can you know the technique behind the "perfect" leg lift unless you try to perform one? You have to be a part of the program before you can really know how good or bad it is.

Accessibility is extremely important to the proper marketing in this business. To be continually successful, you have to know who is coming in and what they are saying about your club. Even if you think they are wrong, they are responding to impressions you gave them. Rather than be self-righteous, you are much better off encouraging their responses and listening to what they say.

We had a problem, for example, with our music. We knew it was good, but the students kept saying they wanted something else. Although they were not specific, they had a complaint. With the idea that the customer is always right, we devised a music suggestion form and gave it to the teachers, staff and students. By involving everyone, we eventually solved the problem and made everyone happy.

This illustrates why marketing does not mean hard-sell advertising, in this field, but a continual search for the right elements. Good advertising should describe the product and refrain from hype. It informs people about the changes in the programs, acknowledges achievements and reports on developments at the studio. Hopefully, if you come in to our studio, it is because you already know what we are about and are intrigued, not because of a lot of false promises or, for that matter, bargain prices. Quality is a bargain in itself and attracts quality.

We also stay on track by continually comparing our day-to-day activities with our purpose. We recently had a problem when we were thinking about designing and manufacturing clothing for our boutique. After thinking about it, however, we realized that while being able to stock and sell clothing that enhances expression is consistent with our purpose, the designing of clothes is not. The solution to the problem was to create another business that fit this particular purpose.

Member recruitment, motivation, and retention

Another key element for ongoing success of an exercise studio is the development of a core group of regulars who generate good word-of-mouth referrals. Regardless of the amount of money spent on the location, whether it is in New York, Los Angeles, Paris or Dubuque, the exercise studio still depends on people. To work, the studio must be like the local bar, a friendly neighborhood place where people drop in because someone knows their name and treats them with respect. Instructors at our studio instinctively reflect that attitude even though they have not been specifically requested to do so.

Once again, keeping your purpose clear will help your instructors maintain a positive attitude, and minimize staff problems. This is a business in which you deal with people who are not wearing makeup or street clothes and are at what I call their "vulnerable best." Because feelings of self-consciousness are running high, clients sense instructor's attitudes immediately.

Legal aspects

You need to understand the laws that pertain to a fitness business in order to guarantee long-range success. Protection of the business and the clientele is as essential as the right staff, music, image and financing. As addressed in the chapter on legal considerations, this is a service business and difficulties can arise when the customer is not totally satisfied with the service. Preventing this dissatisfaction is important but not always possible. Being prepared to deal with these concerns when and if they arise is necessary for ongoing success.

Staffing and budgeting

Employees have direct contact with the clients and are immediate reflections of the studio's purpose, so their happiness is vital to the success of your business. That does not mean you must give them everything they want, because mutual respect depends on each party trusting the other. Make sure their needs are covered, and encourage honest communication at every level.

For that to happen, you must charge your staff members with being part of the process, and then listen to what they say. Have regular staff meetings with prearranged agendas, so they can come prepared and are not surprised by any announcements that affect their lives. End the meeting with an open discussion period during which they can talk about their concerns.

Also be aware of what you need from each other on an individual basis. Give people as much responsibility as they can handle without becoming overwhelmed, and then let them do their jobs without you constantly looking over their shoulders. Have clear job descriptions that explain exactly what you expect from them, and conduct periodic reviews in which you can discuss accomplishments and areas needing improvement. Don't confine the interaction to these reviews, however, and allow for spontaneous discussions when the need arises.

Visibility of owners and management is crucial to success. The staff needs to see and be acknowledged by its bosses. Also they will feel more involved if they see management involved in classes and other operations.

Staff members who feel management and owners have an interest in their work and provide positive reinforcement for a job well done, including economic reinforcement, are likely to do a good job and maintain a positive relationship with the studio. We also make a point, at our studio, of socializing with the staff and spending time with them to find out their strengths and weaknesses. In addition to making us function more like a family, it helps the staff develop to our mutual advantage.

We spent six months training a teacher who was offered a job as an assistant choreographer for the Olympics one week before we were to open. We knew he couldn't turn the offer down, nor would we have wanted him to. When something like this happens to you, all I can say is be thrilled, don't let them feel guilty, and let them go, knowing they can have a home and future support if they need it. By doing this, you will have created a valuable ally.

As far as economic planning goes, an ongoing, comprehensive budget is essential to continued success. Don't be afraid to be conservative but maintain a consistent awareness of the income/outgo. Build into the budget a means for dealing with slow times, raises and other unknowns. It is important to have an accountant familiar with your type of business. Seek someone who is experienced and who will have the interest of the business at heart. Overseeing the total operation is necessary to success. Be sure to review the economic operations on a regular basis.

Replenishing one's energy and satisfaction is also fundamental to ongoing success. Insist that staff take vacations at least once a year. If you don't get away for a week or two every year, you cannot see where you are going, where you have been, or how your actions fit into the larger perspective of your life. By leaving for just a few days, you not only get all these answers, but come back with your commitment reaffirmed.

Professional affiliations

Networking on a professional level is also important to your success. If you are committed to your business, you must also want the field to be successful and be willing to work for this larger success. After all, the more exciting the business climate is, the more opportunity there is for everyone.

To generate that successful business climate, you should be affiliated with professional organizations such as AFAA in order to exchange exciting information, assist in setting standards and policies and gather new knowledge about the field.

These organizations become increasingly important as the business grows. We are currently faced with several vital issues, such as the certification and licensing of teachers. As these issues develop, we will need the resources of a professional organization such as AFAA and the American College of Sports Medicine to look out for our interests.

In addition to these affiliations, we also believe in setting up relationships with the best professionals in related fields. When I have a problem with insurance or a question on body composition and testing, I consult the best professionals I can find.

Since clubs are part of a general community, it is important to have a link with the city council and other civic officials. By networking with these people on business, political and social issues, everyone is assisted, including ourselves.

Summary

There are no secrets to success in the fitness field, only a process of taking one small step at a time. I can best compare this to something our yoga teacher says about the body. "Don't compare yourself to other people, and work at your own pace. Forgive it for having limitations when it doesn't do what you want and acknowledge it when it does. To benefit others the most, don't copy, but put your personal stamp on your efforts. Be patient, and don't expect overnight success."

I would add that you should stay focused in the present and enjoy the process of becoming successful. Look at things that are difficult, such as financial or personnel problems, not as setbacks, but indicators that need to be corrected. And as you do whatever needs to be done, however small, do it as if it were the most important job in the world. Then when it comes time to step back and assess what you have done, you will have an enormous sense of pleasure from seeing the complete fruition of your original purpose.

Chapter 5

Aerobics: Past, Present, and Future

Aerobics and Fitness Association of America and Campbell's Institute for Health and Fitness

"Reach Your Outer Limits: Join the Moon Base Fitness Club;" "Space Aerobics: Your Guide to Fitness." Are these marketing statements just an absurdity or a reflection of the future? Before you decide, consider the following:

- The fitness movement that began in the 1970s has expanded far beyond the original scope of a national interest in health. It has become a way of life for millions, a popular movement deeply ingrained in the consciousness and life-style of a large segment of our society.
- This movement was fostered by a dramatic increase in leisure time and leisure-time activities, by a near obsession with looking good and staying young, and by a growing desire of people to take control of their lives in an age of stress and anxiety.
- Fitness is definitely not a fad. By any standards, fitness is, in John Naisbitt's words, a "megatrend," and will continue to be a major force in America and around the world for the foreseeable future.

What has caused this sudden interest in physical fitness? One of the triggers has been the emerging sensitivity of the baby boom generation to the benefits of well-being. The "me" generation of the 1970s is now more and more committed to living a full, active life with the help of proper eating habits, sensible life-style, and exercise.

Another factor is the current status of disease diagnosis, treatment, and rehabilitation. Health care has come a long way, so far in fact that many diseases that killed large numbers of people only 20–50 years ago now can be cured or arrested. What has occurred as a result is that many more middle-aged and older persons are faced with living a number of years with a chronic health problem. Exercise has been found to have a positive effect on the prevention or treatment of many chronic health problems. Because the possibility of feeling better for longer exists through a positive life-style, many people embrace aerobic exercise as the means to fitness. Therefore, fitness is deeply woven into the fabric of today's life-styles.

One of the dramatic changes brought on by the fitness movement is the increase of physical activity by women. Sweating, pumping iron, and tedious workouts were once limited to the male's domain. With the emergence of women's sports, and other cultural changes, women have taken a leadership role in the active life-style. A recent survey revealed that while women comprise only about 52% of the US population, they hold almost 60% of the memberships in health clubs. Of those women, the most active are those 25-34 years old.

The President's Council on Physical Fitness and Sports reports that 38% of the general women's populace participates "regularly" in organized exercise, and that female participation in organized athletics increased 135% between 1975 and 1985. Looking at the American population as a whole, the Council reports that 65% name exercise as a segment of their daily life-style, compared to just 23% in 1970. A similar study conducted by Campbell Soup Company found that 69% of those surveyed were active. The breakdown revealed the following:

- 8% live a very active life-style, tend to belong to a club and participate in all its different activities, doing it for the good it does
- 9% live a very active life-style, with an interest and involvement in sports and games, athletes for the fun of it
- 32% live a moderately active life-style, choosing to exercise at home
- 20% are different from the rest in that they choose to walk on a daily basis
- the other 31% are spectators only

Another indicator of the growth of the fitness movement is the commitment by a rising number of companies who are sponsoring employee wellness programs. According to the 1984 Yankelovich Monitor, estimates are that for every one dollar spent on fitness programs, three dollars are saved from the cost of caring for the sick.

Future generations will regard aerobic exercise as an everyday necessity—a natural part of life's fundamental activities. As long as there are bodies to be strengthened, there will be spirits to challenge them. And as the human species evolves, the commitment and pursuit of physical fitness will find a permanent place in tomorrow's world.

Predictions for the future of aerobics and fitness include:

- greater cooperation between professional organizations for the education and training of fitness professionals
- a smooth and rapid flow of data from the exercise physiology laboratory to the workplace of fitness training
- public recognition of the aerobic instructor's contribution as an integral part of a society dedicated to maintaining health, with a corresponding elevation in the status of aerobic instructors
- a diversification in the career role of aerobic instructor: aerobic directors, coordinators, aerobic trainers, researchers, as well as the hands-on instructor
- commitment from employers in business and industry to provide scheduled fitness breaks throughout the day for their employees
- the introduction of "stay-well" incentives by insurance companies, schools, corporations, and third-party carriers
- the inclusion of aerobic competition in the Olympics, after comprehensive evaluations of sanctioning guidelines, standardization of judging criteria, and clarification of the skills and techniques involved
- continuous monitoring and upgrading of standardized guidelines and principles of safe and effective exercise demanded by a highly educated, knowledgeable exercising public and researched by an international network of fitness professionals.

No one can predict if the present form of aerobic dance-exercise will be with us for centuries to come. Different variations, innovations, styles, and trends will fade in and out, just as they have since the sport made its earthshaking appearance. However, it is a safe guess that aerobic sports will be here to stay. In addition to the desire to achieve the multiple benefits of aerobic sports, there will always be a desire to include in one's life fitness "for the fun of it." As a highly technical society becomes increasingly complex, people will require a dose of pure and simple aerobic joy.

Appendices

Appendix A

Basic Exercise Program Outline

AFAA recommends the following progression for the instruction of a one-hour freestyle aerobic class.

1. Preclass instruction   [**1 minute**]
2. Warm-up: a balanced combination of static stretching and rhythmic limbering exercises   [**7 minutes**]
3. Standing exercises: exercises from the following groups in order of preference
   - standing leg work (optional)
   - arms, chest, and shoulders   [**4 minutes**]
   - aerobics and postaerobic cool-down   [**20 minutes**]
   - waist work   [**5 minutes**]
4. Floorwork: exercises from the following groups in order of preference
   - outer thigh   [**4 minutes**]
   - buttocks   [**5 minutes**]
   - inner thigh   [**4 minutes**]
   - abdominals   [**5 minutes**]
5. Static stretching   [**5 minutes**]

Appendix B

Correct and Incorrect Exercise Positions

Marti Steele West, BA
Linda Shelton, BA

I. Warm-up stretches: Static stretches and Rhythmic limbering

Do's

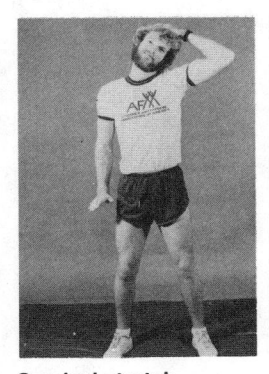

1. Cervical stretch

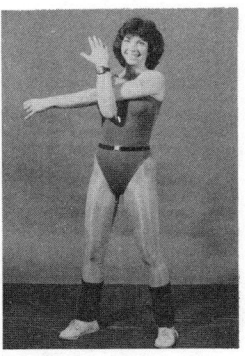

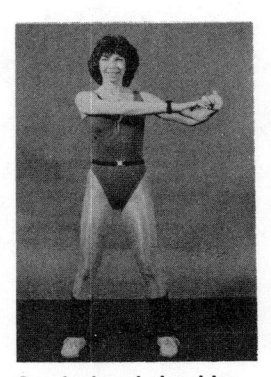

2. Cervical and shoulder stretch

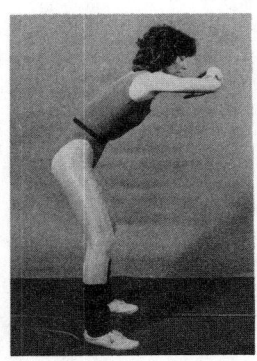

3. Shoulder stretch

4. Upper back stretch

282 CORRECT AND INCORRECT EXERCISE POSITIONS

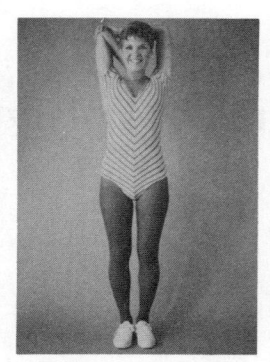

5. Shoulder and triceps stretch

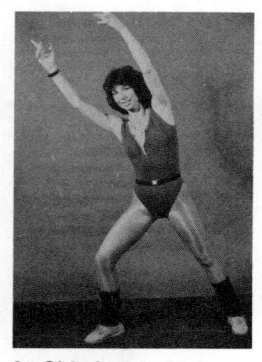

6. Side lunge

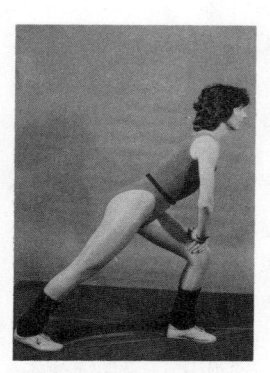

7. Hamstring stretch

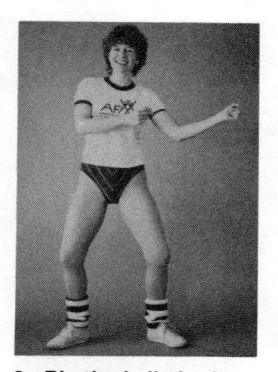

8. Rhythmic limbering

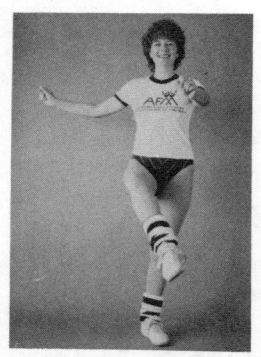

9. Rhythmic limbering

CORRECT AND INCORRECT EXERCISE POSITIONS **283**

Don'ts

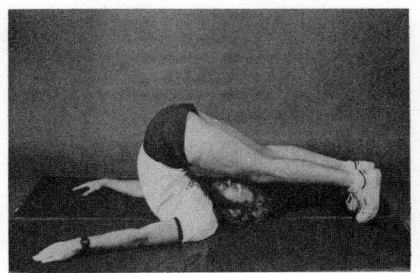

The Plow

Quad rock

II. Posture Alignment

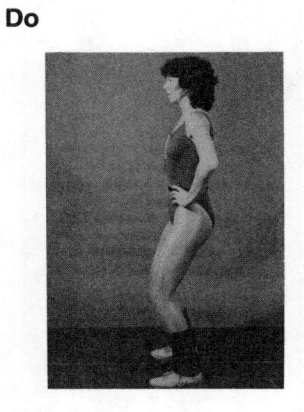

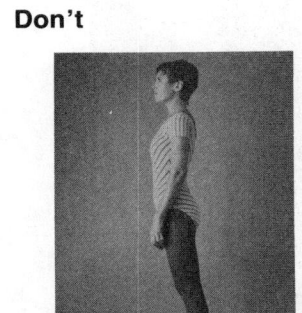

Do

Side view

Don't

Side view

284 CORRECT AND INCORRECT EXERCISE POSITIONS

III. Arms

Do's

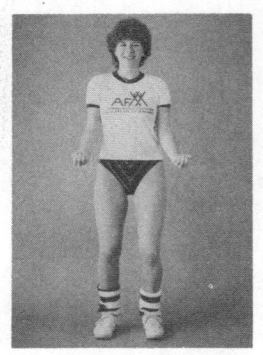

1A and 1B. Bicep curls

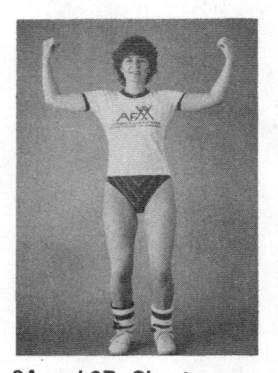

2A and 2B. Chest presses

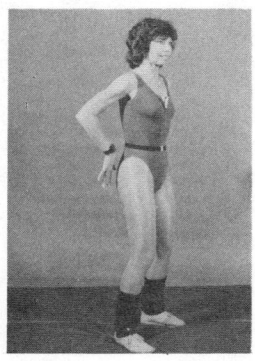

3. Triceps resist left

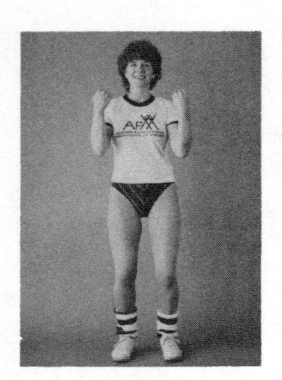

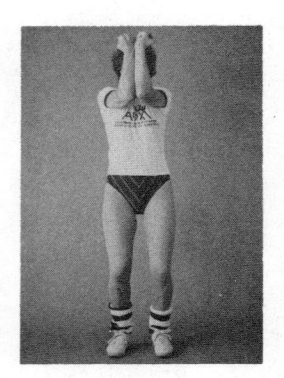

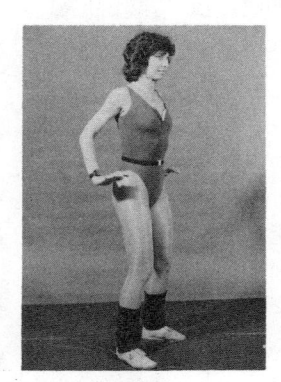

4. Triceps press

CORRECT AND INCORRECT EXERCISE POSITIONS   **285**

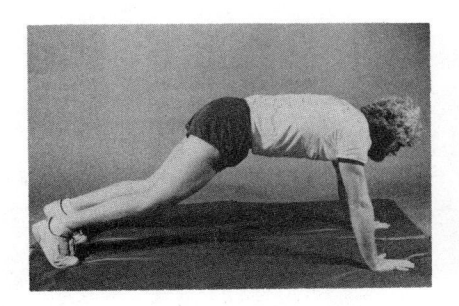

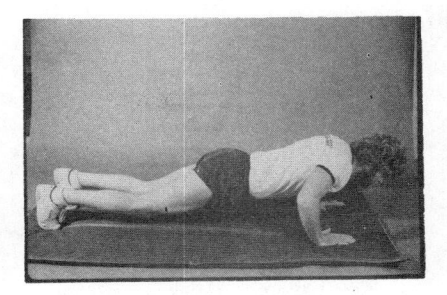

5A and 5B. Push ups

IV. Aerobics

Do's

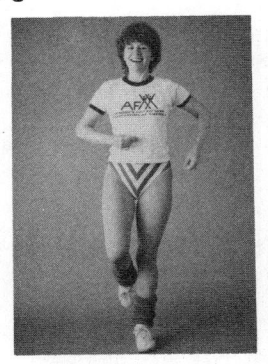

1. Jogging

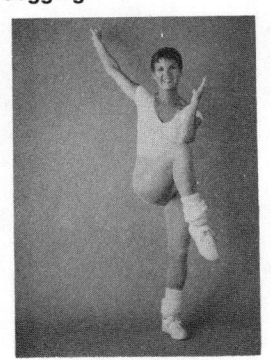

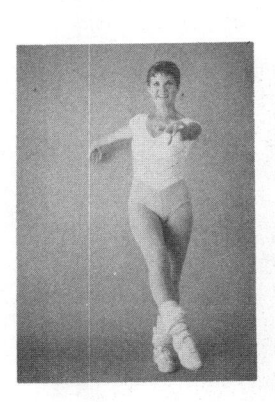

2. Kickouts

3. Alternate elbow to knee

286 CORRECT AND INCORRECT EXERCISE POSITIONS

V. Waist

Do

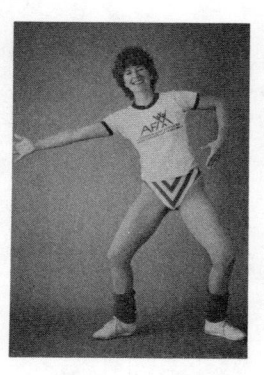

Lateral side bend

Don'ts

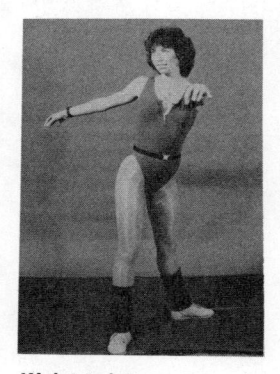

Waist twists

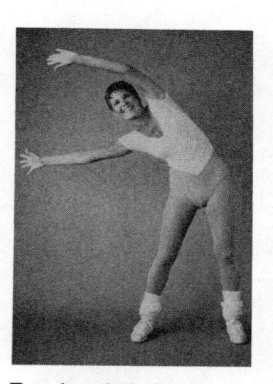

Two-handed side bend

VI. Outer thigh

Do's

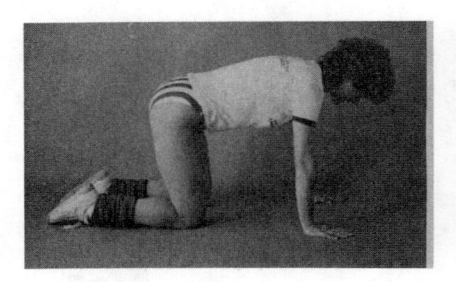

1. Beginning hydrant position

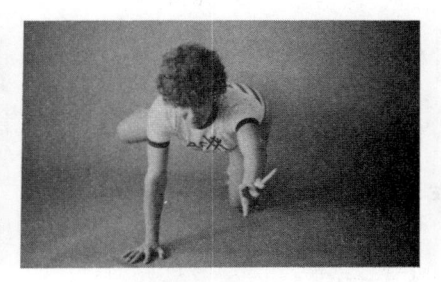

2. Hydrant alignment check

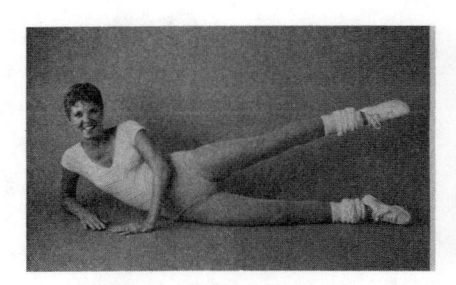

3. Side lying outer thigh lift

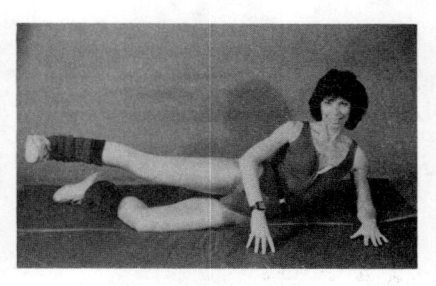

4. Side lying outer thigh lift

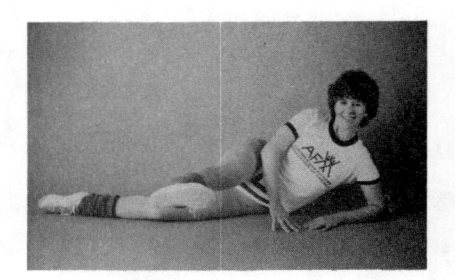

5. Side lying outer thigh lift

288 CORRECT AND INCORRECT EXERCISE POSITIONS

Don'ts

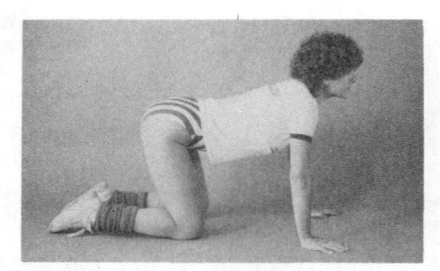

Beginning hydrant position

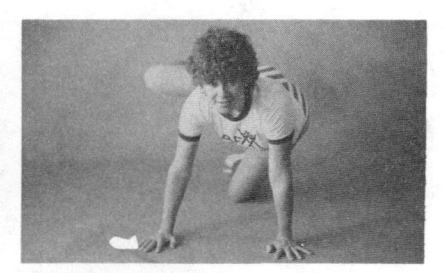

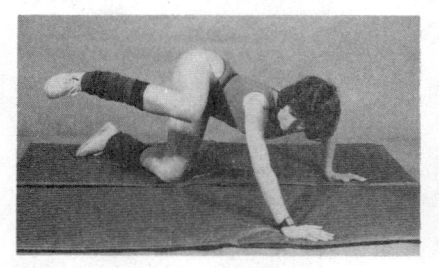

Hydrant

Hydrant

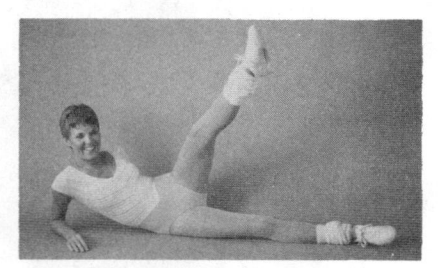

Side lying outer thigh lift

VII. Inner thigh

Do

Inner thigh lift

Don'ts

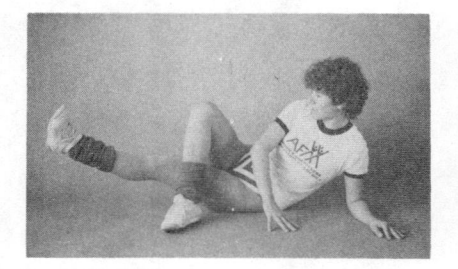

Inner thigh lift

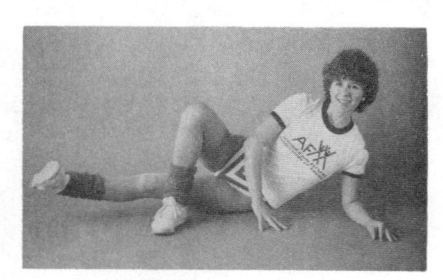

Don'ts

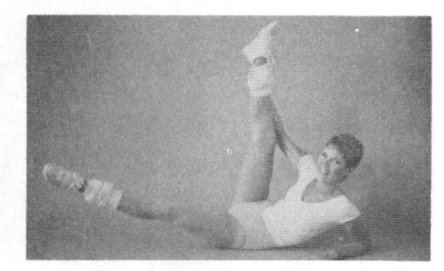

Scissors

VIII. Buttocks

Do's

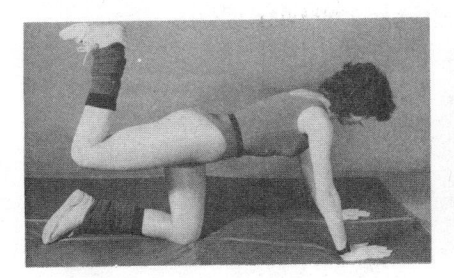

1. Gluteal press

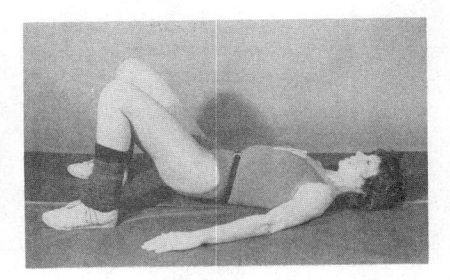

2. Pelvic lift

Don'ts

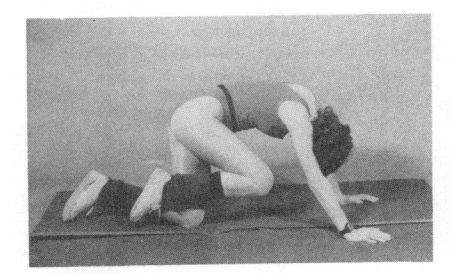

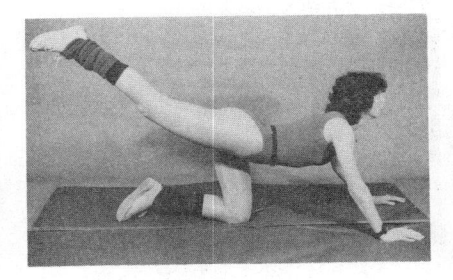

Donkey kicks

Donkey kicks

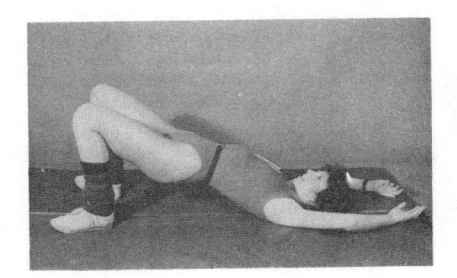

Pelvic lift

290 CORRECT AND INCORRECT EXERCISE POSITIONS

IX. Abdominals

Do's

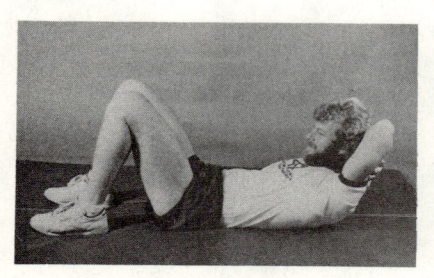

1. Abdominal start position

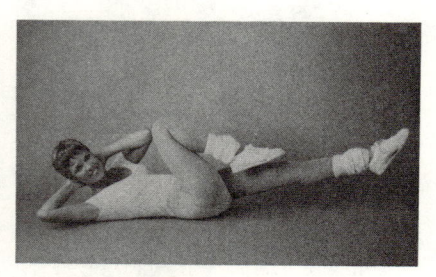

2. Alternate elbow to knee

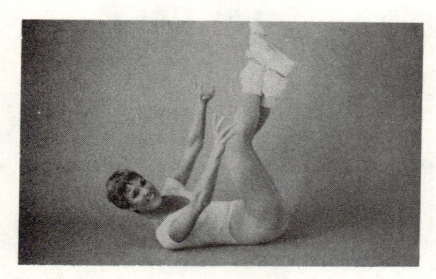

3. Abdominal crunch with twist

Don'ts

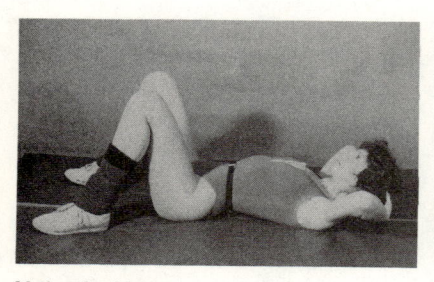

Abdominal incorrect

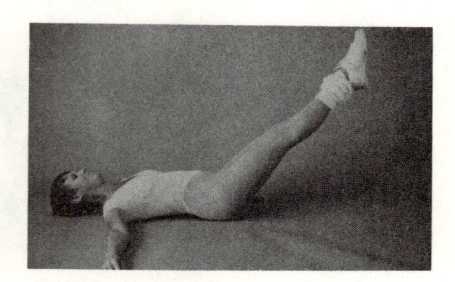

Two-legged lift

X. Cool-down stretches

Do's

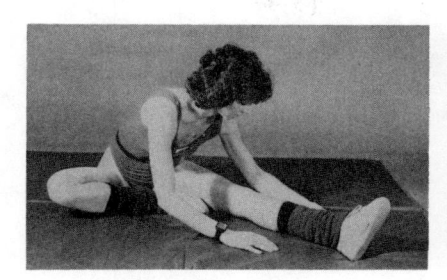

1. Inverted hurdler

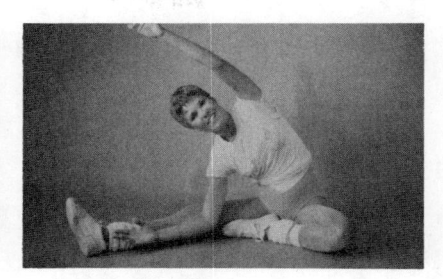

2. Inverted hurdler

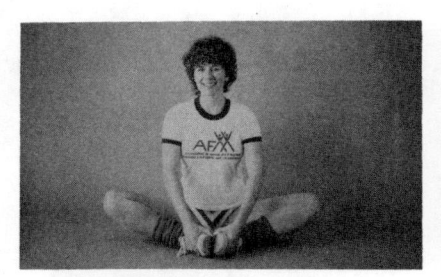

3. Hip adductor stretch

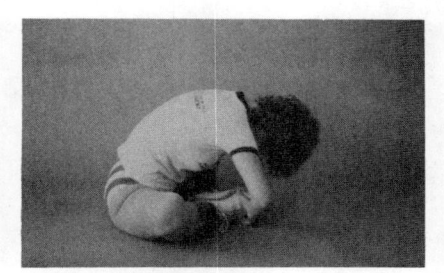

4. Hip adductor stretch

Appendix C

Medical Emergencies: A Treatment Guide for Aerobics Instructors

Gerald P. Whelan, MD, FACEP

Overview of What Each Category Will Cover

What it is
- A brief overview of some of the major medical emergencies that might arise in the course of an aerobic exercise class and how to handle them.

What it is not
- A substitute for certification in Basic Cardiac Life Support (BCLS) by the American Heart Association or the American Red Cross. This certification should be mandatory for all instructors.
- A substitute for basic first aid training (also available from the American Red Cross or other sources), which would be desirable for aerobics instructors.
- A substitute for good old common sense, which should always take precedence over any guidelines (unfortunately not available from any known source other than yourself).

What it looks like
- Familiarize yourself with the signs of each problem area.

What to do
- Read this section over and become familiar with its contents. Review it periodically and keep it available for quick reference.

What not to do
- Consider it a complete source or a substitute for the training mentioned above.

Who to call
- Your local Heart Association or Red Cross to answer any questions you may have or to find out where and when training is available.

How to prevent it
- Areas to consider and discuss with students so emergencies can be avoided.

Medical Emergency

What it is
A sudden injury or unforeseen medical illness that may lead to loss of life, limb, or function if not immediately treated by qualified medical personnel.

What it is not
Any of the host of sports injuries including sprains, strains, or even most fractures, which can and should be referred for treatment to a qualified health care professional and require no intervention on an emergency basis other than termination of exercise, application of ice, or splinting.

What to do
Stay calm, assess the situation, call for qualified help (usually the paramedics) and proceed as outlined in the specific sections below.

What not to do
- Do not panic.
- Do not underestimate a true emergency.
- Do not exceed your own capabilities.
- Do not allow anyone else to treat the victim unless they are properly qualified.
- Do not wait to call for help. If in doubt, err on the side of caution and call.

Who to call
In most communities paramedics or at least trained Emergency Medical Technicians (EMTs) are available to respond by ambulance. Be certain that the phone number is clearly posted near the telephones and know the procedure for calling in an emergency.

How to prevent it
Medical emergencies can best be prevented by stressing to students the necessity for proper medical screening before beginning a vigorous exercise program, by encouraging students to consult with their physicians if they have any chronic medical problems and by stressing the need to individualize their workout and pace themselves. Frequent pulse checks can

let the student know if he or she is overdoing it. The instructor should continuously be monitoring the students for any signs of weakness or trouble in breathing.

Minor sports injuries can best be prevented by adhering to the principles of safe and sane exercise. Major injuries are most often related to problems in the physical plant. Survey for safety. Is the room overcrowded so that students are likely to crash into each other? Are rugs and floor coverings hazardous? Are there sharp corners or exposed mirror edges where students might fall on them? Is the wiring for lights and sound systems up to code?

Cardiopulmonary Arrest

What it is
A complete cessation of pumping action by the heart, most often due to heart attack but can be due to other causes. Untreated, it is uniformly fatal and even delay in treatment may cause permanent brain damage in as little as four to six minutes.

What it is not
It is not a heart attack (see below) nor any other form of loss of consciousness in which the heart continues to function.

What it looks like
- The victim collapses and there is no movement or moaning.
- There is no spontaneous breathing even after the airway has been opened.
- No pulse can be felt. After a brief period, the pupils will enlarge and not react to light.

What to do
Immediately begin cardiopulmonary resuscitation (CPR) and send someone to call the paramedics. CPR must be learned and practiced conscientiously as noted above. For our purposes here, a review of the essentials will be sufficient.

- Establish that the victim is in fact unresponsive.
- Open the airway by tilting the head back.
- Look, listen, and feel for breathing.
- If no breathing, give four quick breaths by the mouth-to-mouth technique, being certain to pinch the nostrils closed.
- Feel for a pulse in the neck, over the carotid artery.
- If no pulse, begin closed chest massage.
- Place the heel of one hand two fingerbreadths above the lowest point of the breastbone, the other hand on top of the first, and compress one and a half to two inches.

- After fifteen compressions, give the victim two more breaths and continue.
- If there are other trained rescuers present, switch over to two-person CPR at a ratio of one breath interposed after every five compressions.
- Continue until paramedics arrive and allow them to assume care.
  If all the foregoing are not completely familiar to you, take a formal CPR training or recertification course immediately.

What not to do
- Do not delay in beginning CPR.
- Do not forget to call for help.
- Do not do CPR on anyone who is breathing or has a pulse.
- Do not quit until help arrives.
- Do not attempt to transport the victim on your own.

Who to call
Paramedics or another emergency rescue squad. *Immediately.*

How to prevent it
Stress the importance of fitness screening to your students before beginning an exercise program, particularly to those over 40 or those with risk factors such as obesity, high blood pressure, diabetes, smoking history, or a strong family history of heart disease. Keep a close eye on such students during classes and if they show signs of fatigue or have trouble breathing, have them stop or slow down.

Heart Attack (Myocardial Infarction)

What it is
Permanent and irreversible damage to a part of the heart muscle due to a blockage of its blood supply. This may result in an irregular heartbeat leading to cardiopulmonary arrest (see above) and sudden death, to progressive failure of the heart's pumping action leading to death hours or days later, or to complete recovery.

What it is not
A whole host of other conditions that may be impossible to recognize without sophisticated medical testing. Hence if there is any question of a heart attack, proceed as if it were the case.

What it looks like
The victim usually complains of chest pain, most often described as pressing or squeezing, like a weight on the chest. There is often difficulty breathing, a cold sweat, and sometimes nausea or even vomiting. The pain may travel down into the arms, but this is not always the case. The victim may appear pale or dusky.

MEDICAL EMERGENCIES

What to do
Immediately stop any exertion. Have the victim sit or lie down, whichever is most comfortable. Give him air and space and loosen his clothing. Call for paramedics and watch the patient closely. If he has a prescription for nitroglycerine tablets and has them with him, let him take one. The greatest immediate danger is that of cardiopulmonary arrest (see above), so be prepared to initiate CPR if indicated.

What not to do
- Do not underestimate the danger.
- Do not walk the victim around and do not allow the victim to go home or to the hospital either by himself or with any well-intentioned but untrained friends.
- Do not give any medication unless it is the patient's own, and he has been instructed in how to take it.

Who to call
The paramedics. *Immediately.*

How to prevent it
Again, stress the importance of medical screening in high-risk people and carefully monitor your students in your classes. If they look bad or report any of the above symptoms, make them stop immediately.

Shortness of Breath (Dyspnea)

What it is
Any situation in which a person has difficulty breathing out of proportion to the degree of exertion, and which persists after stopping exercise. Often, it is associated with a real sense of "air hunger" and panic regarding the inability to get one's breath.

What it is not
- Normal rapid breathing, which is to be expected with exertion and which rapidly resolves with rest.
- Hyperventilation, which is often psychogenic in origin but which may be impossible to differentiate. As usual, if in doubt, proceed as for the worst.

What it looks like
The victim will demonstrate rapid and difficult breathing. The nostrils may be flared, and the ribs may push out with each breath. Depending on the nature of the problem, there may be audible wheezing with each breath (asthma). The victim may appear dusky about the mouth and the nail beds may look dark. There is very often a real and unmistakable look of panic in the victim's eyes.

What to do

Stop any exertion. Sit the victim down but never try to lay him down if he resists. Talk to the victim and have him try to consciously get control of his breathing, to slow it down. If he has a history of asthma or chronic bronchitis or emphysema and has an inhaler with him, let him use it as instructed. If you suspect he may be hyperventilating, try having him rebreathe into a small paper bag. If there is not a rapid and definite response to any of the above, call for help.

What not to do

Do not allow the victim to continue any level of exertion nor to leave, other than by paramedic ambulance, unless the symptoms have completely resolved. The only exception might be a known asthmatic who has had many similar attacks and feels comfortable going to the hospital accompanied by friends or family. Again, never administer any medication not specifically prescribed for that person.

Who to call

Paramedics.

How to prevent it

Monitor your students and have anyone showing severe shortness of breath stop until recovered. Stress to your students regularly the importance of taking medications as prescribed. Asthmatics can and should exercise but only under the care and instructions of a physician.

Fainting (Syncope)

What it is

Loss of consciousness and collapse, usually with return of consciousness after a brief period of time.

What it is not

Cardiopulmonary arrest: there is usually no cessation of breathing or heart function although depending on the cause, the pulse may be either rapid and thready or very slow.

What it looks like

The victim may be partially or completely unresponsive, but breathing continues and a pulse can be felt. Spontaneous movements usually are present.

What to do

Loosen the victim's clothing. Lay him on his back and elevate his legs. A cool towel may be applied to the forehead. If ammonia capsules are available they may be broken and briefly held under the victim's nose. As he awakes, calm him and keep him quiet. Call for help, since the reason for his passing out may require further emergency treatment by a physician.

What not to do
- Do not begin CPR in the presence of breathing or pulse.
- Never attempt to give anything by mouth to an unconscious person.
- Do not allow the victim to resume any exercise or leave without being accompanied by medical personnel.

Who to call
Paramedics

How to prevent it
Stress fitness screening, medical care for any chronic problems and individual pacing with frequent pulse checks. Monitor your students and check anyone who looks weak or wobbly.

Airway Obstruction

What it is
A blockage of the airway interfering with or completely preventing breathing.

What it is not
Shortness of breath (see above) in which the airway itself is clear and the problem is in the lungs.

What it looks like
The victim of partial obstruction may make highpitched crowing noises when trying to take a breath in. The victim of complete obstruction will make no noise and will be unable to speak. In both cases it will be obvious that he is making unsuccessful efforts to get air in and his rib cage may show signs of such strain. If complete obstruction persists for very long the victim will collapse and show no further respiratory effort.

What to do
The treatment of obstructed airways is part of the BCLS courses previously mentioned which should be mandatory for all instructors. Hence, again, only a basic review.
- If the victim is making any noises at all or is able to speak, sit him down, keep him as quiet as possible, and call for help.
- If the victim is conscious but unable to speak or make any noises, proceed as follows:
  - Lean the victim forward and apply four sharp blows between the shoulder blades. (There is some current controversy regarding the use of back blows in the treatment of the obstructed airway. But the

current recommendations of the American Heart Association include them, and in the author's opinion they are of value. Hence, they are recommended here. Students of BCLS classes may also wish to substitute abdominal thrusts for chest thrusts in the above sequences; either is acceptable, although the author favors the chest thrusts.)
- If no relief, grasp the victim from behind with your arms across his lower ribs and apply four sharp squeezes.
- If no relief, repeat back blows and squeezes until victim resumes breathing or collapses.
- If victim has collapsed, place him on his back and open the airway by tilting the head back.
- Look, listen, and feel for breathing.
- If no breathing, attempt mouth-to-mouth breathing.
- If unable to get air into the lungs, roll the victim toward you and apply four sharp blows between the shoulder blades.
- If no relief, place the victim on his back again, turn his head to the side and position your hands as if you were going to do closed chest massage, i.e., the heel of one hand on the lower portion of the breastbone with the other hand on top of the first.
- Give four sharp, downward thrusts on the chest.
- Put your finger in the victim's mouth and sweep out the back of the throat, removing any foreign material that might have been dislodged.
- If unsuccessful, call for help and continue repeating the above sequence until either successful or help arrives.
- If successful and breathing resumes, keep the victim quiet, give nothing by mouth except very small sips of water, and call for help. The victim of such an episode, even if successfully treated, needs further medical evaluation on an emergency basis.

Again, if the above sequence is not completely familiar to you, go back to a formal BCLS course.

What not to do
- Do nothing for the victim of a partial airway obstruction, since the greatest risk is that your efforts will turn a partial obstruction into a complete and potentially fatal one.
- Do not give up before help arrives. As the victim's throat relaxes after collapse, efforts which had been previously unsuccessful may be successful.
- Do not attempt to use any device to remove an object from the airway, unless you have special medical training to do so.

Who to call
The paramedics. It is reasonable to make your initial attempts before calling, but if these are unsuccessful or, as noted above, even if they are successful, the paramedics should be called.

How to prevent it
Simply and completely preventable. Never, ever, allow anyone to have anything in his or her mouth during an aerobic workout, especially chewing gum.

Seizure Convulsion

What it is
An uncontrolled contraction of all the muscles of the body due to a disorganized discharge of impulses from the brain. There is loss of consciousness, and the victim may urinate or defecate during the seizure.

What it is not
- Muscle twitching or spasms in which the person remains conscious.
- Fainting where there is collapse but no muscle contractions.

What it looks like
A seizure may begin with twitching of only one part of the body and progress to a total body seizure, or it may begin all at once. The eyes usually roll upward and often to one side, the back frequently arches, and there may be foaming at the mouth with a gurgling noise. The victim will fall to the floor and not respond.

What to do
The most important thing to remember is that nearly all seizures will stop by themselves after a minute or two. Gently restrain the victim, so that he does not injure himself or anyone else, and wait for the seizure to stop. Whether the seizure stops or not, call for help.

It can be most helpful to the doctor who will subsequently treat the patient, if you can note and remember whether the seizure began on one side and if so which one. Give this information to the paramedics before they leave.

What not to do
Contrary to what you may have been told previously, do not attempt to put anything in the victim's mouth. If he bites his tongue, he will do so at the onset of the seizure and any attempts to push anything into his clenched teeth will only do more damage. Do not try to stop the muscular contractions, simply control them and prevent all-out thrashing.

Who to call
Paramedics. Even if the seizure stops, evaluation in a hospital emergency department is necessary on an emergency basis.

How to prevent it
If any of your students has a known seizure disorder, be certain that they are being treated by a physician and encourage them to take their medications as directed.

Stroke (Cerebrovascular Accident [CVA])

What it is
A blockage of one of the blood vessels leading to a part of the brain, causing that part of the brain to cease to function.

What it is not
A seizure, a fainting spell, a headache.

What it looks like
The victim may have sudden or progressive onset of weakness or even complete paralysis of one side of the body. The face may droop on one side and if the dominant side of the brain is affected, the ability to speak or to understand speech may be impaired or speech may be slurred.

What to do
Make the victim comfortable, try to be reassuring. Call for help.

What not to do
No form of treatment is necessary or possible outside the hospital setting. Remember that although the victim may be unable to speak, he may understand everything that is being said, so be careful of what you say in front of him.

Who to call
Paramedics.

How to prevent it
Again, the best preventive measure is stressing general fitness and qualified medical treatment for high blood pressure or any other chronic medical conditions, particularly in older students.

Palpitations

What it is
A rapid heartbeat, sensed as abnormal by the individual, out of proportion to the degree of exertion and persisting after terminating the

exertion. Often a chronic and recurring problem in people with some types of heart problems.

What it is not
- The normal or even exaggerated rapid heart beat which is clearly related to exertion and resolves with rest or cooling down.
- A heart attack or acute shortness of breath, although both could either cause or be caused by palpitations.

What it looks like
There are no specific symptoms to see, but the victim will report an abnormal fluttering sensation in the chest. There may or may not be associated trouble breathing, lightheadedness, or chest pain. Those who experience palpitations frequently may appear quite comfortable, while those having a first attack will look more frightened than anything else.

What to do
Have the person stop any heavy exertion. A moderate cool-down, such as walking a bit, may be appropriate if the symptoms occurred with maximal exertion. If palpitations persist and are accompanied by shortness of breath, lightheadedness, or chest pain, make the patient comfortable by having him sit or lie down according to his preference and call the paramedics. Watch carefully for signs of cardiopulmonary arrest and be prepared to initiate CPR. If the person has no other symptoms and has had similar episodes before, he can try holding his breath and bearing down hard for 5-10 seconds once or twice. If this is successful, he can probably arrange to see his own doctor but should not resume exercise. If unsuccessful but still with no other symptoms, he should go to a hospital emergency department. If this is a recurrent condition and he is comfortable, whether he goes by ambulance or with friends can be left to his judgment but he obviously should not be allowed to drive.

What not to do
- Do not attempt any treatment if the victim has any other symptoms besides the palpitations, or if he has never had palpitations previously.
- Do not attempt the above treatment more than twice.
- Do not administer any drugs which have not been prescribed to the victim for these episodes.

Who to call
For palpitations with the other symptoms listed, call the paramedics. As indicated, for simple recurring palpitations the individual can exercise some judgment. For palpitations that resolve with or without treatment, no call need necessarily be made.

Electrical Shock

What it is
Contact of the body with a source of electrical energy sufficient to cause muscular contractions, burns, collapse, or cardiopulmonary arrest.

What it is not
A minor contact which produces only slight and transient discomfort or a heat burn due to sparks or fire from a faulty piece of electrical equipment or wiring.

What it looks like
If the victim is still in contact with the source, he may be locked in a state of muscular contraction or twitching and unable to release his grip. If he has fallen free, he may be dazed or in a state of complete collapse and, in some cases, may have sustained cardiopulmonary arrest. There may be evidence of electrical burns at the site of contact and at the site where the current exited the body (may be at some distance from the contact point).

What to do
Before all else, as the rescuer be sure that the victim is no longer in contact with the source before touching him so as to prevent your sustaining the same shock. If he is in contact, have the power turned off if at all possible before attempting rescue. If this is impossible, use a nonconducting material like a wooden pole to push the victim away from the source.

Once free of contact, if the victim is unresponsive, check for signs of cardiopulmonary arrest. If present, immediately begin CPR.

If breathing and pulse are present, keep the victim lying down, make him comfortable, and call for help.

What not to do
- Never touch a victim who is still in contact with the source of the shock.
- Never use any metal or other conducting material in attempts to extricate him.

Who to call
Paramedics. Even if the victim seems to recover, major electrical shock can cause very serious internal injuries and emergency evaluation by a physician is always indicated.

How to prevent it
Be certain that all electrical equipment, music systems, lights, fans, etc., are in good repair and recheck them regularly. Never touch any electrical equipment while standing on a wet surface.

Since the instructor is the one most often using electrical equipment, he is at highest risk. Hence, there is definite value in ensuring that another trained person is present to respond, if the instructor is the victim of this or any medical emergency.

Neck Injury

What it is
A serious injury to the neck involving the vertebral bones with loss of protection or actual injury to the spinal cord. Injury to the spinal cord can lead to permanent paralysis.

What it is not
A simple twist or sprain which may result from overexertion; should be referred for treatment to the student's own physician.

What it looks like
Almost always the result of major injury such as a fall down a flight of stairs, coming down on one's head off a trampoline, or other injuries involving a great deal of force. The victim will usually complain of pain in the neck or pain with any attempts at movement. Numbness or paralysis of the arms or legs will only be present if the spinal cord has been injured.

What to do
Keep the victim absolutely still, particularly the head and neck. If necessary, hold the head with gentle traction until help arrives.

What not to do
- Do not attempt any form of movement and never allow anyone to attempt any manipulation.
- Never assume the injury is minor or stable. An error in the wrong direction can cause one who might have recovered to be turned into a quadriplegic for life!

Who to call
Paramedics. Such victims should only be moved after the neck has been stabilized and immobilized with proper equipment and then only by those trained to do so.

How to prevent it
Discourage any exercise involving force and heights such as trampolines. Be sure stairways are safe and controlled.

Appendix D

Glossary of Terms

Linda Shelton, BA

abduction
Movement away from the midline of the body
acidosis
Too much acid in the blood and body fluids
actin
A contractile protein of muscle fiber
acute
Having a sudden onset, characterized by sharpness, severity, and brief duration
adaptive shortening
Shortening of muscle fibers and decreased range of motion due to inactivity
adduction
Movement toward the midline of the body
adipose tissue
Connective tissue in which fat is stored
adolescent onset obesity
After puberty, when an individual acquires too much fat due to the sudden increase in the number of fat cells
adrenaline (epinephrine)
A hormone secreted by the medulla of the adrenal glands, especially under conditions of stress that induces physiologic symptoms such as accelerated heart rate, increased arterial blood pressure, and increase in blood sugar concentration
adult onset obesity
After age 18, when an individual acquires too much fat due to the increase in the size of his fat cells

aerobic
Means literally, with oxygen, or in the presence of oxygen
aerobic capacity (cardiorespiratory endurance)
The ability of the body to remove oxygen from the air and transfer it through the lungs and blood to the working muscles
aerobic exercise
A method of conditioning the cardiorespiratory system by using a variety of activities that create an increased demand for oxygen over an extended period of time
agonist
A muscle that is a prime mover, directly responsible for a particular action
alkalosis
When the blood has a lower hydrogen ion concentration than normal and an excessive base (bicarbonate ions) in the extracellular fluids
all-or-none law
A muscle contracts to its fullest potential or not at all
amenorrhea
Absence of menstruation
amino acids
Building blocks of protein; organic compounds containing nitrogen, hydrogen, and carbon
amphiarthrodial
A type of articulation joined by hyaline cartilage, classified as either permanent or stationary joints and slightly moveable
anaerobic
Requiring no oxygen; usually short spurt, high energy activities
anaerobic threshold
The point at which the body can no longer meet its demand for oxygen and anaerobic metabolism is accelerated
anemia
A condition in which there is a reduced number of erythrocytes or decreased percentage of hemoglobin in the blood
angina pectoris
Chest pains caused by insufficient supply of oxygen to the heart muscle
anorexia nervosa
A psychological eating disorder, usually seen in young women, who intentionally starve themselves
anoxemia
A deficiency of oxygen in the blood
anoxia
A deficiency of oxygen, most frequently occurring when blood supply to any part of the body is completely cut off

GLOSSARY OF TERMS

antagonist
A muscle that acts in opposition to the action produced by a prime mover

anterior
Front side of an organ or part of the body

aorta
The largest artery in the body that delivers oxygenated blood from the left ventricle to the entire body

aortic stenosis
A narrowing of the valve opening between the lower left chamber of the heart and the aorta

arrhythmia
An abnormal rhythm of the heart beat

arteriole
Small arteries that regulate the flow of blood into the capillaries

arteriosclerosis
Abnormal thickening or hardening of the arteries that causes the artery walls to lose their elasticity

artery
Large vessels with middle smooth muscle layer which carry oxygenated blood away from the heart to the body tissues

atherosclerosis
A type of arteriosclerosis in which the inner layer of the artery wall becomes thick and irregular due to fat deposits, decreasing the inner diameter of the artery

arthritis
Inflammation of the joints

ATP (adenosine triphosphate)
Intracellular carrier of chemical energy produced by the body for muscular work

atrophy
A reduction in size or wasting away of any organ cell, resulting from disease or disuse

autonomic nervous system
Division of the nervous system that functions involuntarily and is responsible for innervating cardiac muscle, smooth muscle, and the glands

axial skeleton
The bones of the head and the trunk: skull, vertebral column, thorax, and sternum

ballistic
Bounce or explosive movement, unsustained

basal metabolic rate (BMR)
The energy requirements necessary for maintenance of life processes such as heart beat, breathing, and cell metabolic activities

bilateral
Affects both sides of the body equally
blood pooling
A condition caused by ceasing vigorous exercise too abruptly so that blood remains in the extremities and may not be delivered quickly enough to the heart and brain
blood pressure
The pressure of the blood in the arteries
bradycardia
Abnormally slow heart rate
bronchus
One of two large passageways between trachea and the lungs
brown fat
Believed to be a more concentrated energy source that can be utilized more efficiently than other forms of fat
bulemia
A psychological eating disorder characterized by food gorging then induced vomiting after eating, as a means of weight control
bursa
A fluid-filled sac or cavity, located in the tissue at points of pressure or friction, mainly around joints
bursitis
Inflammation of the bursa sac, can be an overuse syndrome
calisthenic exercises
Part of a workout that emphasizes specific muscular work, utilizing resistance
calorie
The amount of heat necessary to raise the temperature of 1 gram of water 1°C
cancellous bone
Inner, spongy portion of bone tissue
capillary
Small, thin-walled blood vessels connecting arterial and venous blood systems that allow the exchange of materials between blood and tissues
carbohydrate
Organic compounds containing carbon, hydrogen, and oxygen; when broken down, the main energy source for muscular work and one of the basic foodstuffs
cardiac
Pertaining to the heart
cardiac output
The volume of blood pumped by each ventricle in one minute
carotid pulse
Pulse located on the carotid artery down from the corner of the eye, just under the jawbone; used for taking heart rate

cartilage
White, semi-opaque fibrous connective tissue; cushions and prevents wear on articular surfaces

catecholamine
A hormone that is a neurotransmitter, released under conditions of stress, includes epinephrine and norepinephrine

cervical spine
Refers to the neck; the first seven vertebrae of the spine

cholesterol
A chemical compound found in animal fats and oils; higher levels of cholesterol are often associated with high risk of atherosclerosis

chondromalacia
Softening of condral cartilage on patella (backside); first symptoms usually clicking or grating sound in knee

chronic
Persisting for a long period of time

circumduction
Movement in which the extremity describes a 360° circle

compact bone
Hard portion of bone that forms the diaphysis and epipysis

concentric contraction   p. 29
Isotonic movement in which the muscle shortens

condyle
A rounded projection at the end of a bone that articulates with another bone

connective tissue
Primary tissue characterized by cells separated by intercellular fluid that supports and binds together other tissues and forms ligaments and tendons

coronary arteries
Two main arteries, arising from the aorta, arching down over the top of the heart, and carrying blood to the heart muscle

coronary thrombosis
An obstruction, generally a blood clot, within a coronary artery which hinders the flow of blood to a part of the heart

CPR (cardiopulmonary resuscitation)
First-aid measure to aid an individual suffering from lack of oxygen, conscious or unconscious

cueing
Verbal technique using small words or phrases that describe upcoming exercises or body alignment positions

dendrite
Nerve-cell process that transmits impulse to cell body

diabetes
A hereditary metabolic disease, characterized by an inadequate activity of insulin, affecting the regulation of normal blood glucose levels

diaphysis
Shaft of a long bone, consisting of a hollow cylinder of compact bone that surrounds a medullary cavity

diaphragm
Domelike sheet of skeletal muscle that separates the thoracic and abdominal cavities; contraction during inspiration expands the thoracic (chest) cavity

diathrodial (synovial)
Freely moveable joint with movement limited only by ligaments, muscles, tendons and adjoining bones

diastolic pressure
Blood pressure within the arteries when the heart is in relaxation between contractions

distal
End of any body part that is further from the midline of the body or from point of attachment

diuretic
A drug that stimulates increased renal water excretion

dorsal
Pertaining to the back

dysmenorrhea
Painful menstruation

eccentric contraction
Muscle lengthens while contracting, developing tension as when the muscles oppose the force of gravity

ectomorph
Body type, characterized by frail and delicate bone structure, lean musculature, and usually very little fat

edema
An abnormal accumulation of fluid in body parts or tissues; swelling

electrocardiogram (EKG or ECG)
A graphic record of the electrical activity and heart beat pattern

electrolyte imbalance
Inappropriate concentration of ions in body fluids

embolism
Sudden blocking of artery or vein by a clot brought to its place by the blood current

empty calories
A term used to denote food contributing calories that are void of nutrients, protein, vitamins, and minerals, i.e., alcohol, sugar, fat

GLOSSARY OF TERMS 313

endocrine glands
Ductless glands that empty their secretions directly into the blood stream; these secretions contain specific hormones that influence growth, reproduction, emotion

endomorph
Body type characterized by a large block-shaped body, wider at hips and abdominals, a predominance of fat tissue but not necessarily obese

endorphin
A natural substance that can be produced by the body during extended exercise periods that may exhibit "morphine-like," pain inhibiting qualities

endosteum
Thin, transparent outer layer of the heart wall

enzyme
A protein catalyst that stimulates and accelerates the velocity of chemical changes in the body

epicardium
Thin, transparent outer layer of the heart wall

epiphysis
Enlarged ends of bones where growth centers for long bones are located (epiphyseal plate)

ergometer
An apparatus for measuring workloads by an individual, e.g., bicycle

essential amino acids
The eight amino acids that the body cannot manufacture in sufficient amounts to meet physiologic need

eversion
Rotation of the foot, turning the sole outward

extension
A motion of increasing the angle between two bones; straightening of a muscle previously bent in flexion

fascia
Layer of fibrous tissue under the skin or covering and separating muscles

fasciculi
Bundles of nerve, muscle, or tendon fibers, separated by connective tissue

fat
Stored as adipose tissue in the body, it serves as a concentrated source of energy for muscular work; a compound containing glycerol and fatty acids

fatigue
A diminished capacity for work as a result of prolonged or excessive exertion

fatty acid
See *triglyceride*

fibril
Fine thread-like structures which give cells stability

fibroblast
Connective tissue cell located near collagenous fibers which develop into fibers

fibrous joint
See synarthrodial

fixator
A muscle acting to immobilize a joint or bone; fixes the origin of prime movers so muscle action occurring is exerted at the insertion

flexion
Bending of a joint between two bones that decreases the angle between the two bones

frequency
As related to exercise, how often work is performed

frontal
A plane, vertical to the median line that divides the body into anterior and posterior parts

fructose
A monosaccharide, sometimes known as fruit sugar, that does not stimulate insulin production

glottis
Opening between the vocal cords, entrance to the larynx

glycogen
Form in which digested carbohydrates are stored in the muscles and liver and utilized as energy for aerobic activities

glycogenolysis
Body's breakdown of glycogen to glucose

glycolysis
The breakdown of glucose to simpler compounds such as lactic acid; occurs in muscle

glucose
A simple sugar; form in which carbohydrates are transported in the blood and transported in tissues; other sugars are converted into glucose by enzymes in the body before they can be used as an energy source

HDL
High-density lipoproteins that return unused fat to the liver for disposal; HDL levels are raised by aerobic exercise; are beneficial due to their "removal" effect on harmful lipoproteins

heart attack
Damage (tissue death) of the heart muscle due to blockage of a coronary artery by either an embolus or thrombus

heart failure
Congestion or accumulation of fluid in various parts of the body result from the inability of the heart to pump out all the blood that returns to it

heat exhaustion
The collapse of an individual, characterized by prolonged sweating and inadequate replacement of salt and fluid without failure of the body's heat-regulating system

heat stroke
Acute medical emergency characterized by rectal temperature at 105° or higher and no sweating, caused by failure of the body's heat-regulating system

hemoglobin
Oxygen-carrying protein of red blood cells

herniated disc
A condition that occurs when the nucleus pulposus distends outside of the intervertebral disc, usually quite painful

homeostasis
A state of equilibrium and internal balance of the body

hormone
A chemical agent secreted by the endocrine glands; each affects a specific organ and elicits a specific response

hyaline cartilage
Translucent bluish-white cartilage with a homogeneous matrix, present in joints and respiratory passage, and forms most of the fetal skeleton

hyper
Beyond normal limits, excessive

hyperextension
To increase the angle of a joint past the normal range of motion

hyperplasia
Increase in the number of cells produced in an organ or body tissues

hypertension
High blood pressure; unstable or persistent elevation of blood pressure above normal ranges. 140/90 is in general a high normal blood pressure

hypertrophy
Increase in size of tissue, organ, or cell, independent of general body growth

hyperventilate
Excessive rate and depth of respiration, leading to abnormal loss of carbon dioxide from the blood; can cause dizziness

hypo
Less than normal

hypoglycemia
An abnormally low blood glucose concentration, characterized by a number of symptoms such as dizziness, nausea, headache, heart palpitations, confusion, forgetfulness

insertion
The place or mode of attachment of a muscle; the moveable part of a muscle during action

insulin
The hormone produced in the pancreas which regulates carbohydrate and fat metabolism and causes increased cellular uptake of glucose

intensity
Degree of strength, energy, or difficulty; as related to a workout: the class level

intervertebral disc
Fibrocartilage cushion between the vertebrae

inversion
To turn inward

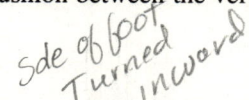

ischemia
A local, usually temporary decrease in blood supply in some part of the body resulting from obstruction of arterial flow

isokinetic
Contraction in which the tension developed by the muscle while shortening at constant speed is maximal over the full range of motion

isometric
Movement against an immovable force; static; a muscle contraction in which the tension increases, but muscle length remains the same

isotonic
A contraction in which a muscle shortens against a force, resulting in movement and performance of work; also referred to as a dynamic or concentric contraction

ketone
A compound formed during the incomplete oxidation of fatty acids

ketosis
An abnormal increase in ketone production and accumulation in the blood; occurs especially in protein-sparing diets or fasting

kinesthetic awareness
Body sense; ability of individuals to "feel" where their bodies are in relation to space

Krebs cycle
A series of chemical reactions occurring in the mitochondria, during which energy is produced from metabolism of carbohydrates, fats and amino acids and the complete oxidation of acetyl CoA is accomplished

kyphosis *hump back*
Abnormal rounding of the thoracic portion of the spine, usually accompanied by rounded shoulders

lactic acid
The byproduct of anaerobic metabolism of glucose or glycogen in muscle

lactose
A disaccharide composed of glucose and galactose; milk sugar

lateral flexion
Movement of head and/or trunk, bending to either side

lateral movement
Any side-to-side movement away from the midline of the body

LDL
Low-density lipoproteins; manufactured in the liver, they circulate throughout the body, making their fat available to all body cells; contain 45% cholesterol

ligament
Bands or sheetlike fibrous tissues that connect bone to bone and reinforce joints from dislocation; they are nonelastic and have limited range of motion

lipid
Fats; organic chemicals made up of carbon, oxygen and hydrogen that are insoluble in water

lordosis
Sway back, increased or excessive lumbar curve

lumbar spine
The largest five vertebrae between the thorax and the pelvis, the area that needs the most protection during exercise

maintenance
When dieting, caloric intake equals caloric expenditure

marrow
A soft, highly vascular and specialized connective tissue found in the medullary cavity of most bones; capable of producing blood cells

maximum heart rate
Theoretical maximum rate at which your heart can beat at your age. 220 minus your age is a formula used to calculate the maximum heart rate in a healthy individual; do not exercise at this rate

maximum oxygen consumption
The highest level of oxygen an individual can consume and utilize per minute

medial
Toward the midline of the body

meniscus
Crescent-shaped fibrocartilage within a joint, i.e., shock absorbers in the knee. A common knee injury caused by trauma or fast rotation movements

mesomorph
  Body type characterized by a solid muscular build
metabolism
  The chemical reaction of a cell or living tissue that transfers usable materials into energy
metatarsalgia
  Pain in the forefoot in the region of the heads of the metatarsals
mitochondria
  Spherical or rod-shaped organelles, found outside the nucleus, that produce energy for cells through cellular respiration
monosaccharide
  Simple sugar, i.e., glucose, fructose, galactose, found in fruits, vegetables, milk, honey, and cane sugar; end-product of all digestible forms of carbohydrates
Morton's syndrome
  A condition where the second toe is longer than the first throwing more weight on the third and fourth toes, causing irritation of the nerves
muscle spindle
  A type of receptor, located among the fibers of a skeletal muscle that responds to muscle contraction (stretch)
muscular endurance
  The ability to perform repetitive work over a prolonged period of time
myelin
  Fatty, white substance forming medullary sheath around nerve
myocardial infarction
  The damaging or death of an area of the heart muscle, resulting from a reduction of blood supply to the area, also called a "heart attack"
myocardium
  The thick, muscular layer forming the heart wall
myofibril
  The longitudinally arranged contractile elements, composed of actin and myosin of a skeletal muscle
myotatic stretch reflex
  The body's automatic protective mechanism against severe injury and abuse. If a muscle is stretched too quickly or with force, the reflex causes the muscle to contract; stretch threshold
negative balance
  In weight control, caloric intake is less than caloric expenditure
neuromuscular
  Pertaining to the relation between nerves and muscles
neuron
  Nerve cell that transmits messages throughout the body

neurotransmitters
Chemical involved in sending message across nerve synapse

nutrients
Substance obtained from food and utilized by the body to promote growth, maintenance and/or repair

orthotics
Material, usually plastic or rubber, that is individually fitted and inserted into everyday shoes to correct foot problems

osteoporosis
Increased softening of the bones, resulting from gradual reduction of bone density; common in older people

overload
Method used to increase the workload beyond the body's normal capacity or to improve and develop muscular strength and endurance

overuse syndrome
Injuries that occur, such as shin splints and tendonitis, from too much activity that places excessive stress on the body

oxidation
The process of oxygen combining with other substances, resulting in heat production and energy

oxygen debt
The amount of oxygen required in the postexercise period in excess of oxygen consumption to reverse the anaerobic reactions during exercise period

peak movements
Large aerobic movements that use both arms and legs simultaneously and require greater amounts of oxygen to be delivered to the muscles

perceived exertion
Techniques where an individual relies on his body senses and reactions to determine work intensity rather than actual measurements

pericardium
Fibrous sac that encloses the heart

periosteum
Double-layered connective tissue covering bone

pH
The symbol for hydrogen ion concentration that indicates the acidity or alkalinity of a solution

plantar
Refers to the sole of the foot

plantar fascitis
Inflammation of the fascia on the ball of the foot caused by overstress and overuse

plaque
Deposits of lipid material mixed with smooth muscle cells and calcium which are lodged in artery walls

PNF
Proprioceptive Neuromuscular Facilitation; a stretching technique in which an individual contracts the same muscle that he wants to stretch

polysaccharide
Carbohydrate form that yields more than two simple sugars upon breakdown, found in cereal grains, roots, bulbs, and tubers. The principle ones are starch, dextrin, glycogen, and cellulose

polyunsaturated fat
A triglyceride in which the fatty acids have two or more points of unsaturation. Contains linoleic acid, an essential nutrient found in vegetable fats

post-aerobic cool down
Rhythmic activities, such as small kicks and walking that provide a transition period between vigorous aerobic work and less aerobically taxing calisthenics or stretching

posterior
Rear

power
Quick movement where the body is propelled either upward or outward; explosive strength; performance of work expressed per unit of time

prime mover
Muscle responsible for a specific movement

pronation
Shifting the body weight to the inside of the foot

prone
Lying face down

propriocepter
Sensor receptors in muscles, joints, and tendons, which give imformation concerning movement and position of the body

protein
A compound composed of carbon, hydrogen, oxygen, and nitrogen, arranged into amino acids linked in a chain, responsible for building and repair of tissue, hormone production, enzyme function

pulmonary artery
The artery extending from the right ventricle of the heart; prime function is to carry venous blood to the lungs for respiration

pulmonary diffusion
Rate of exchange of carbon dioxide and oxygen moving in the lungs

pulmonary ventilation
Movement of air in and out of the lungs

pulse pressure
The difference between the systolic and diastolic blood pressures

radial pulse
Pulse found on the inside of the wrist on the thumb side near the wrist bone

RDA
Recommended Dietary Allowances; percent or amount of calories for proteins, fats, carbohydrates, vitamins, and minerals that should be included in the daily diet

reciprocal innervation
A stretching technique in which an individual contracts the opposite muscle he wants to stretch

recovery heart rate
Heart rate taken at the end of class after a stretch cool-down to gauge when the heart rate has returned to pre-exercise pulse

red blood cell
Erythrocyte; blood cells responsible for oxygen transport

residual volume
The volume of air that remains in the lungs after the deepest possible expiration

respiration
Interchange of oxygen and carbon dioxide between an organism and its environment

resting heart rate
Pulse while still lying down in the morning before arising

rhythmic limbering exercise
Low intensity exercises, performed at a low to moderate pace that help prepare the body for more vigorous exercise by providing an increase in the flexibility of tendons and ligaments, raise muscle temperature, and stimulate muscle function

RICE
Immediate injury treatment: rest, ice, compress, elevate

risk factors
Factors known to be related to disease but cannot be proven to be the actual cause

ROM
Range of motion

rotation
Movements around an axis

sagittal
Plane that divides the body into right and left parts

SAID principle
"Specific adaptations to imposed demand;" training must be relative to the activity for physiological change to take place

saturated fat
A fatty acid carrying the maximum possible number of hydrogen atoms
scanning
Teaching technique of observation; looking for incorrect body alignment and positioning in your class
scoliosis
Abnormal lateral twisting or rotating of the spine
shin splint
Delayed pain on the front or sides of lower legs, caused by inflammation of the fascia connecting to the leg bones or muscle tears
side stitch
Sharp pain in the side, thought to be caused by a spasm in the diaphragm, due to insufficient oxygen supply and improper breathing
smooth muscle
Involuntary muscles consisting of nonstriated, spindle shaped muscle cells, found in the walls of hollow viscera
specificity of training
To improve muscular endurance and strength, applied resistance and range of motion must be specific to the muscle or muscle groups being worked; also applies to endurance training
sphygomanometer
Instrument used to measure arterial blood pressure
spirometer
Instrument used for the collection, measurement, or storage of gas
spot reducing
A popular but false assumption that an individual can "burn" fat only in desired areas
sprain
Wrenching or twisting of a joint in which ligaments are stretched past their normal limits
static stretch
Held, nonbounce muscle contraction in which muscle tension is sustained throughout the stretch
steady state
After the first 3–4 minutes of exercise, oxygen uptake has reached an adequate level to meet the oxygen demand of the tissue; heart rate, cardiac output and pulmonary ventilation have attained fairly constant levels
strain
"Muscle pull;" a stretch, tear or rip of the muscle or adjacent tissue, such as fascia or muscle tendon
strength
Maximum force or tension that a muscle or muscle group can produce against resistance

GLOSSARY OF TERMS 323

stress fracture
Fracture caused by stress, overuse or pathologic weakness of the bone in the foot or leg

striated muscle
Skeletal voluntary muscle that attaches to and moves the skeleton

stroke volume
The volume of blood ejected by each ventricle of the heart during a single systole

subluxation
Dislocation or disarticulation of a joint

submaximal work
Workload performed below maximum heart rate; aerobic exercise is submaximal

supination
Shift the body weight to the outside of the foot

supine
Lying face up

synarthrodial joint
All articulations in which bones are held together tightly by fibrous connective tissue in a nonmoveable fashion, i.e., sacroiliac

synergist
Muscle that combines with another and aids in its action

synovial joint
(See diarthrodial joint)

systolic pressure
The highest level to which arterial blood pressure rises, following the systolic ejection of blood from the left ventricle

target heart rate range
The rate at which the heart is beating to get the optimum aerobic effect; formula for obtaining a target heart rate equals 220 minus your age times 60%-75% is reasonable for a healthy individual to use

tendon
Band of dense fibrous tissue forming the termination of a muscle and attaching muscle to bone with a minimum of elasticity

tendinitis
Continuous, low-grade inflammation of a tendon, with pain on movement; can lead to partial or complete rupture of tendon

thoracic spine
Twelve vertebrae from the neck to lumbar area

tibial torsion
Twisting of the tibia, usually associated with supinated or pronated feet

tonus
A slight, sustained muscle contraction

torque
Amount of twist around an axis

training effects
Physiologic adaptations that occur as a result of aerobic exercise of sufficient intensity, frequency, and duration to produce beneficial changes in the body

transverse
Plane that divides the body into upper and lower halves

triglyceride
A compound composed of glycerol fatty acids; vary in degrees of saturation and stored in the body

unsaturated fats
Contain double bonds between carbon atoms; usually are vegetable rather than animal fat

valsalva maneuver
A dangerous condition that can occur if an individual holds his breath, causing the glottis to close and stomach muscle to contract, forming an unequal pressure in the chest cavity, reduced blood flow to the heart, and insufficient oxygen supply to the brain. Dizziness, temporary loss of consciousness may occur

vasonconstriction
Narrowing of blood vessels as a result of smooth muscle contraction

vasodialation
Dilation of blood vessels due to the relaxation of smooth muscles

vein
Vessel carrying blood toward the heart

ventral
Towards the stomach; anterior or front

ventricle
Blood dispensing chambers of the heart

vertebrae
Bony or cartilaginous segments, separated by discs that form the spinal column

vital capacity
The greatest volume of air that can be forcibly exhaled after the deepest inspiration

warm-up
A balanced combination of static stretch and rhythmic limbering exercises that prepare the body for more vigorous exercise

working heart rate
Heart rate taken at the completion of the aerobic portion of the workout to determine if the individual was in his target zone and at proper intensity for age and physical fitness level